FIRST AID FOR THE USMLE STEP 1

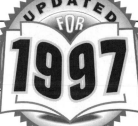

A STUDENT TO 1997 STUDENT GUIDE

VIKAS BHUSHAN, MD

University of California, San Francisco, Class of 1991
University of California, Los Angeles, Diagnostic Radiologist

TAO LE, MD

University of California, San Francisco, Class of 1996
Yale—New Haven Hospital, Resident in Internal Medicine

CHIRAG AMIN, MD

University of Miami, Class of 1996
Orlando Regional Medical Center, Resident in Orthopaedic Surgery

ROSS LEVINE

1997 Student Editor
Johns Hopkins University School of Medicine, Class of 1998

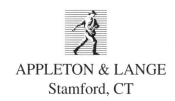

APPLETON & LANGE
Stamford, CT

1997 Contributors

ANTHONY GLASER, MD, PhD
Contributing Author, IMG Section
Medical University of South Carolina, Resident

FREDDY HUANG
Contributing Author, Behavioral Science
University of California, San Francisco, Class of 1998

THONG LE
Contributing Author, Anatomy & Pharmacology
University of Louisville, Class of 1998

ZIQIANG WU
Contributing Author, Biochemistry & Microbiology
University of California, San Francisco, Class of 1998

1997 Associate Contributors

RICK KULKARNI
University of California, San Francisco, Class of 1998

VIPAL SONI
University of California, Los Angeles, Class of 1999

GRACE TORRES
New York Podiatric College, Class of 1998

ANTONIO WONG
University of California, San Francisco, Class of 1998

1997 Faculty Reviewers

DEPARTMENT OF ANATOMY
University of California, San Francisco

WILLIAM GANONG, MD
Lange Professor of Physiology Emeritus
University of California, San Francisco

BERTRAM KATZUNG, MD, PhD
Professor of Pharmacology
University of California, San Francisco

WARREN LEVINSON, MD, PhD
Professor of Microbiology and Immunology
University of California, San Francisco

HENRY SANCHEZ, MD
Assistant Clinical Professor of Pathology
University of California, San Francisco

VIJAY YAJNIK, MD, PhD
Medical Intern
Massachusetts General Hospital

Contents

Preface to the 1997 Edition

With the 1997 edition of *First Aid for the USMLE Step 1,* we continue our commitment to providing students with the most useful and up-to-date preparation guide for the USMLE Step 1. The 1997 edition represents a major revision in many ways and includes:

- Revisions and new material based on student experience with the June and October 1996 administration of the USMLE Step 1.
- A revised and updated guide to efficient exam preparation, including new Step 1 statistics as well as new study and test-taking strategies.
- A new section on what to do if you fail the exam.
- USMLE advice geared toward international medical graduates and osteopathic medical students.
- A new section on First Aid for the Podiatry Student and First Aid for the Student with a Disability.
- More than 800 frequently tested facts and useful mnemonics, including more than 100 new or expanded entries with many new integrative diagrams and tables.
- An updated listing of more than 200 high-yield study topics that highlight key areas of basic science and clinical material emphasized on the USMLE Step 1.
- A completely revised, in-depth guide to more than 200 basic science review and sample examination books, based on a random national survey of thousands of third-year medical students across the country. Includes more than 30 new books and software titles.

The 1997 edition would not have been possible without student and faculty feedback and suggestions. We invite students and faculty to continue sharing their thoughts and ideas to help us improve *First Aid for the USMLE Step 1.* (*See* How to Contribute, p. xv, and User Survey, p. xxiii.)

Los Angeles   Vikas Bhushan
New Haven   Tao Le
Orlando   Chirag Amin
Baltimore   Ross Levine

November 1996

Foreword

The purpose of *First Aid for the USMLE Step 1: A Student-to-Student Guide* is to help medical students and foreign medical graduates review the basic medical sciences and prepare for the United States Medical Licensing Examination, Step 1 (USMLE Step 1). Preparing for this examination can be a stressful, difficult, and costly task. This book helps students make the most of their limited time, money, and energy. As is often the case in medical school, we found that the best advice a student can receive is from other medical students. We also recognized that certain basic science topics and details are "popular" and appear frequently on examinations. With this in mind, *First Aid for the USMLE Step 1* was started in 1989.

As we studied for the NBME Part I, we examined and evaluated scores of review books and thousands of sample questions. We kept track of useful study strategies, frequently tested facts, and helpful mnemonics through a simple computer database. The printed database was first distributed to the medical school class of 1992 at the University of California, San Francisco (UCSF). The next year, a revised edition was self-published under the name *High-Yield Basic Science Boards Review: A Student-to-Student Guide.* This guide was distributed to the UCSF class of 1993 and to numerous faculty and medical students at various institutions.

The title reflects the potential value of this book as the "first" one to get before buying others, and the fact that boards examinations are stressful and unpleasant experiences that students may "aid" each other in overcoming. We feel that this study guide provides a unique and pragmatic approach to the USMLE Step 1 and that it contains useful components not found in current boards review material. *First Aid for the USMLE Step 1* has three major sections:

Section I: Guide to Efficient Exam Preparation is a compilation of general student advice and study strategies for taking the USMLE Step 1.

Section II: Database of High-Yield Facts contains short descriptions of frequently tested facts and concepts as well as mnemonics and diagrams to facilitate learning. It includes a unique summary of subject-by-subject examination emphases as estimated by students who have recently taken the examination.

Section III: Database of Basic Science Review Books is designed to save students time and money by identifying high-quality, reasonably priced review and sample examination books and software. The comments and ratings are based on our analyses and on a nationwide random sampling of third-year medical students.

First Aid for the USMLE Step 1 is not designed to be a comprehensive text or the sole study source for the USMLE Step 1; it is meant as a **guide** to one's preparation for the USMLE Step 1. The material in this book has been written to strengthen one's familiarity with a large number of topics in a short, fact-based review. The authors do not advocate blindly memorizing the lists of facts, and we hope medical students realize that memorization cannot replace an understanding of the concepts that underlie these key points.

Entries in *First Aid for the USMLE Step 1* originated from hundreds of students, foreign medical graduates, and faculty members, who synthesized the facts, notes, and mnemonics from a variety of textbooks, review books, lecture notes, and personal notes. We regret the inability to reference each individual fact or mnemonic owing to the diverse and often anecdotal sources. Although the material has been reviewed by faculty members and medical students, errors and omissions are inevitable. We urge readers to identify errors and suggest improvements. We regret that some students may find certain mnemonics trivializing or offensive. The mnemonics are meant solely as optional devices for learning.

The authors and Appleton & Lange intend to continue updating *First Aid for the USMLE Step 1* so that the book grows in quality and scope and continues to reflect the material covered on the USMLE Step 1. If you have any study strategies, high-yield facts with mnemonics, or book reviews for the next edition, please use the forms included to submit your contributions. (*See* How to Contribute, page xv.) Any student or faculty member who submits material subsequently used in the next edition of *First Aid for the USMLE Step 1* will receive personal acknowledgment in the next edition and one $10 coupon per complete entry, good toward the future purchase of any Appleton & Lange medical book.

Good luck in your studies!!

Acknowledgments

This has been a collaborative project from the start. We gratefully acknowledge the thoughtful comments, corrections, and advice of the many hundreds of medical students, international medical graduates and faculty who have supported the authors in the continuing development of *First Aid for the USMLE Step 1*.

We were originally inspired by two established "student-to-student" guides: Macklis, *Introduction to Clinical Medicine, A Student-to-Student Guide* (Little, Brown), and Betcher, *A Student-to-Student Guide to Medical School: Study Strategies, Mnemonics, Personal Growth* (Little, Brown). An impressive example of what a comprehensive review book can become is Dähnert, *Radiology Review Manual* (Williams & Wilkins).

We acknowledge Dr. Donald Melnick (NBME) and Dr. Peter Ralston (former chairman, USMLE Step 1 Committee) for reviewing the exam preparation guide section of the 1992 and 1996 editions respectively. Thanks to Jeanette Jackson, Beth Sullivan, Thy Nguyen and Grace Torres for their contributions to the Section I Supplement. For reviewing the anatomy section, we thank Dr. Nripendra Dhillon, Dr. Peter Ralston and Dr. Sexton Sutherland from the UCSF Department of Anatomy. For helping us obtain information concerning review books, we thank Joe Libs (Milberry Union Bookstore, UCSF), Sam Morris (Discount Medical Books, San Francisco), Margaret Dawson (Reiter's Scientific & Professional Books, Washington, DC), and Lisa Holster (UCLA Health Sciences Bookstore). Thanks to Noam Maitless for the original book design, Evenson Design Group and Ashley Pound for design revisions, and Design Group Cook for the cover design.

For support and encouragement throughout the process, we are grateful to Karen Bagatelos, Sameer Bhushan, Martina Kreidl, Dr. Sana Khan, Dr. Steve McPhee, Dr. Barbara Gastel, Rosina Samadani, Uzma Samadani, Dr. Eric Schulze, Dr. Daniela Drake, Dr. Lawrence Tierney, Ray Moloney (Paper Book Press), Jonathan Kirsch, Esq., Konrad Fernandez, Jean Williams, Michael Lowe, and the UCSF Office of Medical Student Affairs.

Thanks to our publisher, Appleton & Lange, for offering a coupon for each new contribution used in future editions of this book, and for the valuable assistance of their staff. For enthusiasm, support, and commitment for this ongoing and ever challenging project, thanks to our tireless editor, Marinita Timban. For personal and last minute production support, thanks to our personal copyeditor Andrea Fellows, Jimmy and Bennie Sauls (Rainbow Graphics), and John Williams, Amy Schermerhorn and Anne Fountain (Appleton & Lange).

For submitting major contributions to the 1997 edition, often including dozens of new entries, book reviews or entire annotated books, we give special thanks to Steve Brown (Albany Medical College),

Felix Chien (Kansas City, Missouri), Iris Isip (University of the Philippines), Anthony Lee, Kenny Rudd (Hartford, Connecticut), Sylvia Schmidt (Germany), Rebecca Smith (University of South Carolina), Kohji Suzuki (Tokyo, Japan), Pumipak Tantamjarik (Los Angeles, California), Timothy Tsui (University of Illinois, Chicago) and David Wagar (Portland, Oregon).

For submitting contributions, surveys and suggestions for the 1997 edition we thank Ghulam Abbas, Jennifer Abeles, Laura Adam, Kenneth Adams, Taro Aikawa, Caleb Alexander, Palam Annamalai, Norman Arslanlar, Arthur Baca, Matthew Bacchetta, Rafael Baez, Debra Ball, Victor Baquero, Boone Barrow, Ashish Bassi, Alicia Batson, Jason Bauerschlag, Howard Belkin, Eli Bendavid, Gregory Bernstein, Tim Bhattacharya, Susanne Bobenrieth, Elias Bonaros, Leonid Bouinyi, Kerry Briggs, David Brock, Kimberly Brown, John Cabral, Brian Cadre, Sheila Cain, Emily Chai, Kenneth Chao, Shailendra Chauhan, Richard Chen, Grace Chou, Mary Chou, Art Chow, James Chuang, Mike Chung, Radu Constantinesscuu, Buffy Cook, Keri Davidson, Cara Debley, James Delgado, Loraine Diego, Tiffany Diers, Sol Drapkin, Susan Elbaum, Jean Emilcar, Alan English, Tom Fabricius, Susan Fong, Samuel Frimpong, Evan Garner, Andy Garrett, Brad Gaspard, Jennifer George, Najeeb Ghaussy, Jeanine Grillo, Kira Gritsman, Michael Gruber, Tom Hackett, Robert Hagar, Mirela Halasz, Bert Hartman, Ai-wu He, Joey Hettiarachchy, Laura Horvath, Julie Howard, Hoyt, J. Hsia, Matthias Imoehl, Leo Kabayashi, C. Scott Kammer, Lilly Kao, Veronica Kavorkian, Duane Keitel, Leslee Kelly, Peter Kent, Evan Khan, Leo Kobayashi, Selatin Kraja, Mark Krivopal, Sam Lan, Stephen Lane, Kari Lathrop, Thang Le, Edward Lee, Nancy Lee, Jay Lee, Henry Lin, Mike Liu, Jennifer Logan, Uri Lopatin, M. Lourdes, Kevin Lye, Christopher May, Vikas Mehta, Aaron Michelfelder, Avijit Mitra, Daniel More, Anbin Mu, Anrong Mu, Laura Murvar, Kelly Nations, A. Netalkar, Jose Rivera Nevarez, Henry Nguyen, Tamara Nix, Eliza Oh, Kim Olson, Edward Orlando, Roberto Otero, Shelley Overholt, Michael Parimucha, Kourosh Parsapour, Anil Patel, Ushma Patel, Anil Patel, Ushma Patel, Robert Pearlman, Jim Pilkinton, Jeff Purvis, Quibing Qian, Kevin Raff, Braden Rance, Jennifer Resniek, Matthew Rhames, Netti Riggs, Renard Ruiz, Bridget Sanders, Uzma Samadani, Jasmine Sharma, Brian Shelley, Carol Shi, John Shoosmith, Shannon Sims, Andrius Skucas, Scott Snyder, Evan Sorokin, Brennan Spiegel, David Spiggle, Carl Spiuak, K. Srivatsa, William Steinberg, Andrea Stonecipher, Doug Strobel, Bernard Suarez, Debra Sussman, Jafar Tay, Rachel Tesser, Marc Theilhaber, Lori Travis, Kevin Tseng, Fan-Ying Tseng, Moses Udoh, Eric VanMoorlehem, Anjali Varde, Adil Waheed, Francine Wiest, Mariusz Wirga, Lee Wolfe, Satoru Yamamoto, Bertina Yen, Barbara Young, George Younis, Bin Zhang, and Andru Ziwasimon. We apologize if any names have been omitted or misspelled. Please contact us with any additions or corrections.

Finally, thanks to Ted Hon, one of the founding authors of this book, for his vision in developing this guide on the computer. Eddie Chu and Jeffrey Hansen were also among the founding authors of this book. For major contributions to previous editions, we thank Matthew Voorsanger, John Bethea, Jr., Ketan Kapadia, Lisa Backus, Yi Chieh Shiuey, Shin Kim, Robert Hosseini, Kassem Kahlil, Dax Swanson, Kathleen Liu, Kieu Nguyen, Hatem Abou-Sayed, Shaun Anand, Radhika Sekhri-Breaden, Stephen Gomperts, Sana Khan, Thao Pham, Taejoon Ahn, Alireza Atri, Ross Berkeley, Christine Pham, Judy Shih, David Steensma, Michael Rizen, Kambiz Kosari and Gary Ulaner.

Los Angeles	Vikas Bhushan
New Haven	Tao Le
Orlando	Chirag Amin
Baltimore	Ross Levine

How to Contribute

This version of *First Aid for the USMLE Step 1* incorporates hundreds of contributions and changes suggested by faculty and student reviewers. We invite you to participate in this process.

Please send us your suggestions for:

- New facts, mnemonics, diagrams, or strategies
- High-yield topics that may reappear on future Step 1 exams
- Personal ratings and comments on review books that you have examined

For each entry incorporated into the next edition, you will receive one $10 coupon per entry good toward the purchase of any Appleton & Lange medical book, as well as personal acknowledgment in the next edition. Diagrams, tables, partial entries, updates, corrections, and study hints are also appreciated, and significant contributions will be compensated at the discretion of the publisher. Also let us know about material in this edition that you feel is low yield and should be deleted.

The **preferred** way to submit entries, suggestions, or corrections is via electronic mail, addressed to the authors:

vbhushan@aol.com
taotle@aol.com
chiragamin@aol.com

The preferred way to contact the publisher is via electronic mail, addressed to:

marinita_timban@prenhall.com

For *First Aid for the USMLE Step 1* updates and corrections, visit our internet Website at:

http://www.s2smed.com

Otherwise, please send entries, neatly written or typed or on disk (Microsoft Word), to: First Aid for the USMLE Step 1, 720 Orange St #2, New Haven, CT 06511–9046, Attention: Contributions. Please use the contribution and survey forms on the following pages. Each form constitutes an entry. (Attach additional pages as needed.)

Another option is to send in your entire annotated book. We will look through your additions and notes and will send you Appleton & Lange coupons based on the quantity and quality of any additions that we incorporate into the 1998 edition. Books will be returned upon request. Contributions received by July 15, 1997, receive priority consideration for the 1998 edition of *First Aid for the USMLE Step 1.*

Note to Contributors
All entries are subject to editing and reviewing. Please verify all data and spellings carefully. In the event that similar or duplicate entries are received, only the first entry received will be used. Include a reference to a standard textbook to facilitate verification of the fact. Please follow the style, punctuation, and format of this edition if possible.

Contribution Form I

For entries, mnemonics, facts,
strategies, corrections,
diagrams, etc.

Contributor Name: _____

School/Affiliation: _____

Address: _____

_____

Telephone: _____

E-mail: _____

Topic:

Fact and Description:

Notes, Diagrams, and Mnemonics:

Reference:

Please seal with tape only.
No staples or paper clips.

- (fold here) -

BUSINESS REPLY MAIL
FIRST-CLASS MAIL PERMIT NO. 596 NEW HAVEN CT

POSTAGE WILL BE PAID BY ADDRESSEE

FIRST AID FOR THE USMLE STEP 1
720 ORANGE ST #2
NEW HAVEN CT 06511-9046

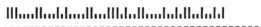

- (fold here) -

Contribution Form II

For high-yield topics for
Section II Supplement

Contributor Name: _____

School/Affiliation: _____

Address: _____

_____

Telephone: _____

E-mail: _____

Please place the subject heading (e.g., Anatomy) on the first line and the high-yield topic on the following two lines.

1. Subject: _____

   Topic: _____

   _____

2. Subject: _____

   Topic: _____

   _____

3. Subject: _____

   Topic: _____

   _____

4. Subject: _____

   Topic: _____

   _____

5. Subject: _____

   Topic: _____

   _____

6. Subject: _____

   Topic: _____

   _____

7. Subject: _____

   Topic: _____

   _____

8. Subject: _____

   Topic: _____

   _____

9. Subject: _____

   Topic: _____

   _____

10. Subject: _____

    Topic: _____

    _____

Please seal with tape only.
No staples or paper clips.

- - - - - - - - - - - - - - - - - - (fold here) -

BUSINESS REPLY MAIL
FIRST-CLASS MAIL PERMIT NO. 596 NEW HAVEN CT

POSTAGE WILL BE PAID BY ADDRESSEE

FIRST AID FOR THE USMLE STEP 1
720 ORANGE ST #2
NEW HAVEN CT 06511-9046

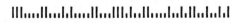

- -
(fold here)

Contribution Form III

For review book ratings for Section III

Contributor Name: _____

School/Affiliation: _____

Address: _____

_____

Telephone: _____

E-mail: _____

We welcome additional comments on review books rated in Section III as well as reviews of texts not rated in Section III. Please fill out each review entry as completely as possible. Please do not leave "Comments" blank. Rate texts using the letter grading scale provided on p. 218, taking into consideration other books on that subject.

1. *Title/Author:* _____   Days needed to read: _____

   Publisher/Series: _____   ISBN Number: _____

   Rating: _____   *Comments:* _____

   _____

   _____

2. *Title/Author:* _____   Days needed to read: _____

   Publisher/Series: _____   ISBN Number: _____

   Rating: _____   *Comments:* _____

   _____

   _____

3. *Title/Author:* _____   Days needed to read: _____

   Publisher/Series: _____   ISBN Number: _____

   Rating: _____   *Comments:* _____

   _____

   _____

   _____

4. *Title/Author:* _____   Days needed to read: _____

   Publisher/Series: _____   ISBN Number: _____

   Rating: _____   *Comments:* _____

   _____

   _____

5. *Title/Author:* _____   Days needed to read: _____

   Publisher/Series: _____   ISBN Number: _____

   Rating: _____   *Comments:* _____

   _____

   _____

Please return by July 15, 1997. You will receive personal acknowledgment and a $10 coupon toward selected Appleton & Lange books for each entry that is used in future editions.

Please seal with tape only.
No staples or paper clips.

- (fold here) -

BUSINESS REPLY MAIL
FIRST-CLASS MAIL PERMIT NO. 596 NEW HAVEN CT

POSTAGE WILL BE PAID BY ADDRESSEE

FIRST AID FOR THE USMLE STEP 1
720 ORANGE ST #2
NEW HAVEN CT 06511-9046

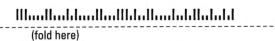

- (fold here) -

User Survey

Contributor Name: _____

School/Affiliation: _____

Address: _____

_____

Telephone: _____

E-mail: _____

What student-to-student advice would you give someone preparing for the USMLE Step 1?

Are you aware of any commercial review courses not listed in Section I: Guide to Efficient Exam Preparation? If yes, which ones? What commercial courses have you been enrolled in, and what were your overall assessments of the courses?

What would you change about the study and test-taking strategies listed in Section I: Guide to Efficient Exam Preparation?

Were there any high-yield facts or topics in Section II that you think were inaccurate or should be deleted? Which ones and why? What would you change or add?

What review books for the USMLE Step 1 are not covered in Section III? Would you change the rating of any of the review books in Section III? If so, which one(s) and why?

What other suggestions do you have for improving *First Aid for the USMLE Step 1*? Any other comments or suggestions? What did you like most about the book?

Please return by July 15, 1997. You will receive personal acknowledgment and a $10 coupon toward selected Appleton & Lange books for material that is used in future editions.

Please seal with tape only.
No staples or paper clips.

-- (fold here) --

BUSINESS REPLY MAIL
FIRST-CLASS MAIL PERMIT NO. 596 NEW HAVEN CT

POSTAGE WILL BE PAID BY ADDRESSEE

FIRST AID FOR THE USMLE STEP 1
720 ORANGE ST #2
NEW HAVEN CT 06511-9046

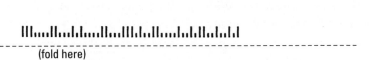

-- (fold here) --

How to Use This Book

Medical students who have used previous editions of this guide have given us feedback on how best to make use of the book.

It is recommended that you begin using this book as early as possible when learning the basic medical sciences. You can use Section III to select first-year course review books and then use those books for review while taking your medical school classes.

Use different parts of the book at different stages in your preparation for the USMLE Step 1. Before you begin to study for the USMLE Step 1, we suggest that you read Section I: Guide to Efficient Exam Preparation and Section III: Database of Science Review Books. **If you are an international medical graduate student, an osteopathic medical student, a podiatry student, or a student with a disability,** refer to the appropriate Section I supplement for additional advice. Devise a study plan and decide what resources to buy. Scanning Section II will give you an initial idea of the diverse range of topics covered on the USMLE Step 1.

As you study each discipline, **use the corresponding high-yield fact section in *First Aid for the USMLE Step 1* as a way of consolidating the material and testing yourself** to see if you have covered some of the frequently tested items. Work with the book to integrate important facts into your fund of knowledge. Using *First Aid for the USMLE Step 1* as a review can serve as both a self-test of your knowledge and a repetition of important facts to learn.

Return to Section II frequently during your preparation and fill your short-term memory with remaining high-yield facts a few days before the USMLE Step 1. The book can serve as a useful way of retaining key associations and high-yield facts fresh in your memory just prior to the examination. Some students choose to skim the book between the two exam days.

Reviewing the book immediately after the exam is probably the best way to **help us improve the book in the next edition.** Decide what was truly high and low yield and **send in the contribution forms or your entire annotated book.**

Guide to Efficient Exam Preparation

INTRODUCTION

Relax.

This section is intended to make your exam preparation easier, not harder. Our goal is to reduce your stress and help you make the most of your study effort by helping you understand more about the United States Medical Licensing Examination, Step 1 (USMLE Step 1). As a medical student, you are no doubt familiar with taking standardized examinations and absorbing large amounts of material. However, in confronting the USMLE Step 1, it is easy to become sidetracked and not achieve your goal of studying with maximum effectiveness. Common mistakes that students make when studying for the boards include the following:

- "Stressing out" due to an inadequate understanding of the test
- Not understanding how scoring is performed and what your score means
- Not using the NBME/USMLE's own publications for maximum benefit
- Starting to study too late
- Using inefficient or inappropriate study methods
- Buying the wrong books or buying more books than you can ever use
- Buying only one publisher's review series for all subjects
- Buying review books too late or never reading them
- Not using practice examinations for maximum benefit
- Not analyzing and improving your test-taking strategies
- Getting bogged down by reviewing difficult topics excessively
- Studying material that is rarely tested on the USMLE Step 1
- Failing to master certain high-yield subjects due to overconfidence

In this section, we offer advice to help you avoid these pitfalls and be more productive in your studies. First, it is important to understand what the examination involves.

USMLE STEP 1—THE BASICS

The purpose of the USMLE Step 1 is to test your understanding and application of important concepts in basic biomedical sciences.[2]

A degree of concern about your performance on the USMLE Step 1 examination is expected and appropriate. However, medical students all too often become unnecessarily anxious about the examination. It is important to take a moment to understand what it involves. As you become more familiar with the USMLE Step 1, you can translate your anxiety into more efficient preparation.

The USMLE Step 1 is the first of three examinations that you must pass in order to become a licensed physician in the United States.[1] The USMLE is a joint endeavor of the National Board of Medical Examiners (NBME) and the Federation of State Medical Boards (FSMB). In previous years, the examination was strictly organized around seven traditional disciplines: anatomy, behavioral science, biochemistry, microbiology, pathology, pharmacology, and physiology. In June 1991, the NBME began administering the "new" NBME Part I examination, which offers a more integrated and multidisciplinary format and more **clinically** oriented questions.

In 1992, the USMLE replaced both the Federation Licensing Examination (FLEX) and the certifying examinations of the NBME.[3] The USMLE now serves as the **single** examination system for United States medical students and international medical graduates seeking medical licensure in the United States.

Format

The USMLE Step 1 is a multiple-choice examination administered over a two-day period (Fig. 1). It consists of four booklets, each containing approximately 180 items. On each day of the examination, one booklet is administered in the morning and one is administered in the afternoon. You are allotted three hours to complete each test booklet. A sample answer sheet and the table of normal

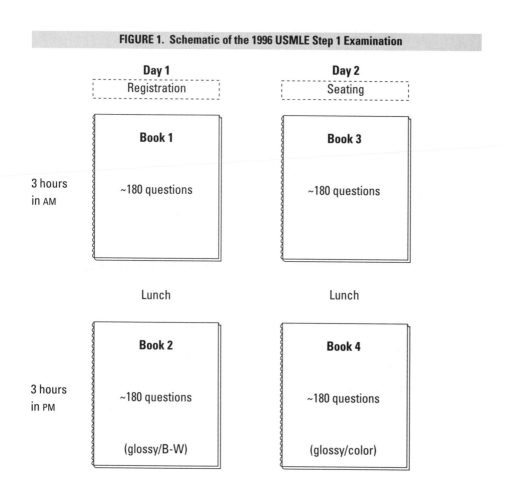

FIGURE 1. Schematic of the 1996 USMLE Step 1 Examination

	Day 1	Day 2
	Registration	Seating
3 hours in AM	**Book 1** ~180 questions	**Book 3** ~180 questions
	Lunch	Lunch
3 hours in PM	**Book 2** ~180 questions (glossy/B-W)	**Book 4** ~180 questions (glossy/color)

laboratory values provided within each booklet are shown in the *USMLE Step 1 General Instructions, Content Outline, and Sample Items.*[4]

Figure 1 should give you a mental image of the exam structure. Note that:

Test booklets vary in difficulty, so do not become discouraged early in the exam.

- Booklets vary in overall difficulty. There does not seem to be a pattern of increasing or decreasing difficulty as you proceed through the exam.
- Subject areas vary randomly from question to question. Many questions incorporate multiple basic science and medical concepts.
- The afternoon booklets are usually printed on high-quality glossy paper and include a number of photographs. In 1996, students reported a black-and-white glossy booklet during the afternoon of the first day and a color glossy booklet during the afternoon of the second day.
- The exam is scored if all four booklets are opened.[5] Otherwise, a notation on the USMLE transcript is made that the examination was incomplete.

Question Types

One-best-answer items are the most commonly used multiple-choice format. They usually consist of a statement or a question followed by a list of three to five options. You are required to select the one best answer among the options. A number of options may be partially correct, in which case you must select the option that best answers the question or completes the statement. A variation of this format employs negatively phrased questions that include negative words such as EXCEPT, LEAST, and NOT.

About half the Step 1 questions begin with a description of a patient.[6]

Clinical vignettes have become a prominent feature of the USMLE Step 1. They consist of a short description of a clinical case or scenario, often including lab values and radiologic images, followed by a question or questions in the one-best-answer format described previously.

Matching sets consist of a list of approximately 4 to 26 items from which you choose the one best answer that corresponds to each of the numbered items or questions located below the list. Once again, a number of options may be partially correct, in which case you must select the option that best answers the question or completes the statement.

Student experience from the June 1996 administration indicates that questions in each booklet are organized by type, starting with the one-best-answer items, followed by negatively phrased one-best-answer items, and ending with matching sets. Although the numerical proportions of question types vary with each booklet, students recall that the one-best-answer items constituted approximately 92% of all questions, while negatively phrased one-best-answer items constituted about 3% and matching sets made up roughly 5% of the questions (Fig. 2).

FIGURE 2. Question Type and Order

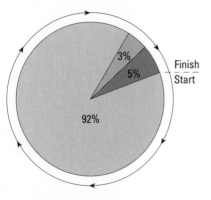

~92% One-best-answer

~3% Negatively phrased one-best-answer

~5% Matching and extended matching

4

FIGURE 3A. Simulated Score Report—Front Page

Doe, John I.
000 Main St.
Any Town, CA 12345

USMLE ID: 0-123-456-7
Test Date: June 1996

The USMLE is a single examination program for all applicants for medical licensure in the United States; it replaces the Federation Licensing Examination (FLEX) and the certifying examinations of the National Board of Medical Examiners (NBME Parts I, II, and III). The program consists of three Steps designed to assess an examinee's understanding of and ability to apply concepts and principles that are important in health and disease and that constitute the basis of safe and effective patient care. Step 1 is designed to assess whether an examinee understands and can apply key concepts of the basic biomedical sciences, with an emphasis on principles and mechanisms of health, disease, and modes of therapy. The inclusion of **Step 1** in the USMLE sequence is intended to ensure mastery of not only the basic medical sciences undergirding the safe and competent practice of medicine in the present, but also the scientific principles required for maintenance of competence through lifelong learning. Results of the examination are reported to medical licensing authorities in the United States and its territories for use in granting an initial license to practice medicine. The two numeric scores shown below are equivalent; each state or territory may use either score in making licensing decisions. These scores represent your results for the administration of Step 1 on the test date shown above.

| PASS | The result is based on the minimum passing score set by USMLE for Step 1. Individual licensing authorities may accept the USMLE-recommended pass/fail result or may establish a different passing score for their own jurisdictions. |

| 200 | This score is determined by your overall performance on Step 1. For recent administrations, the mean and standard deviation for first-time examinees from U.S. medical schools are approximately 205 and 20, respectively, with most scores falling between 165 and 245. A score of 176 is set by USMLE to pass Step 1. The standard error of measurement (SEM)* for this scale is four points. |

| 82 | This score is also determined by your overall performance on the examination. A score of 82 on this scale is equivalent to a score of 200 on the scale described above. A score of 75 on this scale, which is equivalent to a score of 176 on the scale described above, is set by USMLE to pass Step 1. The SEM* for this scale is one point. |

* Your score is influenced by both your general understanding of basic biomedical sciences and the specific set of items selected for this Step 1 examination. The SEM provides an estimate of the range within which your scores might be expected to vary by chance if you were tested repeatedly using similar tests.

Scoring and Failure Rates

Each Step 1 examinee receives a score report that has the examinee's pass/fail status, two test scores, and a graphic depiction of the examinee's performance by discipline and organ system or subject area (Fig. 3). The actual organ system profiles reported may depend on the statistical characteristics of a given administration of the examination.

FIGURE 3B. Simulated Score Report—Back Page

INFORMATION PROVIDED FOR EXAMINEE USE ONLY

The Performance Profile below is provided solely for the benefit of the examinee.
The USMLE will not provide or verify the Performance Profile for any other person, organization,
or agency.

USMLE STEP 1 PERFORMANCE PROFILE

	Lower Performance	Borderline Performance	Higher Performance
Behavioral Sciences			XXXXXXXXXXX
Biochemistry			XXXXXXXXX
Cardiovascular System			XXXXXXXXXXXXX
Gastrointestinal System			XXXXXXXXXXXXXX
General Principles of Health & Disease			XXXXXXX
Gross Anatomy & Embryology		XXXXXXXXXXXXX	
Hematopoietic & Lymphoreticular Systems			XXXXXXXXXXXXXXX
Histology & Cell Biology		XXXXXXXXXXXXX	
Microbiology & Immunology			XXXXXXXXX
Musculoskeletal, Skin, & Connective Tissue			XXXXXXXXXXXXXXXX
Nervous System/Special Senses			XXXXXXXXX
Pathology			XXXX*
Pharmacology			XXXXXXX
Physiology		XXXXXXX	
Renal/Urinary Systems		XXXXXXXXXXXXX	
Reproductive & Endocrine Systems			XXXXXXXXXXX
Respiratory System			XXXXXXXXXX*

The above Performance Profile is provided to aid in self-assessment. The shaded area defines a borderline level of performance for each content area; borderline performance is comparable to a HIGH FAIL/LOW PASS on the total test.

Performance bands indicate areas of relative strength and weakness. Some bands are wider than others. The width of a performance band reflects the precision of measurement; narrower bands indicate greater precision. The band width for a given content area is the same for all examinees. An asterisk indicates that your performance band extends beyond the displayed portion of the scale.

This profile should not be compared to those from other Step 1 administrations.

Additional information concerning the topics covered in each content area can be found in the *USMLE Step 1 General Instructions, Content Description, and Sample Items.*

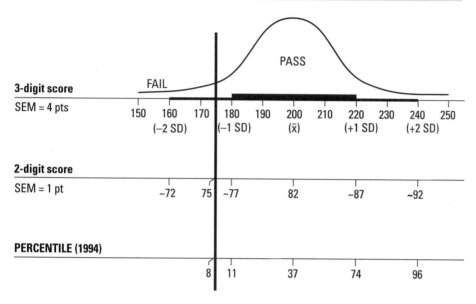

FIGURE 4. Scoring Scales for the USMLE Step 1: Approximate 1994 Equivalencies

3-digit score
SEM = 4 pts

2-digit score
SEM = 1 pt

PERCENTILE (1994)

FIGURE 5. Score to Percentile Conversion[7]

Three-Digit Score	Anchor Group* (%ile)	June '94** (%ile)
244	99	98
240	98	96
235	97	93
230	94	89
225	89	82
220	83	74
215	76	65
210	67	56
205	57	46
200	48	37
195	38	29
190	29	22
185	21	16
180	15	11
176	**11**	**8**
170	7	5
165	4	4
160	3	2
155	2	2

* Anchor Group June 91 2nd-yr US students

** June 94 US and Canadian 1st-time takers

For 1996, USMLE provided two overall test scores based on the total number of items answered correctly on the examination. The first score, the three-digit score, was reported as a scaled score, in which the mean was 208 and the standard deviation was 20 (Fig. 4). (Values were based on the performance of the June 1991 USMLE Step 1 examinee group.) This means that a score of 208 roughly corresponded to the 50th percentile, while a score of 225 roughly corresponded to the 85th percentile.[8] The June 1996 USMLE score report for students did not include any percentile score equivalents. Percentile performance norms for 1994 were provided to medical schools and have been summarized in Figure 5. The second score scale, the two-digit score, defines 75 as the minimum passing score (equivalent to a score of 176 on the first scale). A score of 82 is equivalent to a score of 200 on the first score scale. To avoid confusion, we refer to scores using the three-digit scale with a mean of 208 and a standard deviation of 20.

A score of 176 or higher is required to pass Step 1. The pass/fail standard for Step 1 is predominantly "content-based." The passing mark was determined by reviewing test items and defining a mastery level of performance.[9] In 1995, 94% of all first-time test takers passed the June administration of the USMLE Step 1 (Fig. 6). The mean score for first-time test takers in the United States was 208 for the June 1995 Step 1 exam (Fig. 7).

It is estimated that passing Step 1 corresponds to answering between 55% and 65% of the questions correctly. After extensive review by the USMLE Step 1 committee in 1995, the pass/fail standard of 176 was unchanged and will likely

The mean Step 1 score for US medical students rose from 200 in 1991 to 208 in 1995.

Passing Step 1 is estimated to correspond to answering 55–65% of the questions correctly.

FIGURE 6. Passing Rates for 1995 USMLE Step 1[11]						
	June 1995		September 1995		Total 1995	
	No. Tested	Passing (%)	No. Tested	Passing (%)	No. Tested	Passing (%)
NBME-Registered Examinees						
First-Time Takers	15,707	94	1,147	79	16,854	93
Repeaters	977	56	1,281	47	2,258	51
NBME Total	**16,684**	**92**	**2,428**	**62**	**19,112**	**88**
ECFMG*-Registered Examinees						
First-Time Takers	8,968	55	11,647	55	20,615	55
Repeaters	6,077	31	6,905	28	12,982	29
ECFMG Total	**15,045**	**45**	**18,552**	**45**	**33,597**	**45**

*Educational Commission for Foreign Medical Graduates.

Near the failure threshold, each three-digit scale point is equivalent to about three questions answered correctly.[10]

FIGURE 7. Trends in Performance on USMLE Step 1[12]

	Percent Failing (< 176)	Percent > 225
1991	11	10
1992	9	11
1993	7	14
1994	8	11
1995	8	15

(NBME-registered first-time test takers only)

remain so until the next substantive reevaluation in 1998. Of note is the fact that the USMLE Step 2 passing threshold was recently raised from 167 to 170.

According to the USMLE, medical schools receive a listing of total scores and pass/fail results plus group summaries by discipline and organ systems. Students can withhold their scores from their medical school if they wish. Official USMLE transcripts, which can be sent on request to residency programs, include only total scores, not performance profiles.

The preceding information is based on students' experience with the June 1995 and June 1996 administrations of the USMLE Step 1 and information published by the NBME (refer to the NBME publications listed in Section III). The format and the scoring of the examination are subject to change, and it is best to consult the latest NBME publications and your medical school for the most current and accurate information regarding the examination.

NBME/USMLE Publications
We strongly encourage students to use the free materials provided by the testing agencies (see page 28), to study in detail the following NBME publications, and to retain them for future reference:

- *USMLE Step 1 General Instructions, Content Outline, and Sample Items* (information given free to all examinees)

- *USMLE Bulletin of Information* (information given free to all examinees)
- *Retired NBME Basic Medical Sciences (Part I) Test Items* (**out of print**)
- *Self-Test in the Part I Basic Medical Sciences* (**out of print**)

The *USMLE Step 1 General Instructions, Content Outline, and Sample Items* booklet contains approximately 180 questions that are identical in format and similar in content to the questions on the actual USMLE Step 1. This practice test is one of the best methods for assessing your boards test-taking skills. However, it does not contain enough questions to simulate the full length of the examination, and its content is a very limited sample of the possible basic science material covered. The extremely detailed 25-page Step I Content Outline provided by the USMLE has not proved useful for students studying for the exam. The USMLE even states that "the content outline is not intended as a guide for curriculum development or as a study guide."[13] We concur with this assessment.

The *USMLE Bulletin of Information* booklet accompanies application materials for the USMLE. This publication has detailed procedural and policy information regarding the USMLE, including descriptions of all three Steps, scoring of the exams, reporting of scores to medical schools and residency programs, procedures for score rechecks and other inquiries, policies for irregular behavior, and test dates.

The now-out-of-print *Retired NBME Basic Medical Sciences (Part I) Test Items* contains nearly 1000 "retired" questions, the content of which frequently reappears on the new USMLE Step 1. This publication allows you to assess your performance on basic science topics and to identify areas of weakness. The retired test items include old NBME Part I questions of the K (multiple true/false) and C (A/B/both/neither) variety, neither of which appears on the USMLE Step 1. Although these question **types** are not found on the current version of the boards, the **content** of these questions is still relevant.

Another out-of-print NBME publication very useful to students in preparing for the USMLE Step 1 is the *Self-Test in the Part I Basic Medical Sciences,* with 630 questions drawn from the old NBME Part I item pool. It can be used in the same way as the *Retired NBME Basic Sciences (Part I) Test Items.* There is some overlap in content between the two publications. Unfortunately, these question booklets are **no longer available from the NBME,** and the NBME does not grant permission to reprint these publications to individuals, medical schools, or organizations.[14] Some medical schools, however, still have old copies of these booklets available for their students. Ideally, a copy should be placed on reserve in the medical library. Another source would be third- and fourth-year students who have saved their copies.

The original questions are becoming more difficult to find every year. However, explanatory answers to all 1623 questions in the *Retired* and *Self-Test* booklets are available as an independent publication titled *Underground Step 1 Answers to the NBME Retired and Self-Test Questions.* This book is designed to be read alone or as a study guide to the NBME questions. This publication is by the same authors as *First Aid for the USMLE Step 1* and is available for $22.95 plus shipping and handling at (800) 247-6553 (see page 280 for a review and the inside back cover of this book for more information).

Although the NBME Self-Test and Retired Test Items are both out of print, they remain a good source of practice questions for the USMLE Step 1.

The most productive way to use these study aids is to take the practice examinations and to identify carefully the questions that were missed or that were answered correctly by guessing. Students often find that many missed questions originate from a limited number of seemingly trivial topics (e.g., congenital diseases involving sphingolipid synthesis). It is worthwhile to study these subjects thoroughly, because student experience has shown that the topics covered in these retired questions (trivial or not) **remain predictors** of many topics tested on the new USMLE Step 1.

In summary, the old NBME publications contain many questions that still approximate the style and content of questions appearing on recent USMLE Step 1 examinations. Moreover, some questions remain superior to questions found in most commercial review books currently on the market. Thus, we suggest that you study all questions available from the NBME before taking the examination. Try some questions early to assess your strengths and weaknesses; save some questions for the few weeks before the exam to evaluate your progress.

DEFINING YOUR GOAL

It is useful to define your own personal performance goal when approaching the USMLE Step 1. Your style and intensity of preparation can then be matched to your goal. Your goal may depend on your school's requirements, your specialty choice, your grades to date, and your personal assessment of test importance.

Just Pass the Exam

As mentioned earlier, the USMLE Step 1 is the first of three standardized examinations that you must pass to become a licensed physician in the United States. For many medical schools, passing the USMLE Step 1 is also required before you can continue with your clinical training. The NBME, however, feels that medical schools should not use Step 1 as the sole determinant of being advanced to the third year.[15] If you are headed for a "noncompetitive" residency program and you have consulted advisers and fourth-year medical students in your area of interest, you may feel comfortable with this approach.

Beat the Mean

Although the NBME warns against the misuse of examination scores to evaluate student qualifications for residency positions, some residency program di-

FIGURE 8. Informal Post-Match Survey: Step 1 Goals*		
Just Pass	**Beat the Mean**	**Ace the Exam**
Pediatrics →	Emergency Medicine	Dermatology
Family Practice →	OB/GYN	ENT
Internal Medicine →	←Radiology	Orthopedics
Anesthesiology	General Surgery	Ophthalmology
Psychiatry		

* Based on the 1995 results of 110 respondents to an informal survey distributed to US fourth-year medical students at UCSF, UCLA, the University of Louisville, and the University of Miami. Arrows indicate perceived trends from 1996: → = increasing; ← = decreasing score.

rectors continue to use Step 1 scores to screen applicants.[16] Thus, many students feel it is important to score higher than the national average.

Internship and residency programs vary greatly in their requests for scores. Some simply request your pass/fail status, whereas others request your total score. Some programs have been known to request a photocopy of your score report to determine how well you performed on the individual sections; however, this is unusual. It is unclear how the continuing changes in the USMLE Step 1 examination and score reporting will affect the application process for residency programs. The best sources of bottom-line information are fourth-year medical students who have recently completed the residency application process.

Fourth-year medical students have the best feel for how Step 1 scores factor into residency applications.

First Aid for the USMLE Step 1 has conducted a small informal post-match survey of fourth-year medical students at several US medical schools regarding the use of Step 1 scores. The results are summarized in Figure 8. Use this information only as a rough guide for goal setting. Trends in certain specialties are evolving rapidly (see also Le, Bhushan, Amin: *First Aid for the Match*, and Iserson: *Getting into Residency*).

Some medical students may wish to "beat the mean" for their own personal satisfaction. For these students, there may be a psychological advantage to scoring higher than the national average.

Ace the Exam

Certain highly competitive residency programs, such as those in ophthalmology and orthopedic surgery, have acknowledged the use of Step 1 scores in the selection process. In such residency programs, greater emphasis may be placed on attaining a high score, so students who wish to enter these programs may

Some competitive residency programs use Step 1 scores in their selection process.

11

want to consider aiming for a very high score on the USMLE Step 1. However, use of the USMLE scores for residency selection has been criticized because neither Step 1 nor Step 2 was designed for this purpose.[17] In addition, only a subset of the basic science facts and concepts that are tested is important to functioning well on the wards. Alternatively, some students may wish to score well in order to feel a sense of mastery as they complete the basic science years.

TIMELINE FOR STUDY

Make a Schedule

There are three basic study patterns:

- *the compulsive (months—ace exam)*
- *the crammer (weeks—just pass)*
- *the IMG (months—variable)*

After you have defined your goals, map out a study schedule consistent with your objectives, your vacation time, and the difficulty of your ongoing course-work (Fig. 9). Determine whether you want to spread out your study time or concentrate it into 14-hour study days in the final weeks. Factor in your own history in preparing for standardized examinations (e.g., SAT, MCAT), but re-member that the USMLE Step 1 is longer and covers far more material than other tests you may have taken.

"Crammable" subjects should be covered later and less "cram-mable" subjects earlier.

Another important consideration is when you will study each subject. Some subjects lend themselves to cramming, whereas others demand a substantial long-term commitment. The "crammable" subjects for Step 1 are those for which concise yet relatively complete review books are available. (See Section III for highly rated review and sample examination books.) Behavioral science and physiology are two subjects with concise review books. Three subjects with longer but quite complete review books are microbiology, pharmacology, and biochemistry. Thus, these subjects could be covered toward the end of your schedule, whereas other subjects (anatomy and pathology) require a longer time commitment and could be studied earlier. Practically speaking, spending a given amount of time on a crammable or high-yield subject (partic-ularly in the waning days before the test) generally produces more correct an-swers on the examination than spending the same amount of time on a low-yield subject. Student opinion indicates that knowing the crammable subjects extremely well probably results in a higher overall score than knowing all the subjects moderately well.

Allow time in your study schedule for getting sidetracked by personal emergencies.

If you are having difficulty deciding when to start your test preparation, you may find the reverse-calendar approach helpful. Start with the day of the test and plan backward, setting deadlines for objectives to be met. Where the plan-ning ends on your calendar defines a possible starting point.

Make your schedule realistic, with achievable goals. Many students make the mistake of studying at a level of detail that requires too much time for a compre-hensive review—reading *Gray's Anatomy* in a couple of days is not a realistic goal! Revise your schedule regularly based on your actual progress. Be careful

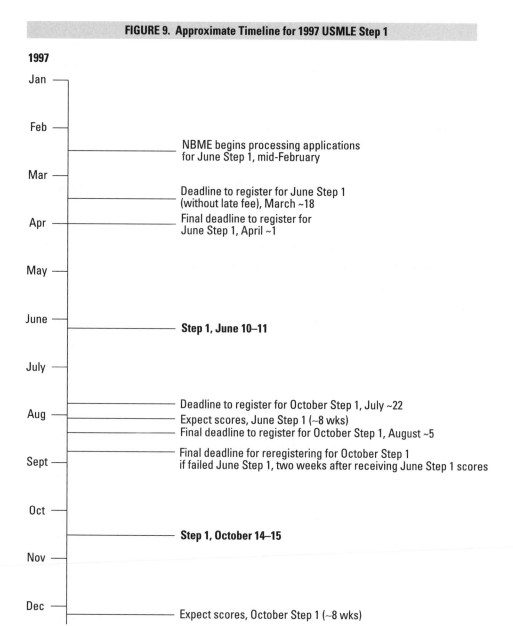

FIGURE 9. Approximate Timeline for 1997 USMLE Step 1

1997

Jan

Feb
— NBME begins processing applications
for June Step 1, mid-February

Mar
— Deadline to register for June Step 1
(without late fee), March ~18

Apr
— Final deadline to register for
June Step 1, April ~1

May

June
— **Step 1, June 10–11**

July

Aug
— Deadline to register for October Step 1, July ~22
— Expect scores, June Step 1 (~8 wks)
— Final deadline to register for October Step 1, August ~5
— Final deadline for reregistering for October Step 1
if failed June Step 1, two weeks after receiving June Step 1 scores

Sept

Oct

— **Step 1, October 14–15**

Nov

Dec
— Expect scores, October Step 1 (~8 wks)

not to lose focus. Beware of feelings of inadequacy when comparing study schedules and progress with your peers. Do not set yourself up for frustration.

You will need time for uninterrupted and focused study. Plan your personal affairs to minimize crisis situations near the date of the test. Allot an adequate number of breaks in your study schedule to avoid burnout. Maintain a healthy lifestyle, with proper diet and exercise. Getting sick before or during the test will not help your cause.

Avoid burnout. You need to reach and maintain peak concentration on exam day.

Year(s) Prior

USMLE asserts that the best preparation for the USMLE Step 1 is "broadly based learning that establishes a strong general foundation of understanding

Buy review books early (first-year) and use while studying for courses.

of concepts and principles in basic sciences."[18] We agree. Although you may be tempted to rely solely on "cramming" in the weeks and months before the test in order to pass, you should not have to. The knowledge gained during your first two years of medical school and even during your undergraduate years provides the groundwork on which to base your test preparation. The majority of your boards preparation should involve resurrecting dormant information stored away during the basic science years. One way to help resurrect this information is to tutor first-year students during your second year. Another strategy is to review related first-year material in your second year. For example, review first-year cardiac physiology and histology while learning second-year cardiac pathology.

Review first year material in parallel with related second-year topics.

We recommend that you buy highly rated review books early in your first year of medical school and use them as you study throughout the two years. When Step 1 comes along, the books will be more familiar and will be personalized to the way in which you learn. It is risky to buy unfamiliar review books in the final two or three weeks.

Talk to third- and fourth-year medical students to familiarize yourself with strengths and weaknesses in your school's curriculum. Identify subject areas in which you excel or with which you have difficulty. Content typically learned in the second year receives more coverage on Step 1 than do first-year topics due to the emphasis placed on integration of basic science information across many courses.[19] Be aware of your school's testing format and determine whether you have adequate exposure to multiple-choice and matching questions.

Month(s) Prior

Review test dates and the application procedure. In 1997, the dates of the USMLE Step 1 are June 10–11 and October 14–15 (Fig. 10). Choose the most appropriate testing site for optimal performance. Many US students simply take the exam at the closest site with all their classmates. A few students report

A major shift to a computer-based Step 1 exam is planned beginning June 1999.

FIGURE 10. Test Dates for the USMLE Step 1, Step 2, and Step 3*

	Step 1	Step 2	Step 3
1997	June 10–11 October 14–15	March 4–5 August 26–27	May 13–14 December 2–3
1998	June 9–10 October 13–14	March 3–4 August 25–26	May 12–13 December 1–2*
1999	June 8–9* October 12–13*	March 2–3* August 24–25*	May 11–12* December 7–8*

1998 and 1999 test dates not yet confirmed. *Indicates exam planned for computer-based administration.

traveling to more distant sites for privacy. Judge for yourself whether you find familiarity reassuring or stressful. If you have any disabilities or "special circumstances," contact the NBME as early as possible to discuss test accommodations (see p. 43, First Aid for the Student with a Disability).

Before you begin to study earnestly, simulate the USMLE Step 1 under "real" conditions to pinpoint strengths and weaknesses in knowledge and test-taking skills. Be sure that you are well informed about the examination and have planned your strategy for studying. Consider what study methods you will use, the study materials you will need, and how you will obtain your materials. Some review books may not be available at your local bookstore, and you may have to order ahead of time to get copies (see list of publisher contacts at the end of Section III). Plan ahead. Get advice from third- and fourth-year medical students who have recently taken the USMLE Step 1. There might be strengths and weaknesses in your school's curriculum that you should take into account in deciding where to focus your efforts. Plan how you might be able to pool resources. You might choose to share books, notes, and study hints with classmates. That is how this book began.

Simulate the USMLE Step 1 under "real" conditions before beginning your studies.

Three Weeks Prior

Two to four weeks before the examination is a good time to resimulate the USMLE Step 1. You may want to do this earlier depending on the progress of your review, but do not do it later, when there will be little time to remedy defects in your knowledge or test-taking skills. Make use of remaining good-quality sample USMLE test questions, and try to simulate the test conditions so that you gain a fair assessment of your test performance. Focus on reviewing the high-yield facts, your own notes, picture books, and very short review books.

In the final two weeks, focus on review and endurance. Avoid unfamiliar material.

One Week Prior

Make sure you have your admission ticket and items necessary for the day of the examination, including five or six #2 pencils, a nonbeeping digital timer, and nonsmudge erasers. Review the site location and test time. Work out how you will get to the test site and what parking and traffic problems you might encounter. Visit the testing site (if possible) to get a better idea of the testing conditions. Determine what you will do for lunch. Make sure you have everything you need to ensure that you will be comfortable and alert at the test site (e.g., seat cushions, earplugs, your favorite talismans). Assess your pre-exam living and sleeping arrangements. Do you have an inconsiderate roommate or a loud neighbor who could possibly disrupt your sleep or concentration several days before the exam? Do you have a raucous bird nesting outside your window? Politely announce your upcoming exam to people in your environment in order to avoid confrontations the night before the test. Take aggressive measures to ensure an environment fit for concentration and sufficient sleep (do not shoot the bird—buy some earplugs). If you really need absolute quiet and have the money, reserve a hotel room for the night(s) before the exam. If you must travel a long distance to the test site, consider arriving the day before and staying overnight with a friend or at a nearby hotel (make early hotel reservations).

One Day Prior

Ensure that you will be comfortable and alert.

Try your best to relax and rest the night before the test. Double-check your admissions and test-taking materials as well as comfort measures as discussed earlier so you do not have to deal with such details the morning of the exam. Do not study any new material. If you feel compelled to study, then quickly review short-term-memory material (e.g., Section II: Database of High-Yield Facts) before going to sleep (the brain does a lot of information processing at night). However, do not quiz yourself, as you may risk becoming flustered and confused. Do not underestimate your abilities. Remember that regardless of how hard you studied, you cannot know everything. There will be things on the exam that you have never even seen before, so do not panic.

Many students report difficulty sleeping the night prior to the exam. Do whatever it takes to ensure a good night's sleep (e.g., massage, exercise, warm milk).

Morning of the Exam

No notes, books, calculators, pagers, recording devices, or alarm timers are allowed. If you must leave, you will be escorted and will not receive extra time.

Wake up at your regular time and eat a normal breakfast. Drink coffee, tea, or soda in moderation, or you may end up wasting exam time on bathroom breaks. Make sure you have your admission ticket, test-taking materials, and comfort measures as discussed earlier. Wear loose, comfortable clothing. Plan for a variable temperature in the testing center. Remember that you will arrive early in the morning, when it may be cool, and you will not leave until late in the afternoon, when it may be warmer. Arrive at the test site a few minutes before the time designated on the admission ticket; however, do not come too early, as this may increase anxiety. Seating will be assigned, but ask to be reseated if necessary. You need to be seated in an area that will allow you to remain comfortable and to concentrate. Some students find that sitting in the very front or the very back of the room is the least distracting. Listen to your proctors regarding any changes in instructions or testing procedures specific to your test site.

Plan bathroom breaks so you do not lose valuable testing time.

Remember that it is natural (and even beneficial) to be a little nervous. Focus on being mentally clear and alert. Avoid panic. When asked to begin each booklet, catch your breath, read the directions carefully, rapidly skim the entire booklet, and then begin. Remember your time budget. If time and the testing center permit, take breaks to stretch and relax.

The lunch break is an excellent opportunity to recover, relax, and reorganize your thoughts. Some students use the break to discuss questions with classmates or to look up information. Some students also recommend reviewing theme topics during lunch and between days one and two. However, do what feels comfortable. If you decide to review the morning session, do not dwell on perceived mistakes. Remain focused and briefly review topics that you feel are likely to reappear.

Certain "theme" topics tend to recur throughout the exam and across both days.

Between the First and Second Days

Try your best to relax. You need the rest to avoid fatigue on the second day. Maintain a positive attitude and do not be discouraged. If you feel absolutely compelled, you can lightly review short-term memory material or "theme" topics heavily tested on the first day. Many students report topics being repeated on the second day. Opinions vary as to the value of looking up topics from the first day. Pros: The topic may be repeated and you may be better prepared. Cons: You may increase your stress and anxiety over questions you believe you have already answered incorrectly.

Do a quick analysis of your test-taking technique and how you might modify it for the second day. Assess whether your pace of answering questions was too slow, too fast, or just right. Again, do whatever it takes to ensure a good night's sleep.

After the Test

Have fun and relax regardless of the outcome. Taking the test is an achievement in itself. Enjoy the free time you have before your clerkships. Once you have recovered sufficiently from the test (or from partying), we invite you to send us your feedback, corrections, and suggestions for entries, facts, mnemonics, strategies, book ratings, and so on (*see* How to Contribute, p. xv). Sharing your experience benefits fellow medical students and foreign medical graduates.

If you pass Step 1, you are not allowed to retake the exam in an attempt to raise your score.

IF YOU THINK YOU FAILED

After the test, many examinees feel that they have failed, and most are at least unsure of their pass/fail status. There are several sensible steps you can take to plan for the future if you do not achieve a passing score. First, save and organize all your study materials, including review books, practice tests, and notes. If you studied from borrowed materials, make sure that you have immediate access to them. Review your school's policy regarding requirements for graduation and promotion to the third year. About one-half of the medical schools accredited by the Liaison Committee on Medical Education require passing Step 1 for promotion to the third year, and two-thirds require passing Step 1 as a requirement for graduation.[20] Even if passing Step 1 is not necessary for promotion to the third year, it is probably best to retake the exam at the next available administration. Weigh your options carefully. Finally, familiarize

FIGURE 11. Pass Rates for USMLE Step 1 Repeaters 1995[22]

Score in June	Percent Passing in October
173–175	82
170–172	76
165–169	57
160–164	29
150–159	11
<150	0
Overall	**57**

yourself with reapplication procedures for Step 1, including application deadlines and upcoming test dates.

USMLE Step 1 results usually arrive in the mail about six weeks after the test administration. If you do not achieve a passing score on the June administration of Step 1, then you have about eight weeks to prepare for the October Step 1. The deadline for the October administration is generally extended two weeks past the June Step 1 score mailings for examinees who fail and wish to repeat the exam.[21]

If you believe that your scores were incorrectly determined, you may request that your answer sheets be rechecked by hand. The resulting scores will be honored. The request must be submitted in writing with a fee to the test administration entity that registered you for the Step 1. The performance profiles on the back of the USMLE Step 1 score report provide valuable feedback concerning your relative strengths and weaknesses (*see* Fig. 3B). Study the performance profiles closely. Set up a study timeline to repair defects in knowledge as well as to maintain and improve what you already know (*see* Timeline for Study, p. 12). Do not neglect high-yield subjects. Finally, it is normal to feel somewhat anxious about retaking the test. However, if anxiety becomes a problem, seek appropriate counseling.

Sixty percent of the NBME-registered first-time takers who failed the June 1995 Step 1 repeated the exam in October. The overall pass rate for that group in October was 57% (down from 64% in 1994). However, pass rates varied widely depending on previous performance on the June 1995 administration (Fig. 11).

Although the NBME allows an unlimited number of attempts to pass the Step 1, both the NBME and the FSMB recommend that licensing authorities allow a minimum of three and a maximum of six attempts for each Step examination.[23] Again, review your school's policy regarding retakes.

IF YOU FAILED

Even if you came out of the exam room feeling that you failed, seeing that failing grade in cold print can be traumatic, and it is natural to feel upset. Different people react in different ways: For some it is a stimulus to buckle down and study harder; for some it "takes the wind out of their sails" for a few days; and for some it may lead to a reassessment of their goals and abilities. For a few, however, failure may trigger weeks or months of sadness, feelings of hopelessness, social withdrawal, and inability to concentrate—in other words, a true clinical depression.

If you are depressed, seek help. As you know from your studies, depression is a common, potentially disabling, and at times even a fatal illness. Depression is also very treatable, and you must use the same resources that you plan to offer your patients. In other words, you must seek treatment, whether from a school counselor, psychiatrist, or psychologist. Do not "treat" yourself with alcohol, illegal drugs, or anything else—you need the same skilled help that anyone else with this problem needs.

Even if your reaction is not so intense, ask yourself the following questions:

- Who says I should never fail? To never experience failure is to be perfect, and it is absurd to expect anyone to be perfect.
- Is failing a true catastrophe? Certainly it would be better if you had not failed. Failing does not mean that you cannot reach your goal of becoming a US licensed physician. Failing an exam is like getting a flat tire while going on a trip: It is annoying and frustrating, but it does not mean that you cannot reach your destination.

As the figures show, the majority of people who fail Step 1 the first time will pass on their second attempt. But be realistic: If you obtained a very low mark, or have already failed several times before, you need to reevaluate not only your study methods but also your goals. Although there are some people who are merely "bad test takers" with the potential to become good physicians, you need to ask yourself if it is really in your best interests to pursue a career that is giving you such a hard time. Remember that you will never run out of exams to take: after Step 1 come Step 2 and Step 3, in-service exams as a resident, specialty board exams at the end of residency, and then possible recertification exams in your specialty every few years.

STUDY METHODS

It is important to have a set of study methods for preparing for the USMLE Step 1. There is too much material to study by random reading and memorization. Experiment with different ways of studying. You do not know how effective something might be until you try it. This is best done months before the test in order to determine what works and what you enjoy. Possible study options include:

- Studying review material in groups
- Creating personal mnemonics, diagrams, and tables
- Taking practice tests alone or in groups
- Attending faculty review sessions
- Making or sharing flashcards
- Reviewing old syllabi and notes

- Making cassette tapes of review material to study during commuting time
- Playing Trivial Pursuit–style games with facts and questions
- Getting away from home for an extended period to avoid distractions and to immerse yourself in studying

Study Groups

A good study group has many advantages. It can relieve stress, organize your time, and allow people with different strengths to exchange information. Study groups also allow you to pool resources and spend less money on review books and sample tests.

There are, however, potential problems with study groups. It is difficult to study with people who have different goals and study paces. Avoid large, unwieldly groups. Otherwise, studying can be inefficient and time-consuming. Some study groups also tend to socialize more than study.

If you choose not to belong to a study group, it may be a good idea to find a support group or study partner simply to keep pace with and share study ideas. It is good to get different perspectives from other students in evaluating what is and is not important to learn. Do not get discouraged by interactions with a few overly compulsive students; everyone studies and learns differently.

Mnemonics and Memorizing

Developing good mnemonics takes time and work.

Cramming is a viable way of memorizing short-term information just before a test, but after one or two days you will find that much of that knowledge has dissipated. For that reason, cramming and memorization by repetition ("brute force") in the weeks before the exam are not ideal techniques for long-term memorization of the overwhelming body of information covered by Step 1. Mnemonics are memory aids that work by linking isolated facts or abstract ideas to acronyms, pictures, patterns, rhymes, and stories—information that the mind tends to store well.[24] The best mnemonics are your own, and developing them takes work. The first step to creating a mnemonic is understanding the information to be memorized. Play around with the information and look for unique features that help you remember it. In addition, make the mnemonic as colorful, humorous, or outlandish as you can; such mnemonics are the most memorable. Effective mnemonics should link the topic with the facts in as specific and unambiguous a manner as possible. In memorizing the mnemonic, engage as many senses as possible by repeating the fact aloud or by writing or acting it out. Keep the information fresh by quizzing yourself periodically with flashcards, in study groups, and so on. Do not make the common mistake of simply rereading highlighted review material. The material may start to look familiar, but that does not mean you will be able to remember it in another context during the exam.

Quiz yourself periodically. Do not simply reread highlighted material.

Review Sessions

Faculty review sessions can be helpful. Review sessions that are geared specifically toward the USMLE Step 1 tend to be more helpful than general review sessions. Open "question and answer" sessions tend to be inefficient and not worth the time. Focus on reviews given by faculty who are knowledgeable in the content and testing format of the USMLE Step 1.

Commercial Courses

Commercial preparation courses can be helpful for some students, but they are expensive and require significant time commitment. They are usually effective in organizing study material for students who feel overwhelmed by the volume of material. Note that the multiweek courses may be quite intense and may thus leave limited time for independent study. Note that some commercial courses are designed for first-time test takers and that others focus on students who are repeating the examination. Some courses focus on international medical graduates who must take all three Steps in a limited amount of time. See page 323 for summarized data and excerpted information from several commercial review courses.

STUDY MATERIALS

Quality and Cost Considerations

Although there is an ever-increasing number of board review books and software on the market, the quality of the material is highly variable. Some common problems:

- Certain review books are too detailed for review in a reasonable amount of time or cover subtopics not emphasized on the exam (e.g., a 400-page histology book).
- Many sample question books were originally written years ago and have not been updated adequately to reflect trends on the revised USMLE Step 1.
- Many sample question books use poorly written questions or contain factual errors in the explanations.
- Explanations for sample questions range from nonexistent to overly detailed.
- Software for boards review is of highly variable quality, may be difficult to install, and may be fraught with bugs.

Review Books

Most review books are the products of considerable effort by experienced educators. There are many, and you must choose which ones to buy based on their relative merits. Although recommendations from other medical students

If a given review book is not working for you, stop using it, no matter how highly rated it may be.

are useful, many students simply recommend whatever books they used without having compared them to other books on the same subject. Do not waste time with very outdated "hand-me-down" review books. Some students blindly advocate one publisher's series without considering the broad range of quality encountered within most series. Weigh different opinions against each other, read the reviews and ratings in Section III of this guide, and choose review books very carefully. You are investing not only money but also your limited study time. Do not worry about finding the "perfect" book, as many subjects simply do not have one, and different students prefer different styles.

There are two types of review books: books that are stand-alone titles and books that are part of a series. The books in a series generally have the same style, and you must decide if that style is helpful for you. However, a given style is not optimal for every subject. For example, charts and diagrams may be the best approach for physiology and biochemistry, whereas tables and outlines may be better for microbiology.

When possible, try to use the same books for medical school exam review and Step 1 review.

Find out which books are up to date. Some new editions represent major improvements, whereas others contain only cursory changes. You should take into consideration how a book reflects the format of the USMLE Step 1. Note that some of the books reviewed in Section III have not been updated adequately to reflect the clinical emphasis and question format of the current USMLE Step 1. Books that emphasize obscure facts and minute details tend to be less helpful for the USMLE Step 1, because there are now fewer "picky" questions and more problem-solving questions.

Texts, Syllabi, and Notes

Use texts and syllabi with care. Many textbooks are generally too detailed for high-yield boards review and include material that is generally not tested on the USMLE Step 1 (e.g., drug dosages, complex chemical structures). Syllabi often reflect the emphasis of the faculty, which may not correspond to the emphasis of the boards. Old class notes have the advantage of presenting material in the way you learned it but suffer from the same disadvantages as syllabi. When using texts or notes, engage in **active learning** by making tables, diagrams, new mnemonics, and conceptual associations whenever possible. Supplement incomplete or unclear material with reference to other appropriate textbooks. Keep a good medical dictionary at hand to sort out definitions.

Do not waste your time with outdated or overly difficult questions.

Practice Tests

Taking practice tests provides valuable information about strengths and weaknesses in your fund of knowledge and test-taking skills. Some students use practice examinations simply as a means of breaking up the monotony of studying and adding variety to their study schedule. Other students study almost solely from practice tests. There is a wide range of quality in available practice material, and it is easy to become frustrated by low-quality sample questions or questions without explanations. Approach sample examinations critically, and do not waste time with low-quality questions until you have exhausted better sources.

After taking a practice test, try to identify concepts and areas of weakness, not just the facts that you missed. Do not panic if you miss a lot of questions on a practice examination. Use the experience to motivate your study and prioritize what areas need the most work.

Use practice tests to identify concepts and areas of weakness, not just facts that you missed.

Use quality practice examinations to improve your test-taking skills. Analyze your ability to pace yourself so that you have enough time to complete each test booklet comfortably. Practice examinations are also a good means of training yourself to concentrate for long periods of time. Consider taking practice tests with a friend or in a small group to increase motivation and simulate more accurately the format and schedule of the real examination. Analyze the pattern of your responses to questions to determine if you have made systematic errors in answering questions. Common mistakes are reading too much into the question, second-guessing your initial impression, and misinterpreting the question.

Students report that many practice exam books have questions that are, on average, shorter and less clinically oriented than the current USMLE Step 1. Many Step 1 questions demand fast reading skills and application of basic science facts in a problem-solving format.

GENERAL STUDY STRATEGIES

The USMLE Step 1 was created according to an integrated outline that organizes basic science material in a multidisciplinary approach. Broad-based knowledge is more important than in prior years, so the old adage "Just study bugs, drugs, and biochem" is not enough to ensure that you do well on the USMLE Step 1. The exam is designed to test basic science material and its application to clinical situations. About half of the questions include clinical situations, although some are very brief.

In spite of the change in the organization of the subject matter, the detailed Step 1 content outline provided by the USMLE has not proved useful for students. We feel that it is still best to approach the material along the lines of the seven traditional disciplines. In Section II, we provide suggestions on how to approach the material within each subject. We also list some topics that are often neglected.

Practice questions that include case histories or descriptive vignettes are helpful in preparing yourself for the clinical slant of the USMLE Step 1. We suggest going through a number of quality practice questions from NBME publications or updated review books to get a feel for what is expected of you, but do not get bogged down in studying case histories. It is not necessary to memorize all normal laboratory values, because they are printed on the insides of both the front and back covers of all test booklets. Approaching the USMLE Step 1 along the lines of the disciplines outlined in Section II (especially the high-yield areas) has proved to be the most productive method of studying among students in our survey.

TEST-TAKING STRATEGIES

Practice and perfect test-taking skills and strategies well before the test date.

Your test performance is influenced by both your fund of knowledge and your test-taking skills. You can increase your performance by considering each of these factors. Test-taking skills and strategies should be developed and perfected well in advance of the test date so you can concentrate on the test itself. We suggest you try the following strategies to see if they might work for you.

Pacing

You have 180 minutes to complete approximately 180 questions (down from 185). This works out to 60 questions per hour and about 60 seconds per question. We recommend that you aim for an average of 55 seconds per question, or approximately 66 questions per hour. This allows you to have about 15 minutes at the end of the examination to verify answers and to go over any particularly difficult questions that you may have guessed or skipped. Some students prefer to mark a temporary answer on all skipped questions in case they do not have time to return. You may find that some question types (e.g., extended matching) may require less time to process than others. Dealing with such question types first prevents you from leaving quickly answerable questions unanswered.

An old NBME analysis of previous board examinations revealed that some students left a few items unanswered in the first examination book of the first morning.[25] This indicates that pacing yourself may be especially important when working on the first booklet. Make the necessary pacing adjustments as you work on each booklet. Pacing errors leading to unanswered questions have been known to occur even among students who were considered to be very well prepared.

Dealing with Each Question

There are several established techniques for efficiently approaching multiple-choice questions. See what works for you. All questions can be identified as easy, workable, or impossible. Your goal should be to answer all easy questions, to work out all workable questions in a reasonable amount of time, and to make quick and intelligent guesses on all impossible questions. Most students read the stem and turn immediately to the choices. Other students try to avoid distractor traps by covering up the choices when reading the stems; they think of their own best answer and then compare it to the available choices. Try both techniques on practice exams and see what works best for you.

In general, when you eliminate an incorrect choice on a question, mark it out to avoid rereading it unnecessarily. If you are unsure about a choice, place a question mark by it. When you think you have determined the best answer, circle it and mark your answer sheet accordingly.

Difficult Questions

Questions on the USMLE Step 1 require varying amounts of time to answer. Some problem-solving questions take longer than simple, fact-recall questions. Because of the exam's clinical emphasis, you may find that many of the questions appear workable but take more time than is available. It can be tempting to dwell on these types of questions for an excessive amount of time because you feel you are on the verge of "figuring it out." Resist this temptation and budget your time. Answer the question with your best guess, make a mark signifying "tentative" on your booklet or answer sheet, and come back to the question after you have completed the rest of the booklet. This keeps you from inadvertently leaving any blank questions in your efforts to beat the clock. Remember to save a few minutes at the end to remove all stray marks from the answer sheet and to make sure that all questions have been answered.

Do not dwell excessively on questions that you are on the verge of "figuring out." Make your best guess and move on.

Inevitably, there will be some questions for which you will not have a clue (i.e., impossible questions). Do not be disturbed by these questions. Guess and move on. As a medical student, you are used to scoring well on standardized examinations (otherwise you would not be in medical school), so the USMLE Step 1 may be your first experience with facing lots of questions to which you do not know the answer. Prepare yourself for this. After narrowing down the answers as best you can, have a plan for guessing so that you do not waste time. Remember that you are not expected to know all the answers.

Another reason for not dwelling too long on any question is that certain questions may be **experimental** or may be **printed incorrectly.** Not all questions are scored. Some questions serve as "embedded pretest items" that do not count toward your overall score.[26] Students have also noted several printing errors in past USMLE Step 1 examinations. The lesson here is that you should not waste too much time with ambiguous or "flawed" questions. The reason you are having difficulty with the question may lie in the question itself, not with you!

Look for the basic science principle or fact behind the clinical vignette.

Clinical Vignettes

Although half the questions on the Step 1 have a clinical slant, do not be intimidated. Most clinical vignettes are simply basic science problems presented in the context of a clinical scenario. Look for the underlying basic science principle or fact when you encounter a clinical vignette. Some students suggest adopting an aggressive approach toward longer vignettes. This would include reading the question first, skimming over the answers, and then working back through the clinical history, laboratory data, and diagnostic studies as needed. Practice interpreting graphs, clinical data, and photographic images to boost your speed. Some clinical vignettes can be answered directly without reviewing the preliminary material. Some students report value in selectively reviewing introductory clinical medicine books, pathophysiology books, and USMLE Step 2 review books that emphasize clinical presentation of disease.

Batch Fill-in

Most students mark their answer sheets after answering each question. However, constantly shifting back and forth between the test booklet and the answer sheet can break concentration and impart a small but significant time penalty. Batch fill-in separates the tasks of answering the questions and transcribing the answers. First, mark the answers clearly in the margin of the test booklet as you do each question, and then carefully transcribe two pages' worth of answers onto the answer sheet before turning the page. Batch fill-in may improve your concentration by keeping your eyes focused on the booklet and help you develop a good question–answer rhythm. (You may want to revert to transcribing answers question by question toward the end of each test session.) In addition, some students recommend using a dull pencil to fill in the answer sheet because it may be faster. Batch fill-in does not work for everyone; do not use batch fill-in unless you have practiced it extensively.

Margin Marking

Feel free to write in the test booklet and circle or underline key phrases. Draw diagrams or make notes concerning specific facts when encountering case histories or descriptive vignettes. Focus on specific "buzzwords" within the clinical histories. If you find it helpful, circle important directions and repeated words in the answers. Many students mark the possible answers as "T," "F," or "?" to work out difficult questions.

Guessing

There is **no penalty** for wrong answers. Thus, no answer sheet should be turned in with unanswered questions. A hunch is probably better than a random guess. If you have to guess, we suggest guessing an answer you recognize over one that is totally unfamiliar. If you have studied the subject and do not recognize a particular answer, then it is more likely a distractor than a correct answer. Remember, however, that distractors are carefully written and edited to appear reasonable to all but the most competent examinees. Unlike many other standardized tests, such as the SAT, questions do not appear to increase in difficulty as you progress through each booklet.

The conventional wisdom regarding "reconsidering" answers is do not change answers that you have already marked unless there is a convincing and logical reason to do so—in other words, go with your first hunch. You can test this strategy for yourself by keeping a running total of the questions on which you seriously considered changing your answer when taking practice exams. Experience eventually tells you when to trust your first hunches.

Fourth-Quarter Effect (Avoiding Burnout)

Pacing and endurance are important. Practice helps develop both. Even if a number of examinees leave an examination session early, especially in the last session of the last day, do not leave prematurely. Use any extra time at the end to return to unresolved questions or carefully recheck your answers. Do not be too casual in your review or you may overlook serious mistakes. Many students report that near the end of a booklet they suddenly remember facts that help answer questions they had guessed on earlier.

Do not leave the test too early. Carefully review your answers if possible.

Remember your goals, and keep in mind the effort you have devoted to studying compared with the small additional effort needed to complete and check over the examination. Every point you earn is to your advantage. The difference between passing and an average score is far fewer questions than you might think—about 25% of students who failed were within 15 questions of passing.

The "Glossy" Booklets

The "glossy" booklets contain many questions with accompanying gross and microscopic photographs. Two such booklets appeared in the June 1996 exam. Student experience shows that some of these questions can be answered correctly independent of the photograph.

Do not panic if you are unfamiliar with a particular photograph.

Types of photographs include gross pathology (e.g., hydatidiform mole, cardiac valve vegetations), histopathology (e.g., liver cirrhosis, myocardial infarction, glomerulonephritis), blood smears (e.g., target cells, basophilic stippling), dermatopathology (e.g., lupus, Lyme disease, basal cell carcinoma), and imaging (e.g., CT anatomy, cerebral angiogram, plain film fractures).

IRREGULAR BEHAVIOR

During 1995, more than 75 individuals were reported by proctors to be suspicious of "irregular behavior," including continuing to work after being asked to stop, taking notes, talking with other examinees, looking at other examinees, falsifying score reports, and memorizing, reproducing, and disseminating test items. If a determination of irregular behavior is made, a permanent annotation is made on the individual's USMLE record.[27]

TESTING AGENCIES

National Board of Medical Examiners (NBME)
Department of Licensing Examination Services
3750 Market Street
Philadelphia, PA 19104-3190
(215) 590-9700
http://www.nbme.org

Educational Commission for Foreign Medical Graduates
3624 Market Street, Fourth Floor
Philadelphia, PA 19104-2685
(215) 386-5900 or (202) 293-9320
Fax: (215) 386-9196
http://www.ecfmg.org

Federation of State Medical Boards
400 Fuller Wiser Road, Suite 300
Euless, TX 76039-3855
(817) 571-2949
Fax: (817) 868-4099
http://www.fsmb.org

USMLE Secretariat
3750 Market Street
Philadelphia, PA 19104-3190
(215) 590-9600

REFERENCES

1. Bidese, Catherine M., *U.S. Medical Licensure Statistics and Current Licensure Requirements 1995,* American Medical Association, 1995 (ISBN 0899707270).
2. National Board of Medical Examiners, *Part I Examination Guidelines and Sample Items, 1991,* Philadelphia, 1990.
3. National Board of Medical Examiners, *Bulletin of Information and Description of National Board Examinations, 1991,* Philadelphia, 1990.
4. Federation of State Medical Boards and National Board of Medical Examiners, *United States Medical Licensing Examination: 1995 Step 1 General Instructions, Content Outline, and Sample Items,* Philadelphia, 1994.

5. Federation of State Medical Boards and National Board of Medical Examiners, *United States Medical Licensing Examination: 1995 Bulletin of Information,* Philadelphia, 1994.

6. "Report on 1995 Examinations," *The National Board Examiner,* Winter 1996, Vol. 43, No. 1, pp. 1–4.

7. National Board of Medical Examiners, *Performance Norms for the June 1994 USMLE Step 1,* Philadelphia, 1994.

8. "Highlights of the 1991 Annual Meeting: Standard Setting System, Score Reporting and Examinee Feedback Plan, USMLE Implementation Plans," *The National Board Examiner,* Spring 1991, Vol. 38, No. 2, pp. 1–6.

9. Swanson, David B., Case, Susan M., Melnick, Donald E., et al., "Impact of the USMLE Step 1 on Teaching and Learning of the Basic Biomedical Sciences," *Academic Medicine,* September Supplement 1992, Vol. 67, No. 9, pp. 553–556.

10. O'Donnell, M.J., Obenshain, S. Scott, and Erdmann, James B., "I: Background Essential to the Proper Use of Results of Step 1 and Step 2 of the USMLE," *Academic Medicine,* October 1993, Vol. 68, No. 10, pp. 734–739.

11. "Report on 1995 Examinations," *op. cit.,* Vol. 43, No. 1, pp. 1–4.

12. National Board of Medical Examiners, *Summary of Examinee Performance,* Philadelphia, 1995.

13. FSMB and NBME, *USMLE: 1993 Step 1 General Instructions, Content Outline, and Sample Items, op. cit.*

14. http://www.nbme.org/usmleex.htm

15. Swanson et al., *op. cit.*

16. Iserson, K., *Getting into Residency,* Tucson, AZ, Galen Press, 1996 (ISBN 1883620104).

17. Case, Susan M., and Swanson, David B., "Validity of NBME Part I and Part II Scores for Selection of Residents in Orthopaedic Surgery, Dermatology, and Preventive Medicine," *Academic Medicine,* February Supplement 1993, Vol. 68, No. 2, pp. S51–S56.

18. FSMB and NBME, *USMLE: 1993 Step 1 General Instructions, Content Outline, and Sample Items, op. cit.*

19. Swanson et al., *op. cit.*

20. "Report on 1995 Examinations," *op. cit.*

21. National Board of Medical Examiners, *United States Medical Licensing Examination: 1993 Application Instructions for Step 1 and Step 2,* Philadelphia, 1992.

22. "Report on 1995 Examinations," *op. cit.*

23. Swanson et al., *op. cit.*

24. Robinson, Adam, *What Smart Students Know,* New York, Crown Publishers, 1993 (ISBN 0517880857).

25. National Board Examinations, "Preliminary Report on June 1988 Part I Performance," *The National Board Examiner,* Fall 1988, Vol. 35, No. 4, p. 3.

26. O'Donnell et al., *op. cit.*

27. http://www.usmle.org/97/irreg.htm

NOTES

Special Situations

International Medical Graduate (IMG) is the term now used to describe any student or graduate of a non-US or non-Canadian medical school, regardless of whether he or she is a US citizen. The old term "Foreign Medical Graduate" (FMG) was replaced because it was misleading when applied to US citizens attending medical schools outside the United States.

The IMG's Steps to Licensure in the United States

In order to become licensed to practice in the United States, an IMG must go through the following steps (not necessarily in this order). These steps must be completed by all IMGs even if you are already a practicing physician and have completed a residency program in your own country:

- Complete the basic sciences program of your medical school (equivalent to the first two years of US medical school).

- Take the USMLE Step 1. You can do this while still in school or after graduating, but your medical school must certify that you have completed the basic science part of your school's curriculum in order to be eligible.

- Complete the clinical clerkship program of your medical school (equivalent to the third and fourth years of US medical school).

- Take the USMLE Step 2. If you are still in medical school, you must be certified by your school that you are within one year of graduating to be allowed to take Step 2.

- Take the Educational Commission for Foreign Medical Graduates (ECFMG) English test (or an equivalent to the Test of English as a Foreign Language recognized by the ECFMG).

- Graduate with your medical degree.

- Once you have passed Step 1, Step 2, and the English test, you must obtain an ECFMG certificate; you can get this from ECFMG (see following) after you have sent them a copy of your degree, which they will verify with your medical school. This can take eight weeks or more. The ECFMG certificate is required for you to obtain a position in an accredited residency program; some programs do not allow you to apply unless you already have this certificate.

- The ECFMG has announced that applicants who have not met all of the requirements for ECFMG certification on or before June 30, 1998 will be required to pass the Clinical Skills Assessment (CSA) exam (see following) in order to obtain an ECFMG certificate.

- Apply for residency positions in your field of interest, either directly or through the National Residency Matching Program ("the Match"). You do not need to have an ECFMG certificate, to have graduated, or to have passed any USMLE Step or the English test in order to apply for residen-

cies, either directly or through the Match, but you do need to have passed
all the examinations necessary for ECFMG certification (i.e., Step 1, Step 2, English test) by a certain deadline (in 1997, this is February 21) in order to be entered into the Match itself. If you have not passed all these exams, you will be automatically withdrawn from the Match.

- Obtain a visa to allow you to enter and work in the United States if you are not already a US citizen or green card holder (permanent resident).

- Some states require IMGs to obtain an educational/training/limited medical license that allows them to practice as a resident in the state in which their residency program is located. The residency program may assist you with this application. Note that medical licensing is the prerogative of each individual state, not of the federal government, and that states vary in the exact laws about licensing (although all 50 states recognize the USMLE).

- Take USMLE Step 3 during your residency, and then obtain a full medical license. Note that as an IMG you will not be able to take Step 3 and obtain an independent license until you have completed one, two, or three years of residency, depending on which state you live in. However, even if you live in a state that requires two or three years of residency in order to take Step 3, you can still take Step 3 and then obtain a license in another state. Once you have a license in any one state you are permitted to practice in federal facilities such as VA hospitals and in Indian Health Service facilities in any state. This can open the door to "moonlighting" opportunities. For details on individual state rules, write to the licensing board in the state in question or contact the FSMB (see following).

- Complete your residency and then take the appropriate specialty board exams in order to become board certified (e.g., internal medicine, surgery). If you already have a specialty certification in your home country (e.g., in surgery, cardiology), some specialty boards may grant you six months' or one year's credit toward your total residency time.

USMLE Step 1 and the IMG

The USMLE Step 1 is administered by the ECFMG at approximately 78 examination centers in North America and around the world in June and September of each year. USMLE Step 1 is often the first, and for most IMGs the most challenging, hurdle to overcome. The USMLE is a standardized licensing system that gives IMGs a level playing field (it is the same exam series taken by US graduates, even though it is administered by the ECFMG rather than by the NBME). This means that pass marks for IMGs, for both Step 1 and Step 2, are determined by a statistical process that is based on the scores of US medical students in 1991. In general, to pass Step 1, you will probably have to score higher than the bottom 8–10% of US and Canadian graduates in Step 1. However, in 1995, only 55% of ECFMG candidates passed Step 1 on their first attempt, compared with 93% of US and Canadian medical students and graduates.

Developing good test-taking strategy is especially critical for the IMG.

A good Step 1 score is key to a strong IMG application.

As an IMG, you must do as well as you can on Step 1 in particular. Probably no one ever feels totally ready to take Step 1, but nearly all IMGs require a period of serious study and preparation to reach their potential. A poor score on Step 1 is a distinct disadvantage when applying for most residencies. Remember that if you pass Step 1, you cannot retake it to try to improve your score. Your goals should be to beat the mean, because you can then confidently assert that you have done better than average for US students. Good Step 1 scores lend credibility to your residency application.

Do commercial review courses help improve your scores? Reports vary, and these courses can be expensive. Many IMGs decide to try the USMLE on their own first and then consider a review course only if they fail. But many states require that you pass within three attempts, so you do not have many chances. (For more information on review courses, see pp. 323–329.)

The Other Exams and the IMG

- **USMLE Step 2.** In the past, this examination had a reputation for being much easier than Step 1, but this no longer seems to be the case for both IMGs and US medical students. In August 1995, 56% of ECFMG candidates passed on their first attempt, compared with 94% of US and Canadian candidates. Because this is a clinical sciences exam, cultural and geographic considerations play a greater role than they do in Step 1. For example, if your medical education gave you a lot of exposure to malaria, brucellosis, and malnutrition, but little to alcohol withdrawal, child abuse, and cholesterol screening, you must do some work to familiarize yourself with topics that are more heavily emphasized in US medicine. Also, you must have a basic understanding of the legal and social aspects of US medicine, because you will be asked questions about communicating with and advising patients.

Native English–speaking IMGs are also required to take the language test.

- **The English language test.** All IMGs must take an English test, irrespective of citizenship (including US-born US citizens) and native language. Although this exam can appear absurd to the native English speaker, it is generally considered to be a fair and appropriate test. It does not involve any use of medical knowledge or medical terminology; in the first part, candidates listen to tape recordings of typical English conversations and are asked simple questions to assess their comprehension. In the second part, written sentences are presented in which candidates are asked to choose an appropriate replacement for a missing word that is both grammatically correct and meaningful. This test is strictly pass–fail; there is no numerical grade. If English is not your native language, you must assess your English ability. The test is generally not difficult for those who feel comfortable having ordinary and natural conversations with Americans. Having lived in or visited the United States for an extended period is almost always an advantage for the foreign-born IMG seeking US licensure.

- **Clinical Skills Assessment (CSA).** Applicants for ECFMG certification will be required to pass the ECFMG **Clinical Skills Assessment (CSA)**, which incorporates a Test of Spoken English. In addition applicants must pass the basic medical and clinical science examinations and the ECFMG English test. This additional assessment will require that the examinee to demonstrate proficiency on components of clinical skills such as history taking, physical examination, organization and interpretation of clinical data, as well as interpersonal skills and oral English. Applicants will be required to pass the CSA if they have not met all of the requirements for ECFMG certification on or before June 30, 1998, as set forth in the applicable edition of the ECFMG *Information Booklet.*

To be eligible to take the CSA, applicants must be either a **student** officially enrolled in a medical school listed in the current edition of the *World Directory of Medical Schools* published by the World Health Organization and within 12 months of completion of the full didactic curriculum **or** must be a **graduate** of a medical school which was listed in the *World Directory* at the time of graduation. In addition, all applicants for the CSA must have passed the required basic medical and clinical science examinations and the ECFMG English test or Test of English as a Foreign Language (TOEFL) under the current ECFMG policies. Graduates of foreign medical schools who currently hold a Standard ECFMG Certificate or who will meet all of the current requirements for certification by June 30, 1998, will *not* be required to take the CSA but will be eligible to do so. However, such applicants will not be issued a new Standard ECFMG Certificate.

The CSA will be administered throughout the year on a daily basis in a single ECFMG test center in Philadelphia, Pennsylvania. In it, candidates are required to demonstrate their skills in the course of ten half-hour interactions with each of ten standardized "patients," all of whom are specially trained actors. The exam lasts five hours and is conducted over an entire morning or an entire afternoon session. Each "patient" grades each student. The interaction is not watched by any observers, but it will be video- and audio-taped in case any problems or disputes arise later. You must pass the CSA to enter the residency Match.

The ECFMG Clinical Skills Assessment (CSA) will include a number of clinical problems that physicians in programs of graduate medical education in the United States will likely encounter. Specifically, it will consist of clinical encounters with standardized patients during which the examinee will be asked to obtain a focused history, perform a relevant physical examination and communicate initial diagnoses and a management plan to the standardized patients. Following the clinical encounter with each patient, a written exercise will be administered to the examinee in the form of a

There is a big difference between textbook learning of a language and actually being immersed in the culture that goes with it.

patient progress note. The standardized patients are individuals who are trained to portray clinical problems that may include positive findings. They are trained to document and evaluate the clinical skills performance of the examinee and other related behaviors such as interpersonal skills.

Passing this exam demonstrates your ability to use English in the practice of clinical medicine with patients. This exam requires that you demonstrate proficiency in English conversation in the context of doctor–patient encounters. Fluency, intelligible pronunciation, and organized history and physical exam skills are likely to be keys to success.

The ECFMG Clinical Skills Assessment will be implemented beginning July 1, 1998. Additional information will be made available later in 1997.

Resources for the IMG

- ECFMG
  3624 Market Street, Fourth Floor
  Philadelphia, PA 19104-2685
  (215) 386-5900 or (202) 293-9320
  Fax: (215) 386-9196

  This number is answered only between 9:00 AM and 12:30 PM, and between 1:30 PM and 5:00 PM Monday through Friday EST. The ECFMG often takes a long time to answer the phone and is often busy at peak times of the year, and there is then a long voice-mail message to listen to, so it is better to write or fax early rather than rely on a last-minute phone call. Do not contact the National Board of Medical Examiners. All IMG exam affairs are conducted by the ECFMG. The ECFMG publishes the *Handbook for Foreign Medical Graduates* and *Information Booklet* on ECFMG certification and the USMLE program; the latter gives details of dates and locations of forthcoming USMLE, CSA, and English tests for IMGs, together with application forms. It is free of charge and is also available from the public affairs offices of US embassies and consulates worldwide, as well as from Overseas Educational Advisory Centers. Single copies of the handbook may also be ordered by faxing a request to (215) 387-9963.

- Federation of State Medical Boards
  400 Fuller Wiser Road, Suite 300
  Euless, TX 76039-3855
  (817) 868-4000
  Fax: (817) 868-4099

  FSMB publishes Exchange, Section I, which gives detailed information on examination and licensing requirements in all US jurisdictions. The 1996–1997 edition costs $25. (Texas residents must add 7.75% state sales tax.) To obtain publications, write to Federation Publications at the above address. All orders must be prepaid by a personal check drawn on a US bank, a cashier's check, or a money order payable to the Federation. Foreign orders must be accompanied by an international money order or the equivalent, payable in US dollars through a US bank or a US affiliate of a foreign bank. For Step 3 inquiries, the telephone number is (817) 868-4000, and the fax number is (817) 868-4099.

- Some of the Step 1 commercial review courses listed in Section III are conducted outside the United States. Write or call the course providers for details.

- The ECFMG has a home page on http://www.ecfmg.org with the complete ECFMG Information Booklet available online. Late announcements (e.g., dates of mailing out score reports) are also made on this site.

- The FSMB has a home page at http://www.fsmb.org

- The Internet news groups misc.education.medical and bit.listsery.medforum can be valuable forums to exchange information on licensing exams, residency applications, and so on.

- Some immigration information for IMGs is available from the various sites of Siskind, Susser, Haas & Chang, a firm of attorneys specializing in immigration law, on the following websites, which include a searchable index and a free e-mail subscription to immigration law bulletins:
  http://www.telalink.net/~gsiskind/bulletin.html
  http://www.visalaw.com/~gsiskind/95feb/2feb95.html
  http://www.telalink.net/~gsiskind/95feb/2feb95.html
  http://www.americanlaw.com/q&a28.html

- International Medical Placement Ltd., a US company specializing in recruiting foreign physicians to work in the United States, has a site at http://www.cyberdeas.com/imp. This site includes ordering information for several publications by FMSG, Inc., including USMLE Study Guides and residency matching information, and details of USMLE lecture courses offered by the author of these publications, Dr. Stanley Zaslau. It also has information on seminars held by the company in foreign countries for physicians thinking of moving to the United States.

- *The International Medical Graduates' Guide to U.S. Medicine: Negotiating the Maze* by Louise B. Ball (199 pages; ISBN 1-883620-16-3).

Galen Press
PO Box 64400
Tucson, AZ 85728-4400
(800) 442-5369 (United States and Canada)
(520) 577-8363
Fax: (520) 520-6459

Price: $28.95 plus $3.00 shipping and handling, add $2.95 for priority mail (US dollars); Arizona residents add 7% sales tax.

This book has a lot of detailed information, and is particularly strong on the intricacies of immigration law as it applies to foreign citizen IMGs who wish to practice in the United States—although this is a rapidly changing field, and some of this information is probably out of date already. However, much of the book's contents may be irrelevant for any one person, as many chapters are geared toward specific situations (e.g., how to sponsor a relative, how a small American town may try to sponsor a foreign physician, how a US faculty member can sponsor a foreign clinical research fellow), and there is considerable duplication across chapters.

Bottom line: Great for foreign citizens who need help in understanding how to "negotiate the maze" of medical immigration regulations, but not necessarily high-yield for many other IMGs.

FIRST AID FOR THE OSTEOPATHIC MEDICAL STUDENT

NBOME Part I—The Basics

The National Board of Osteopathic Medicine Examination (NBOME) is the osteopathic version of the USMLE. Osteopathic students must pass Parts I and II in order to graduate. In 1995, the NBOME introduced a new assessment tool called the Comprehensive Osteopathic Medical Licensing Examination (COMLEX). Similar to the NBOME that it will replace, COMLEX is to be administered in three Levels. The new examinations will be phased over a three-year period (Fig. 12). In 1995, only the Level III exam was administered; by 1997 all three Levels of COMLEX will be administered. COMLEX will then be the only exam offered. A stated goal of this program is to get all states to recognize this examination as equivalent to the USMLE and to allow DO candidates to use this examination for licensing.

FIGURE 12. Test Dates for NBOME and COMLEX

	Level I	COMLEX	June 3–4 October 14–15
1997	Level II	COMLEX	March 11–12 October 14–15
	Level III	COMLEX	February 18–19 June 10–11

Like the Step 1, the NBOME Part I is a multiple-choice examination given over two days. It consists of four booklets, each containing approximately 150 questions. You are allotted 240 minutes for each booklet. In order to sit for Level I, you must have successfully completed at least 75% of the second-year curriculum.

The exam consists of one-best-answer questions, negatively phrased best answer questions, and matching sets. Questions are often organized with clinical case vignettes that consist of short cases with three to six associated questions. In the June 1995 administration of the NBOME Part I, there were approximately seven clinical vignettes per booklet. In addition to the seven traditional basic science subjects covered by the USMLE Step 1, the NBOME Part I also tests osteopathic principles. Several students who took both exams in 1996 reported that the USMLE was a "much better written" exam, but also "more difficult" than the NBOME.

For all three Levels, raw scores are converted to a score ranging from 5 to 995. For Part I and Level II, a score of 400 is required to pass. For Level III, a score of 350 is required. The COMLEX uses the same conversion scales. Scores are usually mailed eight weeks after the test date. In 1995, 88% of all first-time test takers passed the June administration of the NBOME Part I. The mean score on the June 1995 exam was 488. If you pass an NBOME or COMLEX examination, you are not allowed to retake that test to improve your grade. If you fail, there is no limit to the number of times you can retake the exam in an effort to pass.

The NBOME and the USMLE

Aside from dealing with the NBOME Part I, you must decide if you will also take the USMLE Step 1. We recommend that you consider taking the USMLE in addition to the NBOME for the following reasons:

- **If you are applying to allopathic residencies.** Although there is growing acceptance of NBOME certification by allopathic residencies, some allopathic programs prefer or require passage of the USMLE Step 1; including academic programs and programs in competitive specialties. Fourth-year DO students who have already matched can tell you what programs and specialties are looking for USMLE scores.
- **If you plan to practice in Texas, Louisiana, or North Carolina.** These states require that osteopathic physicians pass the USMLE system to obtain a license for practice. However, these states may also have reciprocating agreements with other states that accept the NBOME. There, you might be licensed in another state and then petition to have your license transferred.

- **If you are unsure regarding your postgraduate training plans.** Certainly, successful passage of both the NBOME Part I and USMLE Step 1 will provide you with the greatest range of options when applying for internship and residency training.

Unfortunately, taking both exams can be trying. Students planning to take both exams in June 1997 have to deal with the USMLE Step 1 one week after taking the NBOME Part I. In October, Step 1 and Part I examination dates conflict. An alternative would be to take Part I or Step 1 in June and wait until October to sit for the other exam. The clinical classwork that most DO students receive during the summer of their third year (as opposed to starting clinical clerkships) is considered helpful in integrating the basic science knowledge for the NBOME or the USMLE.

Preparing for the NBOME

Student experience suggests that you should start studying for the NBOME four to six months before the test date. An early start will allow you to devote up to a month per subject. The recommendations made in Section I regarding study and testing methods, strategies, and resources hold true for the NBOME as well. In addition, you should seek resources which review osteopathic principles, such as the Student Osteopathic Medical Association's (SOMA's) "blue book" or Greenman's *Principles of Manual Medicine.* The SOMA blue book has been out of print for several years, so try to get a copy from a third-year student. Take full advantage of the *Examination Guidelines and Sample Exam* distributed by the NBOME. This publication and additional information can be obtained by writing:

NBOME
2700 River Road, Suite 607
Des Plaines, IL 60018

Apart from the osteopathic principles, the NBOME and USMLE exams are similar in scope, content, and emphasis. Both exams often require that you apply and integrate knowledge over several areas of basic science in order to answer a question. Likewise, your preparation for both exams should be very similar. However, students who have taken both exams report that the NBOME makes greater use of "buzzwords" (e.g., "rose spots" in typhoid fever), whereas the USMLE often avoids buzzwords in favor of straight descriptions of clinical findings or symptoms (e.g., rose-colored papules on the abdomen instead of "rose spots"). In 1996, many students reported an emphasis on overall pharmacology and microbiology.

The National Board of Podiatric Medical Examiners (NBPME) tests (see Fig. 13 for examination dates) are designed to assess whether a candidate possesses the knowledge required to practice as a minimally competent entry-level podiatrist. In all states that recognize them, the NBPME examinations are used as part of the licensing process governing the practice of podiatric medicine. Individual states use the examination scores differently; therefore, DPM candidates should refer to the information in the *NBPME Bulletin of 1997 Examinations.*

Candidates performing at extreme levels are passed or failed at 90 minutes.

The NBPME Part I is generally taken after the completion of the second year of podiatric medical education. Unlike the USMLE Step 1, there is no behavioral science section. The exam does sample the seven basic science disciplines: general anatomy; lower extremity anatomy; biochemistry; physiology; medical microbiology and immunology; pathology; and pharmacology. Questions covering these content areas are interspersed throughout the test.

Your NBPME Appointment

In early spring, your college registrar will have you fill out an application for the NBPME Part I. After receipt of your application and registration fees, you will be mailed the *NBPME Bulletin of 1997 Examinations.* It gives you a list of Sylvan Learning Centers across the country that are participating in the computer-based testing format. You must find the location nearest you and set up an appointment to take the examination. We suggest that you do this as soon as you receive your *NBPME Bulletin* because the reservation slots fill up quickly, especially in the home cities of the seven podiatric medical schools.

On the day of the exam, arrive at the testing center at least 30 minutes before your scheduled appointment. At that time, you will be registered, escorted to a computer terminal, and given a tutorial to acquaint you with the exam format. At the end of the examination, you will be asked to complete a survey regarding your computer-based testing experience.

Computer-Based Testing (CBT)

The NBPME Part I is delivered as a Computerized Mastery Test (CMT). The format is multiple choice. Each candidate is administered a base test of 90 ques-

FIGURE 13. 1997 NBPME Examination Dates

Part 1	July 10–11 (Registration Deadline—May 2)
Part 1 (retake)	September 11–12 (Registration Deadline—August 8)

tions. The maximum time permitted for this base test is 90 minutes. Following the base test, candidates performing at extreme levels (high or low) are passed or failed immediately. Candidates with an intermediate level of performance are administered additional testlets (consisting of 15 questions each) permitting them additional opportunity to demonstrate minimal competence. The maximum time allowed for each additional testlet is 15 minutes. You should try your best on each question, marking any questions that you would like to review should time permit. There is no penalty for guessing. No more than 180 questions are administered to a candidate.

Interpreting Your Score

On completion of the NBPME Part I, a pass/fail decision is reported on the computer. You need a scaled score of at least 75 to pass. Eighty-five percent of first-time test takers pass the NBPME Part I. In computing the scaled score, the number of questions vary from candidate to candidate; however, this is taken into consideration along with the number of questions answered correctly. Approximately two weeks after the examination, you will receive your official score report by mail. Passing candidates receive a message of congratulations, but no numerical score is reported. Failing candidates receive a report with one score between 55 and 74 in addition to diagnostic messages intended to help identify strengths or weaknesses in particular content areas. If you fail the NBPME Part I, you must retake the entire examination at a later date. There is no limit to the number of times you can retake the exam.

Preparation for the NBPME Part I

Students suggest that you begin studying for the NBPME Part I at least three months prior to the test date. Each of the colleges of podiatric medicine conducts a series of board reviews. Ask a third-year student which review sessions are most informative. As with the USMLE Step 1, the suggestions made in Section 1 regarding study and testing methods can be applied to the NBPME as well. This book should be used as a supplement and not as the sole source of information.

Know everything about lower extremity anatomy.

Approximately 24% of the NBPME Part I focus is lower extremity anatomy. Students should rely on the notes and material that they received from their class. Remember, lower extremity anatomy is the podiatrist's specialty—everything is important. Do not forget to study osteology. Keep your old tests and look through old lower extremity class exams because each of the podiatric colleges submits questions from its own exams. This gives you a better understanding of the types of questions that may be asked.

As with the USMLE, the NBPME requires that you apply and integrate knowledge over several areas of basic science in order to answer a question. Students report that many questions emphasize clinical presentations; however, the facts in this book are very helpful in recalling the different diseases and organisms. DPM candidates should expand on the high-yield pharmacology section and study antifungal drugs and treatment protocols for *Pseudomonas,* candidiasis, erythrasma, and so on. The high-yield section focusing on pathology is very useful; however, additional emphasis on diabetes mellitus and all its secondary manifestations should not be overlooked. Students should also focus on classic podiatric dermatopathologies, gout, and arthritis.

A sample set of questions is found in the *NBPME Bulletin of 1997 Examinations.* If you do not receive a *NBPME Bulletin* or if you have any questions regarding registration, fees, test centers, authorization forms, and score reports, please contact your college registrar or:

National Board of Podiatric Medical Examiners (NBPME)
PO Box 6516
Princeton, NJ 08541-6516
(609) 951-6335

Best of luck!

FIRST AID FOR THE STUDENT WITH A DISABILITY

The following material is excerpted from the NBME World Wide Web site (http://www.nbme.org/testacco.htm) and is copyright © 1996 by The Federation of State Medical Boards of the United States, Inc., and the National Board of Medical Examiners.®

Requesting Test Accommodations in USMLE for a Disability
How do I request test accommodations for Steps 1 and 2 of USMLE?

It is helpful to obtain a "Guidelines and Questionnaire" booklet. The booklet provides the procedures for requesting accommodations and for documenting your disability and your need for accommodations.

If you are a student or graduate of an LCME- or AOA-accredited medical school in the United States or Canada, you must write to or telephone the National Board of Medical Examiners:

NBME
Office of Test Accommodations
3750 Market Street
Philadelphia, PA 19104-3190
Telephone: (215) 590-9509

If you are a student or graduate of a foreign medical school, you must contact the Educational Commission for Foreign Medical Graduates to obtain this information:

ECFMG
3624 Market Street, 4th Floor
Philadelphia, PA 19104-2685
USA
Telephone: (215) 386-5900

Be specific about your disability and your individual needs.

How can I receive extra time to take the Steps?

Extra time is one of many accommodations that might be necessary for an examinee with a disability. The Americans with Disabilities Act (ADA) requires that individuals with a disability be provided with "equal access" to the testing program. Therefore, the purpose of accommodations is to "cancel" the effect of the disability, not to provide some extra help in passing an examination.

Because the same types of impairments often vary in severity and often restrict different people to different degrees or in different ways, each request is considered individually to determine the effect of the impairment on the life of the individual and whether a particular accommodation is even appropriate for that person.

Where do I send my request for test accommodations if I am taking Step 1 or Step 2 through the NBME?

Be sure to send your request—and all other documentation, questions, or other information concerning test accommodations—only to the following address:

NBME
Office of Test Accommodations
3750 Market Street
Philadelphia, PA 19104-3190

Do **not** enclose your request or other test accommodation material with your NBME Step 1 and 2 application for registration. If you do not receive a confirmation of your request within two weeks, please call the NBME Office of Test Accommodations at (215) 590-9509 to verify that it was received.

If I am requesting an accommodation from the NBME on Step 1 or Step 2, when should I send in my request and documentation?

In order to allow the necessary time to review your request, please submit your request with all testing results and documentation as soon as you know you will be requesting accommodations for an examination. Your request and accompanying documentation must be postmarked no later than the *final application deadline* for the examination. The final application deadline is listed with the NBME registration materials for each examination administration. Requests for test accommodations cannot be processed by the NBME if postmarked after the deadline.

Can my evaluator or my medical school send in my request for test accommodations?

No. A request for accommodations, by law, must be initiated by the individual with a disability. Also, in order to protect your confidentiality, the NBME does not provide information concerning your request to third parties.

How does the NBME determine what is an appropriate accommodation for USMLE?

As part of the documentation, the examinee's evaluator should recommend appropriate accommodations to ease the impact of the impairment on the testing activity. Professional consultants in learning disabilities, attention deficit disorder, and various other psychiatric and physical conditions review the documentation and recommendations of evaluators to help match the type of assistance with the demonstrated need. The NBME consults with the examinee to determine what accommodations have been effectively used in the past.

If I apply for test accommodations on USMLE, does my disability evaluation have to be up to date?

For someone with a continuing history of accommodation, which would likely include high school and college, as well as medical school, current testing is usually not necessary if objective documentation of the past accommodations is provided. However, the impact of the disability may change over time and new testing may be necessary to demonstrate the current level of impairment and resulting need for accommodation. You will be advised if updated testing is needed.

What are some reasons my request for accommodations might not be approved?

- Insufficient documentation of a need for accommodation. Conditions such as learning disabilities and ADHD are permanent and lifelong. A diagnosis requires an objective history of chronic symptoms from childhood to adulthood as well as evidence of significant impairment currently.

- Lack of presence of a moderate to severe level of impairment attributable to the disorder.

- The identified difficulty is not considered to be a disability under the law, i.e., slow reading without evidence of an underlying language processing disorder; language difficulties as a result of English as a second language.

Once my request for accommodations has been approved, do I need to arrange for accommodations the next time I register for a Step?

An examinee with a disability must provide notification of a request each time accommodations are required. For NBME examinees, a letter requesting accommodations must be sent to the Office of Test Accommodations and must be postmarked no later than the *final published deadline* for the test administration. The letter must also state whether there is any change in the accommodations required and, if so, documentation of the needed change must be provided.

Accommodations are **not** automatic, even if they have been approved for previous Step administrations.

NOTES

Database of High-Yield Facts

Anatomy
Behavioral Science
Biochemistry
Microbiology
Pathology
Pharmacology
Physiology

The 1997 edition of *First Aid for the USMLE Step 1* contains a revised and expanded database of basic science material that student authors and faculty have identified as high-yield for boards review. The facts are loosely organized according to the seven traditional basic medical science disciplines (anatomy, behavioral science, biochemistry, microbiology, pathology, pharmacology, and physiology). Each discipline is then divided into smaller subsections of loosely related facts. Individual facts are generally presented in a three-column format, with the **Title** of the fact in the first column, the **Description** of the fact in the second column, and the **Mnemonic** or **Special Note** in the third column.

Some facts do not have a mnemonic and are presented in a two-column format. Others are presented in list or tabular form in order to emphasize key associations. The database structure is useful for reviewing material already learned. This section is not ideal for learning complex or highly conceptual material for the first time. At the end of each basic science section we list supplementary high-yield topics that have appeared on recent exams in order to help focus your additional review.

The Database of High-Yield Facts is not comprehensive. Use it to complement your core study material and not as your primary study source. The facts and notes have been condensed and edited to emphasize the essential material, and as a result each entry is "incomplete." Work with the material, add your own notes and mnemonics, and realize that not all memory techniques work for all students.

We update Section II annually to keep current with new trends in boards content as well as to expand our database of high-yield information. However, we must note that inevitably many other very-high-yield entries and topics are not yet included in our database.

We actively encourage medical students and faculty to submit entries and mnemonics so that we may enhance the database for future students. We also solicit recommendations of alternate tools for study that may be useful in preparing for the examination, such as diagrams, charts, and computer-based tutorials (*see* How to Contribute, page xiii.)

Disclaimer

The entries in this section reflect student opinions of what is high-yield. Owing to the diverse sources of material, no attempt has been made to trace or reference the origins of entries individually. We have regarded mnemonics as essentially in the public domain. All errors and omissions will be gladly corrected if brought to the attention of the authors, either through the publisher or directly by e-mail.

Anatomy

Several topics fall under this heading, including embryology, gross anatomy, histology, and neuroanatomy. Studying all anatomy topics in great detail is generally a low-yield approach. However, do not ignore anatomy altogether. Review what you have already learned and what you wish you had learned. Do not memorize all the small details. Many questions require you to identify a structure on anatomic cross-section, electron micrograph, or photomicrograph.

When studying, try to stress clinically important material. For example, be familiar with gross anatomy that is related to traumatic injuries (e.g., fractures, sensory and motor nerve deficits), procedures (e.g., lumbar puncture), and common surgeries (e.g., cholecystectomy). There are also many questions on the exam involving x-rays, CT scans, and MR scans. Many students suggest browsing through a well-illustrated general radiology atlas, pathology atlas, and histology atlas by just reading the captions and looking at the pictures. Focus on learning basic anatomy at key levels in the body (e.g., sagittal brain MRI; axial CT midthorax, abdomen, and pelvis). Basic neuroanatomy, especially pathways, has good yield. Basic embryology (especially congenital malformations) has good yield and is worth reviewing.

Cell Type
Embryology
Gross Anatomy
Histology
Neuroanatomy
High-Yield Topics

Erythrocyte

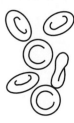

Anucleate, biconcave → large surface area: volume ratio → easy gas exchange (O_2 and CO_2). Source of energy = glucose (90% anaerobically degraded to lactate, 10% by HMP shunt). Survival time = 120 days. Membrane contains the chloride-bicarbonate antiport important in the "physiologic chloride shift," which allows the RBC to transport CO_2 from the periphery to the lungs for elimination.

Eryth = red; *cyte* = cell.
Erythrocytosis = polycythemia = increased number of red cells
Anisocytosis = varying sizes
Poikilocytosis = varying shapes
Reticulocyte = baby erythrocyte

Leukocyte

Types: granulocytes (basophils, eosinophils, neutrophils) and mononuclear cells (lymphocytes, monocytes). Responsible for defense against infections. Normally 4,000–10,000 per microliter.

Leuk = white; *cyte* = cell.

Basophil

Mediates allergic reaction. <1% of all leukocytes. Bilobate nucleus. Densely basophilic granules containing heparin (anticoagulant), histamine (vasodilator) and other vasoactive amines, and SRS-A (**S**low-**R**eacting **S**ubstance of **A**naphylaxis).

Basophilic = staining readily with *basic* stains.

Mast cell

Mediates allergic reaction. Degranulation = release of histamine, heparin, and eosinophil chemotactic factors. Can bind IgE to membrane. Mast cells resemble basophils structurally and functionally but are not the same cell type.

Masten = fatten.
Involved in Type I hypersensitivity reactions. Cromolyn sodium prevents mast cell degranulation.

Eosinophil

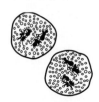

1%–6% of all leukocytes. Bilobate nucleus. Packed with large eosinophilic granules of uniform size. Defends against helminthic and protozoan infections. Highly phagocytic for antigen–antibody complexes.

Eosin = a dye; *philic* = loving.
NAACP:
N = neoplastic
A = asthma
A = allergic processes
C = collagen vascular diseases
P = parasites

Neutrophil

Acute inflammatory response cell. 40%–75% WBCs. Phagocytic. Multilobed nucleus. Large, spherical, azurophilic 1° granules (called lysosomes) contain hydrolytic enzymes, lysozyme, myeloperoxidase.

Hypersegmented polys are seen in vit. B_{12}/folate deficiency.

| Monocyte | 2%–10% of leukocytes. Large. Kidney-shaped nucleus. Extensive "frosted glass" cytoplasm. Differentiates into macrophages in tissues. | *Mono* = one; single; *cyte* = cell |

Monocyte

2%–10% of leukocytes. Large. Kidney-shaped nucleus. Extensive "frosted glass" cytoplasm. Differentiates into macrophages in tissues.

Mono = one; single; *cyte* = cell

Lymphocyte

Small. Round, densely staining nucleus. Small amount of pale cytoplasm. B lymphocytes produce antibodies. T lymphocytes manifest the cellular immune response as well as regulate B lymphocytes and macrophages.

B lymphocyte

Part of humoral immune response. Arises from stem cells in bone marrow. Matures in marrow. Migrates to peripheral lymphoid tissue (follicles of lymph nodes, white pulp of spleen, unencapsulated lymphoid tissue). When antigen is encountered, B cells differentiate into plasma cells and produce antibodies. Has memory. Can function as antigen-presenting cell (APC).

B = **B**one marrow or **B**ursa of Fabricius (in birds).

Plasma cells

Off-center nucleus, clock-face chromatin distribution, abundant RER and well-developed Golgi apparatus. B cells differentiate into plasma cells, which can produce large amounts of antibody specific to a particular antigen.

Multiple myeloma is a plasma cell neoplasm.

T lymphocyte

Mediates cellular immune response. Originates from stem cells in the bone marrow, but matures in the thymus. T cells differentiate into cytotoxic T cells (MHC I, CD8), helper T cells (MHC II, CD4), suppressor T cells, delayed hypersensitivity T cells.

T is for **T**hymus. **CD** is for **C**luster of **D**ifferentiation. **MHC** × **CD** = **8** (e.g., 2 × 4 = 8).

Macrophage

Phagocytizes bacteria, cell debris, and senescent red cells and scavenges damaged cells and tissues. Long life in tissues. Macrophages differentiate from circulating blood monocytes. Activated by γ-IFN. Can function as APC.

Macro = large; *phage* = eater.

Airway cells

Ciliated cells extend to the respiratory bronchioles; goblet cells extend only to the terminal bronchioles.
Type I cells (97% of alveolar surfaces) line the alveoli.
Type II cells (3%) secrete pulmonary surfactant (dipalmitoylphosphatidylcholine), which lowers the alveolar surface tension.

All the mucus secreted can be swept orally (ciliated cells run deeper).
A lecithin:sphingomyelin ratio of > 1.5 in amniotic fluid is indicative of fetal lung maturity.

Juxtaglomerular apparatus (JGA)

JGA = JG cells (modified smooth muscle of afferent arteriole) and macula densa (Na^+ sensor, part of the distal convoluted tubule). JG cells secrete renin (leading to ↑ angiotensin II and aldosterone levels) in response to ↓ renal blood pressure, ↓ Na^+ delivery to distal tubule, and ↑ sympathetic tone. JG cells also secrete erythropoietin.

JGA defends glomerular filtration rate via the renin-angiotensin system.
Juxta = close by.

Microglia

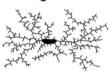

CNS phagocytes. Mesodermal origin. Not readily discernible in Nissl stains. Have small irregular nuclei and relatively little cytoplasm. In response to tissue damage, transform into large ameboid phagocytic cells.

HIV-infected microglia fuse to form multinucleated giant cells in the CNS.

Oligodendroglia

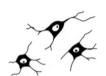

Function to myelinate multiple CNS axons. In Nissl stains, they appear as small nuclei with dark chromatin and little cytoplasm. Predominant type of glial cell in white matter.

These cells are destroyed in multiple sclerosis.

Schwann cells

Function to myelinate PNS axons. Unlike oligodendroglia, many Schwann cells myelinate a single PNS axon. Schwann cells promote axonal regeneration.

Acoustic neuroma is an example of a schwannoma.

Cones

For bright, acute vision (color, concentrated in fovea). Comprise inner and outer segments connected by 9 + 0 modified cilium; outer segment disks continuous with plasma membrane. Contain iodopsin pigment, red-green-blue specific.

Cones are for **C**olor, and their outer segments are **C**ontinuous (with the plasma membrane, unlike rods). Cones have a sharp tip (acuity).

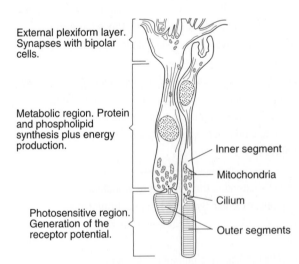

External plexiform layer. Synapses with bipolar cells.

Metabolic region. Protein and phospholipid synthesis plus energy production.

Photosensitive region. Generation of the receptor potential.

Inner segment

Mitochondria

Cilium

Outer segments

Rods

For night vision (no color; many more than cones; none in the fovea). Comprise inner and outer segments connected by 9 + 0 modified cilium; outer segment disks not continuous with plasma membrane. Rods contain rhodopsin pigment.

Rods have **Rhod**opsin.

Rods have high sensitivity due to multiple rods synapsing on one bipolar cell (convergence).

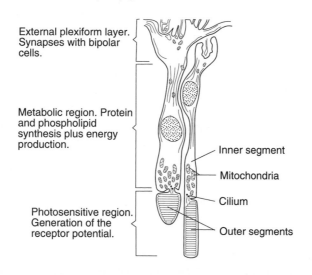

External plexiform layer. Synapses with bipolar cells.

Metabolic region. Protein and phospholipid synthesis plus energy production.

Inner segment

Mitochondria

Cilium

Photosensitive region. Generation of the receptor potential.

Outer segments

ANATOMY—EMBRYOLOGY

Umbilical cord

Contains 2 umbilical arteries, which return deoxygenated blood from the fetus, and 1 umbilical vein, which supplies oxygenated blood from the placenta to the fetus.

Embryologic derivatives

Ectoderm — Epidermis (including hair, nails), nervous system, adrenal medulla, pituitary.

Mesoderm — Connective tissue, muscle, bone, cardiovascular structures, lymphatics, urogenital structures, and serous linings of body cavities (e.g., peritoneal), spleen, adrenal cortex.

Endoderm — Gut tube epithelium and derivatives (e.g., lungs, liver, pancreas, thymus, thyroid, parathyroid).

Notochord — Induces ectoderm to form neuroectoderm (neural plate). Its postnatal derivative is the nucleus pulposus of the intervertebral disc.

Early development

Rule of 2s for 2nd week

2 germ layers (bilaminar disc): epiblast, hypoblast.
2 cavities: amniotic cavity, yolk sac.
2 components to placenta: cytotrophoblast, syncytiotrophoblast.

Rule of 3s for 3rd week

3 germ layers (gastrula): ectoderm, mesoderm, endoderm.

The epiblast (precursor to ectoderm) invaginates to form primitive streak. Cells from the primitive streak give rise to both intraembryonic mesoderm and endoderm.

Neural crest derivatives

ANS, dorsal root ganglia, melanocytes, chromaffin cells of adrenal medulla, enterochromaffin cells, pia, celiac ganglion, Schwann cells, odontoblasts, parafollicular cells (of thyroid).

Dura is of mesodermal origin.

Aortic arch derivatives	1st = part of maxillary artery. 2nd = stapedial artery and hyoid artery. 3rd = common carotid artery and proximal part of internal carotid artery. 4th = on left, aortic arch; on right, proximal part of right subclavian artery. 6th = proximal part of pulmonary arteries and (on left only) ductus arteriosus.	4th arch (4 limbs) = systemic. 6th arch = pulmonary and the pulmonary to systemic shunt (ductus arteriosus).
Fetal erythropoiesis	Fetal erythropoiesis occurs in: 1. Yolk sac (3–8 wk) 2. Liver (6–30 wk) 3. Spleen (9–28 wk) 4. Bone marrow (28 wk onward)	**Y**oung **L**iver **S**ynthesizes **B**lood.
Fetal-postnatal derivatives	1. Umbilical vein—ligamentum teres hepatis 2. Umbilical arteries—medial umbilical ligaments 3. Ductus arteriosus—ligamentum arteriosum 4. Ductus venosus—ligamentum venosum 5. Foramen ovale—fossa ovalis 6. Allantois—urachus—median umbilical ligament 7. Notochord—nucleus pulposus	Urachal cyst or sinus is a remnant of the allantois (urine drainage from bladder).
Branchial apparatus	Branchial clefts are derived from ectoderm. Branchial arches are derived from mesoderm and neural crests. Branchial pouches are derived from endoderm.	**CAP** covers outside from inside (**C**lefts = ectoderm, **A**rches = mesoderm, **P**ouches = endoderm)
Branchial arch 1 derivatives	Meckel's cartilage: mandible, malleus, incus, sphenomandibular ligament. Muscles: muscles of mastication (temporalis, masseter, lateral and medial pterygoids), mylohyoid, anterior belly of digastric, tensor tympani, tensor veli palatini. Nerve: CN V_3	
Branchial arch 2 derivatives	Reichert's cartilage: stapes, styloid process, lesser horn of hyoid, stylohyoid ligament. Muscles: muscles of facial expression: stapedius, stylohyoid, posterior belly of digastric. Nerve: CN VII	
Branchial arch 3 derivatives	Cartilage: greater horn of hyoid. Muscles: stylopharyngeus. Nerve: CN IX	Think of pharynx: stylo**pharyngeus** innervated by glosso**pharyngeal** nerve.

Branchial arches 4 to 6 derivatives	Cartilages: thyroid, cricoid, arytenoids, corniculate, cuneiform. Muscles (4th arch): most pharyngeal constrictors, cricothyroid, levator veli palatini. Muscles (6th arch): intrinsic muscles of larynx. Nerve: 4th arch–X 6th arch–X (recurrent laryngeal branch)	Arch 5 makes no major developmental contributions.
Branchial arch innervation	Arch 1 derivatives supplied by CN V_2 and V_3. Arch 2 derivatives supplied by CN VII. Arch 3 derivatives supplied by CN IX. Arch 4 derivatives supplied by CN X.	
Branchial cleft derivatives	1st cleft develops into external auditory meatus. 2nd through 4th clefts form temporary cervical sinuses, which are obliterated by proliferation of 2nd arch mesenchyme.	Persistent cervical sinus can lead to a branchial cyst in the neck.

Ear development

	Bones	Muscles	Miscellaneous
	Incus/malleus—1st arch	Tensor tympani (V_3)—1st arch	External auditory meatus—1st cleft
	Stapes—2nd arch	Stapedius (VII)—2nd arch	Eardrum, eustachian tube—1st pouch

Pharyngeal pouch derivatives	1st pouch develops into middle ear cavity, eustachian tube, mastoid air cells. 2nd pouch develops into epithelial lining of palatine tonsil. 3rd pouch (dorsal wings) develops into inferior parathyroids. 3rd pouch (ventral wings) develops into thymus. 4th pouch develops into superior parathyroids. 5th pouch houses the ultimobranchial bodies, which become the C cells of the thyroid.	1st pouch contributes to endoderm-lined structures of ear. 3rd pouch contributes to 3 structures (thymus, L and R inferior parathyroids). Ultimobranchial bodies arise from neural crest cells but migrate into 5th pouch.
Thymus	Site of T-cell maturation. Encapsulated. From epithelium of 3rd branchial pouches. Lymphocytes of mesenchymal origin. Cortex is dense with immature T cells; medulla is pale with mature T cells and epithelial reticular cells. Positive and negative selection occurs at the corticomedullary junction.	Think of the **T**hymus as "finishing school" for **T** cells. They arrive immature and "dense" in the cortex; they are mature in the medulla.
Thyroid development	Thyroid diverticulum arises from floor of primitive pharynx, descends into neck. Connected to tongue by thyroglossal duct, which normally disappears but may persist as pyramidal lobe of thyroid. Foramen cecum is normal remnant of thyroglossal duct.	

Intermediate filament	Permanent structure. Long fibrous molecules with 10-nm diameter. Linked to plasma membrane at desmosomes by desmoplakin. Very insoluble. No cytoplasmic pool of monomeric subunits. Intermediate filaments are tissue specific.	
Epithelial cells	Contain cytokeratin.	
Connective tissue	Contains vimentin.	
Muscle cells	Contain desmin.	
Neuroglia	Contain glial fibrillary acidic proteins (GFAP).	
Neurons	Contain neurofilaments.	
Nucleus	Contains nuclear lamin.	
Nissl bodies	Nissl bodies (in neurons) = rough ER; not found in axon or axon hillock. Synthesize enzymes (e.g., ChAT) and peptide neurotransmitters.	
Functions of Golgi apparatus	1. Distribution center of proteins and lipids from ER to the plasma membrane, lysosomes, and secretory vesicles 2. Modifies N-oligosaccharides 3. Adds O-oligosaccharides to serine and threonine residues 4. Proteoglycan assembly from proteoglycan core proteins 5. Sulfation of sugars in proteoglycans and of selected tyrosine on proteins 6. Addition of mannose-6-phosphate on specific lysosomal proteins, which targets the protein to the lysosome	I-cell disease is caused by the failure of addition of mannose-6-phosphate to lysosome proteins, causing these enzymes to be secreted outside the cell instead of being targeted to the lysosome.
Rough endoplasmic reticulum (RER)	Rough ER is the site of synthesis of secretory (exported) proteins and of N-linked oligosaccharide addition to many proteins.	Mucus-secreting goblet cells of the small intestine are rich in RER.
Smooth endoplasmic reticulum (SER)	SER is the site of steroid synthesis and detoxification of drugs and poisons.	Liver hepatocytes and steroid-hormone–producing cells of the adrenal cortex are rich in SER.
Sinusoids of liver	Irregular "capillaries" with round pores 100–200 nm in diameter without diaphragm. No basement membrane. Not a barrier to macromolecules of plasma (full access to surface of liver cells through space of Disse).	
Sinusoids of spleen	Long, vascular channels in red pulp. With fenestrated "barrel hoop" basement membrane. Macrophages found nearby.	T cells are found in the PALS and the red pulp of the spleen. B cells are found in follicles within the white pulp of the spleen.

Anatomy

Pancreas endocrine cell types	Islets of Langerhans are collections of endocrine cells (most numerous in tail of pancreas). α = glucagon; β = insulin; δ = somatostatin. Islets arise from pancreatic buds.	

Adrenal cortex zones

Zona **G**lomerulosa	Aldosterone (outer layer).	**GFR** corresponds with **s**alt
Zona **F**asciculata	Cortisol (middle layer).	(Na$^+$), **s**ugar (glucocorti-
Zona **R**eticularis	Both cortisol and some androgens such as DHEA (inner layer).	coids), and **s**ex (androgens). "The deeper you go, the sweeter it gets."

Adrenal medulla	Chromaffin cells are only cells in the body that secrete epinephrine and norepinephrine.	Pheochromocytoma = most common tumor of the adrenal medulla in adults. Neuroblastoma = most common in children. Pheochromocytoma causes episodic hypertension; neuroblastoma does not.
Types of secretion	Merocrine (eccrine) = by exocytosis (i.e., proteins). Apocrine = secretion with loss of cytoplasm from apical side (i.e., sweat). Holocrine = secretion with destruction of the cell (i.e., products of sebaceous glands).	*Apo*crine = *Api*cal cytoplasm. *Holo*crine = *Whole* cytoplasm.
Brunner's glands	Secrete alkaline mucus. Located in submucosa of duodenum (the only GI submucosal glands). Duodenal ulcers cause hypertrophy of Brunner's glands.	**BAGS: B**runner's **A**lkaline **G**lands, **S**ubmucosal.

Lymph node

A secondary lymphoid organ that has many afferents, one or more efferents. Encapsulated. With trabeculae. Functions are nonspecific filtration by macrophages, storage/proliferation of B and T cells, Ab production.

Follicle

Site of B-cell localization and proliferation. In outer cortex. 1° follicles are dense and dormant. 2° follicles have pale central germinal centers and are active.

Medulla

Consists of medullary cords (closely packed lymphocytes and plasma cells) and medullary sinuses. Medullary sinuses communicate with efferent lymphatics and contain reticular cells and macrophages.

Paracortex

Houses T cells. Region of cortex between follicles and medulla. Contains high endothelial venules into which T and B cells enter from blood. In an extreme cellular immune response, paracortex becomes greatly enlarged. Not well developed in patients with DiGeorge's syndrome.

Peyer's patch

Unencapsulated lymphoid tissue found in lamina propria and submucosa of intestine. Covered by single layer of cuboidal enterocytes (no goblet cells) with specialized M cells interspersed. M cells take up antigen.

IgA production in gut

Stimulated B cell leaves Peyer's patch and travels through lymph and blood to lamina propria of intestine, where it differentiates to IgA-secreting plasma cell. IgA receives protective secretory piece, then is transported across epithelium to gut to deal with intraluminal Ag.

Think of **IgA,** the **I**ntra-**g**ut– **A**ntibody. And always say, "secretory IgA."

Hypothalamus: functions	**T**hirst and water balance (supraoptic nucleus). **A**denohypophysis control via releasing factors. **N**eurohypophysis releases hormones synthesized in hypothalamic nuclei. **H**unger (lateral nucleus) and satiety (ventromedial nucleus). **A**utonomic regulation (anterior hypothalamus regulates parasympathetic activity), circadian rhythms (suprachiasmatic nucleus). **T**emperature regulation: Posterior hypothalamus—heat production when cold. Anterior hypothalamus—coordinates cooling when hot. **S**exual urges and emotions (septate nucleus).	The hypothalamus wears **"TAN HATS."** If you zap your **ventromedial** nucleus, you grow **ven**trally and **medial**ly (hyperphagia and obesity). **L**ittle (**L**ateral) food makes you hungry. If you zap your **P**osterior hypothalamus, you become a **P**oikilotherm (cold-blooded snake).
Posterior pituitary (neurohypophysis)	Receives hypothalamic axonal projections from supraoptic (ADH) and paraventricular (oxytocin) nuclei.	Oxytocin: *oxys* = quick; *tocos* = birth.
Functions of thalamic nuclei	Lateral geniculate nucleus = visual. Medial geniculate nucleus = auditory. Ventral posterior nucleus, lateral part = proprioception, pressure, pain, touch vibration of body. Ventral posterior nucleus, medial part = facial sensation, including pain. Ventral anterior/lateral nuclei = motor.	**L**ateral to **L**ook. **M**edial for **M**usic.
Limbic system: functions	Responsible for **F**eeding, **F**ighting, **F**eeling, **F**light, and sex.	The famous **5 F**s.
CNS/PNS supportive cells	**A**strocytes—physical support, repair, K$^+$ metabolism. **M**icroglia—phagocytosis. **O**ligodendroglia—central myelin production. **S**chwann cells—peripheral myelin production. **E**pendymal cells—inner lining of ventricles.	**"A MOSE** (like 'most') wonderful array of neural supportive cells."

HIGH-YIELD FACTS

Anatomy

Blood–brain barrier	Formed by three structures: 1. Arachnoid 2. Choroid plexus epithelium 3. Intracerebral capillary endothelium Glucose and amino acids cross by carrier-mediated transport mechanism. Nonpolar/lipid–soluble substances cross more readily than polar/water–soluble ones.	Other barriers include: 1. Blood–bile barrier 2. Blood–testis barrier 3. Blood–PNS barrier Example: L-dopa, rather than dopamine, is used to treat parkinsonism because dopamine does not cross blood-brain barrier.
Chorea	Sudden, jerky, purposeless movements. Characteristic of basal ganglia lesion (e.g., Huntington's disease).	*Chorea* = dancing (Greek). Think choral dancing.
Athetosis	Slow, writhing movements, especially of fingers. Characteristic of basal ganglia lesion.	*Athetos* = not fixed (Greek). Think snakelike.
Hemiballismus	Sudden, wild flailing of one arm. Characteristic of subthalamic nucleus lesion.	Half ballistic (as in throwing a baseball).
Tremors: cerebellar versus basal	Cerebellar tremor = intention tremor. Basal ganglion tremor = resting tremor.	Basal = at rest (Parkinson's disease).

Cerebral cortex functions

Brain lesions

Area of lesion	Consequence	
Broca's area	Motor (expressive) aphasia	**BRO**ca's is **BRO**ken speech.
Wernicke's area	Sensory (fluent) aphasia	**W**ernicke's is **W**ordy but makes no sense.
Amygdala (bilateral)	Klüver-Bucy syndrome (hyperorality, hypersexuality, disinhibited behavior)	
Frontal lobe	Frontal release signs (e.g., personality changes and deficits in concentration, orientation, judgment)	
Right parietal lobe	Spacial neglect syndrome (agnosia of the contralateral side of the world)	
Reticular activating system	Coma	
Mamillary bodies (bilateral)	Wernicke–Korsakoff's encephalopathy (confabulations, anterograde amnesia).	

Cavernous sinus

CN III, IV, V_1, V_2, VI all pass through the cavernous sinus. Only CN VI is "free-floating." Also contains cavernous portion of internal carotid artery.

The nerves that control extraocular muscles (plus V_1 and V_2) pass through the cavernous sinus.

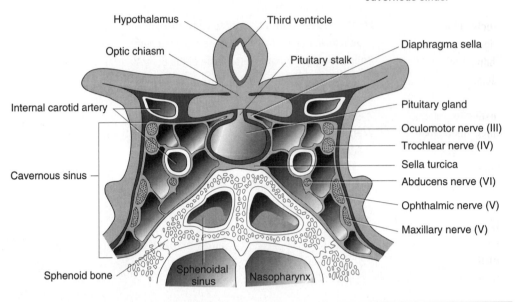

Labels: Hypothalamus, Third ventricle, Optic chiasm, Pituitary stalk, Diaphragma sella, Internal carotid artery, Pituitary gland, Oculomotor nerve (III), Trochlear nerve (IV), Sella turcica, Cavernous sinus, Abducens nerve (VI), Ophthalmic nerve (V), Maxillary nerve (V), Sphenoid bone, Sphenoidal sinus, Nasopharynx

Foramina: middle cranial fossa

1. Optic canal (CN II, ophthalmic artery, central retinal vein)
2. **S**uperior orbital fissure (CN III, IV, V_1, VI, ophthalmic vein)
3. Foramen **R**otundum (CN V_2)
4. Foramen **O**vale (CN V_3)
5. Foramen spinosum (middle meningeal artery)

All structures pass through sphenoid bone. Divisions of CN V exit owing to **S**tanding **R**oom **O**nly (**S**uperior orbital fissure, foramen **R**otundum, foramen **O**vale).

Foramina: posterior cranial fossa

1. Internal auditory meatus (CN VII, VIII)
2. Jugular foramen (CN IX, X, XI, jugular vein)
3. Hypoglossal canal (CN XII)
4. Foramen magnum (spinal roots of CN XI, brain stem, vertebral arteries)

All structures pass through temporal or occipital bones.

Extraocular muscles and nerves

Lateral **R**ectus is CN VI, **S**uperior **O**blique is CN IV, rest are CN III.

The "chemical formula" LR_6SO_4; rest is CN III.

Internuclear ophthalmoplegia

Lesion in the **M**edial **L**ongitudinal **F**asciculus (MLF). Results in medial rectus palsy on attempted lateral gaze. Nystagmus in abducting eye. Convergence is normal. MLF syndrome is seen in many patients with multiple sclerosis.

Cranial nerves

		Function	Type	
Olfactory	I	Smell	**S**ensory	**S**ome
Optic	II	Sight	**S**ensory	**S**ay
Oculomotor	III	Eye movement, pupil constriction, accommodation, eyelid opening	**M**otor	**M**arry
Trochlear	IV	Eye movement	**M**otor	**M**oney
Trigeminal	V	Mastication, facial sensation	**B**oth	**B**ut
Abducens	VI	Eye movement	**M**otor	**M**y
Facial	VII	Facial movement, anterior 2/3 taste, lacrimation, salivation (submaxillary and submandibular salivary glands)	**B**oth	**B**rother
Vestibulocochlear	VIII	Hearing, balance	**S**ensory	**S**ays
Glossopharyngeal	IX	Posterior 1/3 taste, swallowing, salivation (parotid gland), monitoring carotid body and sinus	**B**oth	**B**ig
Vagus	X	Taste, swallowing, palate elevation, talking, thoracoabdominal viscera	**B**oth	**B**rains
Accessory	XI	Head turning, shoulder shrugging, talking	**M**otor	**M**atter
Hypoglossal	XII	Tongue movements	**M**otor	**M**ost

Cranial nerves and passageways

Cribriform plate	I
Optic canal	II
Superior orbital fissure	III, IV, V$_1$, VI
Foramen rotundum	V$_2$
Foramen ovale	V$_3$
Internal auditory meatus	VII, VIII
Jugular foramen	IX, X, XI
Hypoglossal canal	XII

Visual field defects

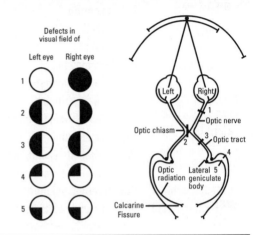

Defects in visual field of

Left eye   Right eye

1. Right anopsia
2. Bitemporal hemianopsia
3. Left homonymous hemianopsia
4. Left upper quadrantic anopsia (right temporal lesion)
5. Left lower quadrantic anopsia (right parietal lesion)

KLM sounds: kuh, la, mi

Kuh-kuh-kuh tests palate elevation (CN X—vagus).
La-la-la tests tongue (CN XII—hypoglossal).
Mi-mi-mi tests lips (CN VII—facial).

Say it aloud.

Vagal nuclei

Nucleus **S**olitarius — Visceral **S**ensory information (e.g., taste, gut distention, etc.).

Nucleus a**M**biguus — **M**otor innervation of pharynx, larynx, and upper esophagus.

Dorsal motor nucleus — Sends autonomic (parasympathetic) fibers to heart, lungs, and upper GI.

Lesions and deviations

CN XII lesion (LMN): tongue deviates **toward** side of lesion.
CN V motor lesion: jaw deviates **toward** side of lesion.
Unilateral lesion of cerebellum: patient tends to fall **toward** side of lesion.

Spinal cord and associated tracts

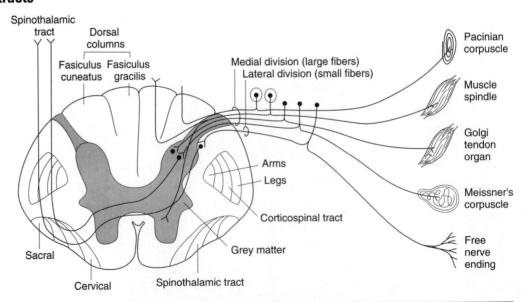

Dorsal column organization	In dorsal columns, lower limbs are inside to avoid crossing the upper limbs on the outside. Fasciculus gracilis = legs. Fasciculus cuneatus = arms.	Dorsal column is organized like you are, with hands at sides—arms outside and legs inside. *Gracilis* (Latin) = graceful, slender, like ballerina's legs.
Brown-Séquard syndrome	Hemisection of spinal cord. Findings below the lesion: 1. Ipsilateral motor paralysis and spasticity (pyramidal tract) 2. Ipsilateral loss of tactile, vibration, proprioception sense (dorsal column) 3. Contralateral pain and temperature loss (spinothalamic tract)	
Lower motor neuron (LMN) signs	LMN injury signs: atrophy, flaccid paralysis, absent deep tendon reflexes. Fasciculations may be present.	**Lower** MN ≈ everything **lower**ed (less muscle mass, **decreased** muscle tone, **decreased** reflexes, **down**going toes).
Upper motor neuron (UMN) signs	UMN injury signs: little atrophy, spastic paralysis, hyperactive deep tendon reflexes, possible positive Babinski.	**Upper** MN ≈ everything **up** (tone, DTRs, toes).

Spindle muscle control

Reflex arc	Muscle spindle stretch stimulates Ia afferents. Ia stimulates alpha motor neurons of agonist muscle to contract extrafusal muscle fibers.
Gamma loop	Gamma motor neurons from CNS contract intrafusal muscle fibers → stretch spindle → reflex arc → stimulate alpha motor neuron. Responsible for maintaining tone.

Brachial plexus

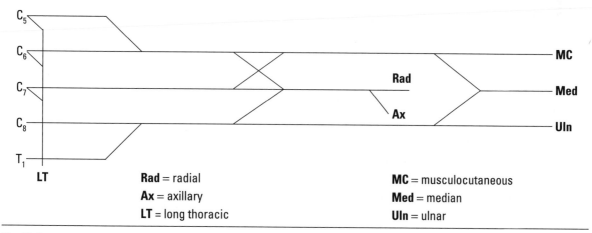

Rad = radial	**MC** = musculocutaneous
Ax = axillary	**Med** = median
LT = long thoracic	**Uln** = ulnar

Radial nerve	Known as the "great extensor nerve." Provides innervation of the **B**rachoradialis, **E**xtensors of the wrist and fingers, **S**upinator, and **T**riceps.	Radial nerve innervates the **BEST**! To **s**upinate is to move as if carrying a bowl of **soup**.

Myotome "dances" (perform while reciting aloud)

Arm:
- **C5** —abduct arm
- **C678**—adduct arm
- **C56** —flex elbow
- **C78** —extend elbow
- **C6** —pronate/supinate
- **C67** —flex/extend wrist
- **C78** —flex/extend fingers
- **T1** —abduct/adduct fingers

Leg:
- **L123** —flex, adduct, medially rotate hip
- **L34** —extend knee
- **L45** —dorsiflex and invert ankle
- **L5,S1**—evert ankle
- **S12** —plantar flex

Cervical rib

An embryologic defect; can compress subclavian artery and inferior trunk of brachial plexus (C8, T1), resulting in:
1. Atrophy of the thenar and hypothenar eminences
2. Atrophy of the interosseous muscles
3. Sensory deficits on the medial side of the forearm and hand
4. Disappearance of the radial pulse upon moving the head toward the opposite side

---

Facial lesion

Central facial

Paralysis of the contralateral facial muscles except the frontalis and orbicularis oculi muscles. Because the motor neurons supplying the frontalis and orbicularis oculi muscles receive bilateral cortical innervation, the muscles are not paralyzed by lesions involving one motor cortex or its corticobulbar pathways.

Bell's palsy

Peripheral facial paralysis.
Can occur idiopathically.
Seen as a complication in diabetes, tumors, sarcoidosis, AIDS, and Lyme disease.
Bell's phenomenon—when an attempt is made to close the eyelid, the eyeball on the affected side may turn upward.
Complete destruction of the facial nucleus itself or its branchial efferent fibers (facial nerve proper) paralyzes all ipsilateral facial muscles.

Clinical reflexes

Biceps = C5 nerve root.
Triceps = C7 nerve root.
Patella = L4 nerve root.
Achilles = S1 nerve root.
Babinski = dorsiflexion of the big toe and fanning of other toes; sign of upper motor neuron lesion.

Embryology

1. Development of the heart, lung, liver, kidney (i.e., what are the embryologic structures that give rise to these organs?).
2. Etiology and clinical presentation of important congenital malformations (e.g., neural tube defects, cleft palate, tetralogy of Fallot, tracheoesophageal fistula, horseshoe kidney).
3. Development of the central nervous system (e.g., telencephalon, diencephalon, mesencephalon).
4. Derivatives of the foregut, midgut, and hindgut.
5. Derivatives of the somites, and malformations associated with defects in somite migration.
6. Fetal circulation (path of oxygenated and deoxygenated blood, fetal circulatory structures and their adult derivatives).
7. Changes in the circulatory/respiratory system on the first breath of a newborn.

Gross Anatomy

1. Anatomic landmarks in relation to medical procedures (e.g., direct and indirect hernia repair, lumbar puncture, pericardiocentesis).
2. Anatomic landmarks in relation to major organs (e.g., lungs, heart, kidneys).
3. Common injuries of the knee (including clinical examination), hip, shoulder, and clavicle; paying attention to the clinical deficits caused by these injuries (e.g., shoulder separation, hip fracture).
4. Clinical features and anatomic correlations of specific brachial plexus lesions (e.g., waiter's tip, wrist drop, claw hand, scapular winging).
5. Clinical features of common peripheral nerve injuries (e.g., common vs. deep peroneal nerve palsy, radial nerve palsy).
6. Etiology and clinical features of common diseases affecting the hands (e.g., carpal tunnel syndrome, cubital tunnel syndrome, Dupuytren's contracture).
7. Anatomic basis for the blood–testis barrier.
8. Major blood vessels and collateral circulatory pathways of the gastrointestinal tract (e.g., collaterals between the superior and inferior mesenteric arteries).
9. Bone structures (metaphysis, epiphysis, diaphysis); linear (epiphysis) and annular (diaphysis) bone growth.

Histology

1. Histology of the respiratory tract (i.e., can you differentiate between the bronchi, terminal bronchioles, respiratory bronchioles, and alveoli?).
2. Structure, function, and electron microscopic (EM) appearance of major cellular organelles and structures (e.g., lysosomes, peroxisomes, glycogen, mitochondria, ER, Golgi apparatus, nucleus, nucleolus).
3. Structure, function, and EM appearance of cell–cell junctional structures (e.g., tight junctions, gap junctions, desmosomes).
4. Histology of lymphoid organs (e.g., lymph nodes, tonsils, thymus, spleen).
5. Resident phagocytic cells of different organisms (e.g., Langerhan's cells, Kupffer cells, alveolar macrophages, microglia).

HIGH-YIELD FACTS

Anatomy

6. Histology of muscle fibers and changes seen with muscle contraction (sarcomere structure, different bands, rigor mortis).
7. Bone ossification (intramembranous vs. endochondral).

Neuroanatomy

1. Etiology and clinical features of important brain, cranial nerve, and spinal cord lesions (e.g., brain stem lesions and "crossed signs," dorsal root lesions).
2. Production, circulation, and composition of cerebrospinal fluid.
3. Neuroanatomy of hearing (central and peripheral hearing loss).
4. Extra-ocular muscles (which muscle abducts, adducts, etc.).
5. Structure and function of a chemical synapse (e.g., neuromuscular junction).
6. Major neurotransmitters, receptors, second messengers, and effects.
7. Blood supply of the brain (anterior, middle, posterior cerebral arterial areas, "watershed" areas) and neurologic deficits corresponding to various vascular occlusions).
8. Functional anatomy of the basal ganglia (e.g., globus pallidus, caudate, putamen).
9. Anatomic landmarks near the pituitary gland.
10. Brain MRI/CT, including morphologic changes in disease states (e.g., Huntington's chorea, MS, aging).
11. Clinical exam of pupillary light reflex: pathway tested, important anatomic lesions.

Radiology

1. X-rays; plain films.
   a. skull (e.g., fractures).
   b. PA and lateral chest films, including important landmarks (costodiaphragmatic recess, major blood vessels, and abnormalities seen with different diseases (consolidation, pneumothorax, cardiomegaly).
   c. abdominal films, including vasculature (locate important vessels in contrast films) and other important structures.
   d. joint films (e.g., shoulder, wrist, knee, vertebrae); including important injuries/diseases (e.g., osteoarthritis, herniated disc).
2. CT/MRI studies.
   a. brain cross-sections (e.g., hematomas, brain lesions, extra-ocular muscles).
   b. chest cross-section (e.g., superior vena cava, aortic arch, heart).
   c. abdominal cross-section (e.g., liver, kidney, pancreas, aorta).

Behavioral Science

A heterogeneous mix of epidemiology/biostatistics, psychiatry, psychology, sociology, psychopharmacology, and more falls under this heading. Many medical students do not study this discipline diligently because the material is felt to be "easy" or "common sense." In our opinion, this is a missed opportunity. Each question gained in behavioral science is equal to a question in any other section in determining the overall score. At many medical schools, this material is not covered in a single course. Many students feel that some behavioral science questions are less concrete and require awareness of social aspects of medicine. For example: If a patient does or says something, what should you do or say back? Basic biostatistics and epidemiology are very learnable and high yield. Be able to apply biostatistical concepts such as specificity and predictive values in a problem-solving format.

Epidemiology
Ethics
Life Cycle
Physiology
Psychiatry
Psychology
High-Yield Topics

HIGH-YIELD FACTS

Behavioral Science

Prevalence versus incidence	Prevalence is total number of cases in a population at a given time. Incidence is number of new cases in a population per unit time.	**Incidence** is new **incidents.**
Sensitivity	Number of true positives divided by number of all people with the disease. False negative ratio is equal to 1 − sensitivity.	**PID** = **P**ositive **I**n **D**isease (note that PID is a sensitive topic).
Specificity	Number of true negatives divided by number of all people without the disease. False positive ratio is equal to 1 − specificity.	**NIH** = **N**egative **I**n **H**ealth.

Predictive value

Positive predictive value	Number of true positives divided by number of people who tested positive for the disease. The probability of having a condition, given a positive test.
Negative predictive value	Number of true negatives divided by number of people who tested negative for the disease. The probability of not having the condition, given a negative test. Unlike sensitivity and specificity, predictive value is dependent on the prevalence of the disease. The higher the prevalence of a disease, the higher the positive predictive value of the test.

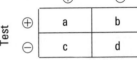

$$\text{Sensitivity} = \frac{a}{a+b}$$

$$\text{Specificity} = \frac{d}{b+d}$$

$$\text{PPV} = \frac{a}{a+b}$$

$$\text{NPV} = \frac{d}{c+d}$$

Odds ratio and relative risk

Odds ratio	Approximates the relative risk if the prevalence of the disease is not too high. Used for retrospective studies (e.g., case-control studies). OR = ad / bc
Relative risk	Disease risk in exposed group/disease risk in unexposed group. Used for cohort studies.

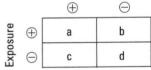

$$RR = \frac{\left[\dfrac{a}{a+b}\right]}{\left[\dfrac{c}{c+d}\right]} \qquad \text{Attributable Risk} = \left[\dfrac{a}{a+b}\right] - \left[\dfrac{c}{c+d}\right]$$

Standard deviation versus error	n = sample size, σ = standard deviation, SEM = standard error of the mean, SEM = $\sigma/\sqrt{n}$ Therefore, SEM < σ and SEM ↓ as n ↑.	If distribution is normal (Gaussian), then $\pm 1\,\sigma$ contains 68% of values, $\pm 2\,\sigma$ contains 95% of values, and $\pm 3\,\sigma$ contains 99.7% of values.
Distribution: skew, bimodal	Terms that describe statistical distributions: Normal ≈ Gaussian ≈ bell-shaped. (Mean = median = mode.) Bimodal is simply two humps. Positive skew is asymmetry with tail on the right. Negative skew has tail on the left.	Positive skew = tail on more positive side (mean > median > mode). Negative skew = tail on more negative side (mean < median < mode).
Precision vs. accuracy	Precision is: 1. The consistency and reproducibility of a test (reliability) 2. The absence of random variation in a test Accuracy is the trueness of test measurements.	Random error = reduced precision in a test. Systemic error = reduced accuracy in a test.
Reliability and validity	Reliability = reproducibility (dependability) of a test. Validity = whether the test truly measures what it purports to measure. Appropriateness of a test.	Test is reliable if repeat measurements are the same. Test is valid if it measures what it is supposed to measure.
Correlation coefficient (r)	r is always between −1 and 1. Absolute value indicates strength of correlation. Pearson coefficient is used when values are evaluated directly. Spearman (rank) coefficient is used when values are placed in rank order and ranks are analyzed. Coefficient of determination = r^2.	Spear**men** stand in ranks.
***t*-test versus ANOVA versus χ^2**	*t*-test checks difference between two means. ANOVA analyzes variance of three or more variables. χ^2 checks difference between two or more percentages or proportions of categorical outcomes (not mean values).	*t*-test = compare means. **ANOVA = AN**alysis **O**f **VA**riance of three or more variables. χ^2 = compare percentages (%) or proportions.
Confidence intervals	Standard 95% confidence interval is an interval that has a 95% probability of containing the true mean.	The smaller the interval, the more precise the estimate.
Meta-analysis	Pooling data from several studies to achieve greater statistical power.	Cannot overcome limitations of individual studies or bias in study selection.

HIGH-YIELD FACTS

Behavioral Science

Case-control study	Observational study. Sample chosen based on presence (cases) or absence (controls) of disease. Information collected about risk factors.	Often retrospective.
Cohort study	Observational study. Sample chosen based on presence or absence of risk factors. Subjects followed over time for development of disease.	The Framingham heart study was a large prospective cohort study.
Clinical trial	Experimental study. Compares therapeutic benefit of 2 or more treatments.	Highest quality study.

Statistical hypotheses

Null (H_0)	Hypothesis of no difference (e.g., there is no association between the disease and the risk factor in the population).	
Alternative (H_1)	Hypothesis that there is some difference (e.g., there is some association between the disease and the risk factor in the population).	

Reality

Study results	H_1	H_0
H_1	Power $(1 - \beta)$	α
H_0	β	

Type I error (α)	Stating that there **is** an effect or difference when there really is not (to mistakenly accept the experimental hypothesis and reject the null hypothesis). α is the probability of making a type I error and is equal to p (usually $< .05$). p = probability of making a type I error.	If $p < .05$, then there is less than a 5% chance that the data will show something that is not really there. α = you "saw" a difference that did not exist—for example, convicting an innocent man.
Type II error (β)	Stating that there **is not** an effect or difference when there really is (to fail to reject the null hypothesis when in fact H_0 is false). β is the probability of making a type II error.	β = you did not "see" a difference that does exist—for example, setting a guilty man free. $1 - \beta$ is "power" of study, or probability that study will see a difference if it is there.
Power	Probability of rejecting null hypothesis when it is in fact false. It depends on: 1. Total number of end points experienced by population 2. Difference in compliance between treatment groups (differences in the mean values between groups)	If you increase sample size, you increase power. There is power in numbers. Power = $1 - \beta$.

Premature infants	Defined as under 2500 g or 34 wk. Have greater physical and emotional problems. Complications of prematurity include low birth weight, infections, respiratory distress syndrome, necrotizing enterocolitis, and persistent fetal circulation.	
Fetal alcohol syndrome	Newborns of mothers who consumed significant amounts of alcohol (teratogen) during pregnancy have a higher incidence of congenital abnormalities, including pre- and post-natal developmental retardation, microcephaly, facial abnormalities, limb dislocation, and heart and lung fistulas. Mechanism may include inhibition of cell migration. The number one cause of congenital malformations in the United States.	

Apgar score (at birth)

Score 0–2 at 1 and 5 min in each of five categories:
1. Heart rate (0, <100, 100+)
2. Respiratory effort (0, irregular, regular)
3. Muscle tone (limp, some, active)
4. Reflex irritability (0, grimace, grimace + cough)
5. Color (blue/pale, trunk pink, all pink)

10 is perfect score.

After Virginia **Apgar,** a famous neonatologist.
A = **A**ppearance (color)
P = **P**ulse
G = **G**rimace
A = **A**ctivity
R = **R**espiration

Heroin addiction

Approximately 500,000 US addicts. Heroin is schedule I (not prescribable). Evidence of addiction is narcotic abstinence syndrome (dilated pupils, lacrimation, rhinorrhea, sweating, yawning, irritability, and muscle aches). Also look for track marks (needle sticks in veins). Related diagnoses are hepatitis, abscesses, overdose, hemorrhoids, AIDS, and right-sided endocarditis.

Naloxone (Narcan) and naltrexone competitively inhibit opioids.
Methadone (long-acting oral opiate) for heroin detoxification or long-term maintenance.

Reportable diseases

Only some infectious diseases are reported, including AIDS (but not HIV positivity), chickenpox, gonorrhea, hepatitis A and B, measles, mumps, rubella, salmonella, shigella, syphilis, tuberculosis.

Leading causes of death in the US by age

Infants	Congenital anomalies, sudden infant death syndrome, short gestation/low birth weight, respiratory distress syndrome, maternal complications of pregnancy.	AIDS is leading cause of death between the ages of 25 and 44.
Age 1–14	Injuries, cancer, congenital anomalies, homicide, heart disease.	
Age 15–24	Injuries, homicide, suicide, cancer, heart disease.	
Age 25–64	Cancer, heart disease, injuries, stroke, suicide.	
Age 65+	Heart disease, cancer, stroke, COPD, pneumonia.	

Disease prevention

1°—Prevent disease occurrence (e.g., vaccination).

2°—Early detection of disease (e.g., Pap smear).

3°—Reduce disability from disease (e.g., exogenous insulin for diabetes).

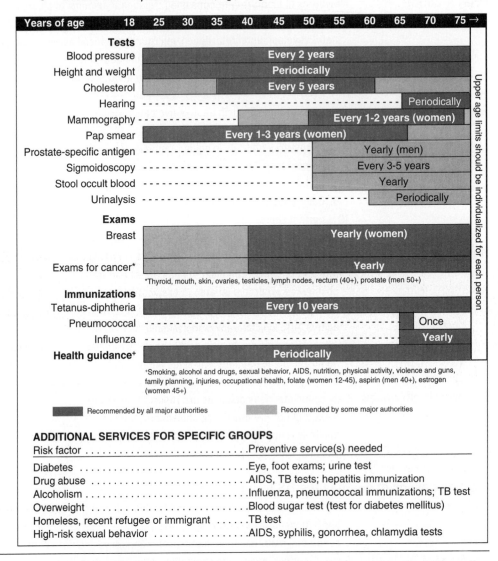

Years of age	18	25	30	35	40	45	50	55	60	65	70	75 →

Tests

Blood pressure — Every 2 years

Height and weight — Periodically

Cholesterol — Every 5 years

Hearing — Periodically

Mammography — Every 1-2 years (women)

Pap smear — Every 1-3 years (women)

Prostate-specific antigen — Yearly (men)

Sigmoidoscopy — Every 3-5 years

Stool occult blood — Yearly

Urinalysis — Periodically

Exams

Breast — Yearly (women)

Exams for cancer* — Yearly

*Thyroid, mouth, skin, ovaries, testicles, lymph nodes, rectum (40+), prostate (men 50+)

Immunizations

Tetanus-diphtheria — Every 10 years

Pneumococcal — Once

Influenza — Yearly

Health guidance+ — Periodically

+Smoking, alcohol and drugs, sexual behavior, AIDS, nutrition, physical activity, violence and guns, family planning, injuries, occupational health, folate (women 12-45), aspirin (men 40+), estrogen (women 45+)

Upper age limits should be individualized for each person

■ Recommended by all major authorities   ■ Recommended by some major authorities

ADDITIONAL SERVICES FOR SPECIFIC GROUPS

Risk factor	Preventive service(s) needed
Diabetes	Eye, foot exams; urine test
Drug abuse	AIDS, TB tests; hepatitis immunization
Alcoholism	Influenza, pneumococcal immunizations; TB test
Overweight	Blood sugar test (test for diabetes mellitus)
Homeless, recent refugee or immigrant	TB test
High-risk sexual behavior	AIDS, syphilis, gonorrhea, chlamydia tests

Elderly population in year 2000

In year 2000, estimated US population = 300,000,000. 35 million > 65 y old. Greatest increase in those > 85 y old.

In year 2000, 13% of US population > 65 y old.

Risk factors for suicide completion

White, male, alone, prior attempts, presence and lethality of plan, medical illness, alcohol or drug use, on 3 or more prescription medications.

Common surgeries

Dilation and curettage, hysterectomy, tonsillectomy, sterilization, hernia repair, oophorectomy, cesarean section, cholecystectomy.

Most done on women.

Divorce statistics	US has highest rate. Teenage marriages at high risk. More common when religions are mixed. Peaks at second/third year of marriage. Higher with low SES. Unrelated to industrialization. Divorcees remarry very frequently.	
Drug agencies	**FDA** = **F**ood and **D**rug **A**dministration (safety and efficacy of drugs). **DEA** = **D**rug **E**nforcement **A**dministration (security of controlled substances). **NIDA** = **N**ational **I**nstitute of **D**rug **A**buse (education, prevention).	**FDA** = protection. **DEA** = prosecution. **NIDA** = prevention.
Medicare, Medicaid	Medicare and Medicaid are federal programs that originated from amendments to the Social Security Act. Medicare Part A = hospital; Part B = supplemental. Medicaid is federal and state assistance for those on welfare or who are indigent.	Medi**care** is **care** for the elderly. Medi**caid** is **aid** for the poor.

BEHAVIORAL SCIENCE—ETHICS

Futility	If medical situation is futile, physician may refuse patient's or family's request for intervention or may spare the patient an invasive intervention. Strict futility defined: 1. Intervention does not make sense pathophysiologically 2. Maximal treatment is failing 3. The intervention has already failed the patient 4. Intervention will not achieve the goals of care	
Autonomy	Obligation to respect patients as individuals and to honor their preferences in medical care.	
Informed consent	Legally requires: 1. Discussion of pertinent information 2. Obtaining the patient's agreement to the plan of care 3. Freedom from coercion	Patients must understand the risks, benefits, and alternatives, which include no intervention.
Exceptions to informed consent	1. Patient lacks decision-making capacity (not legally competent) 2. Implied consent in an emergency 3. Therapeutic privilege—withholding information when disclosure would severely harm the patient or undermine informed decision-making capacity 4. Waiver—patient waives the right of informed consent	
Decision-making capacity	1. Patient makes and communicates a choice 2. Patient is informed 3. Decision is stable over time 4. Decisions consistent with patient's values and goals 5. Decisions not a result of delusions or hallucinations	The patient's family cannot require that a doctor withhold information from the patient.

Advance directives

If medical situation is not futile but the patient is not capable of making an informed decision, is there an advance directive outlining the patient's wishes? If an advance directive does not exist, a physician may appoint and work with a surrogate decision maker.

Oral advance directive

Incapacitated patient's prior oral statements commonly used as guide. Problems arise from variance in interpretation of these statements. However, if patient was informed, directive is specific, patient makes a choice, and decision is repeated over time, the oral directive is more valid.

Written advance directive

1. Living wills—Patient directs physician to withhold or withdraw life-sustaining treatment if the patient develops a terminal disease or enters a persistent vegetative state.
2. Durable power of attorney—Patient designates a surrogate to make medical decisions in the event that the patient loses decision-making capacity. Patient may also specify decisions in clinical situations. More flexible than a living will.

Nonmaleficence

"Do no harm." However, if benefits of an intervention outweigh the risks, a patient may make an informed decision to proceed.

Beneficence

Physicians have a special ethical responsibility to act in the patient's best interest (physician is a fiduciary). Patient autonomy may conflict with beneficence. If the patient makes an informed decision, ultimately the patient has the right to decide.

Confidentiality

Confidentiality respects patient privacy and autonomy. Disclosing information to family and friends should be guided by what the patient would want. The patient may also waive the right to confidentiality (e.g., insurance companies).

Exceptions to confidentiality

1. Potential harm to third parties is serious
2. Likelihood of harm is high
3. No alternative means exist to warn or to protect those at risk
4. Third party can take steps to prevent harm

Examples include:

1. Infectious diseases—physicians may have a duty to warn public officials and identifiable people at risk
2. The Tarasoff decision—law requiring physician to protect potential victim from harm; may involve breach of confidentiality
3. Child and/or elder abuse
4. Impaired automobile drivers
5. Suicidal/homicidal patient
6. Domestic violence

Malpractice

Civil suit under negligence requires:

1. Physician breach of duty to patient
2. Patient suffers harm
3. Breach of duty causes harm

The **4 Ds: D**ereliction of **D**uty **D**irectly led to **D**amage

Anaclitic depression	Anaclitic depression = depression in an infant owing to continued separation from caregiver. Can result in failure to thrive. Infant becomes withdrawn and unresponsive.	*Ana* = against; *clitic* = lean.
Regression in children	Children regress to younger behavior under stress: physical illness, punishment, birth of a new sibling, tiredness. An example is bedwetting in a child when hospitalized.	
Infant deprivation effects	Long-term deprivation of affection results in: 1. Decreased muscle tone 2. Poor language skills 3. Poor socialization skills 4. Lack of basic trust 5. Anaclitic depression Severe deprivation can result in infant death.	Studied by René Spitz. The **4 Ws: W**eak, **W**ordless, **W**anting (socially), **W**ary. Deprivation for longer than 6 months can lead to irreversible changes.
Jean Piaget stages	Cognitive stages (intellectual development): 0–2 y: **S**ensorimotor 2–7 y: **P**reoperational (egocentric thinking) 7–11 y: **C**oncrete operational (conservation of volume) 11+ y: **F**ormal operational (abstract concepts)	**S**lowly, **P**iaget's **C**hildren **F**orm.
Erik Erikson stages	Stages of psychological development in which individual is confronted with major "tasks": 0–1 y: trust versus mistrust 1–3 y: autonomy versus shame/doubt 3–6 y: initiative versus guilt 6–12 y: industry versus inferiority 12–20 y: identity versus role confusion 20–30 y: intimacy versus isolation 30–65 y: generativity versus self-absorption 65+ y: ego integrity versus despair	Cutoff years are 1, 3, 6, 12, 20, 30, 65 (≈doubling).

HIGH-YIELD FACTS

Behavioral Science

Developmental milestones	Approximate Age	Milestone
Infant	3 mo	Holds head up
	4–5 mo	Rolls front to back, sits when propped
	7 mo	Sits alone, orients to voice
	7–9 mo	Stranger anxiety
	15 mo	Walking, few words
Toddler	12–24 mo	Object permanence
	18–24 mo	Rapprochement
	24–30 mo	Parallel play
	24–36 mo	Core gender identity
Preschool	30–36 mo	Toilet training
	3 y	Group play
	4 y	Cooperative play
School age	6–11 y	Development of conscience (superego), same-sex friends, identification with same-sex parent
Adolescence (puberty)	11 y (girls) 13 y (boys)	Abstract reasoning (formal operations)

Kübler-Ross dying stages

Denial, **A**nger, **B**argaining, **G**rieving, **A**cceptance.

Death **A**rrives **B**ringing **G**rave **A**djustments.

Grief

Normal bereavement characterized by shock, denial, guilt and somatic symptoms. Typically lasts 6 mo–1 yr.

Pathologic grief includes excessively intense or prolonged grief, or grief that is delayed, inhibited or denied.

BEHAVIORAL SCIENCE—PHYSIOLOGY

Endorphins and enkephalins

Both have opiate-like activities, are blocked by naloxone, lose activity over time.

Enkephalins are pentapeptides (small).

β-endorphin (31 amino acids) is derived from POMC.

Endorphin = **End**ogenous **m**orphine. Also, Morpheus was the god of sleep.

Neurotransmitter changes with disease

Depression—decreased NE and serotonin (5-HT).

Alzheimer's dementia—decreased ACh.

Huntington's disease—decreased GABA, decreased ACh.

Bipolar affective disorder—decreased serotonin (5-HT).

Schizophrenia—increased dopamine.

Parkinson's disease—decreased dopamine.

Frontal lobe functions

Concentration, **O**rientation, **L**anguage, **A**bstraction, **J**udgment, **M**otor regulation, **M**ood.

Lack of social judgment is most notable in frontal lobe lesion.

COLA-JMM

Hypothalamic nuclei

Satiety	Ventromedial nucleus controls appetite.	Ablating **ventromedial** nucleus will cause you to grow **ventra**lly and **medial**ly (you get fat).
Hunger	Lateral nucleus	

Sleep stages

	Description	Waveform
0—eyes open	Awake, alert, active mental concentration	Beta (highest frequency, lowest amplitude)
0—eyes closed	Awake	Alpha
1 (5%)	Light sleep	Theta
2 (45%)	Deeper sleep	Sleep spindles and K-complexes
3–4 (25%)	Deepest, non-REM sleep; sleepwalking; night terrors, bedwetting (slow-wave sleep)	Delta (lowest frequency, highest amplitude)
REM (25%)	Dreaming, loss of motor tone, possibly memory processing function, erections, $\uparrow$ brain O_2 use	Beta

1. Serotonergic predominance of raphe nucleus key to initiating sleep
2. Norepinephrine reduces REM sleep
3. Extraocular movements during REM due to activity of PPRF (parapontine reticular formation/conjugate gaze center)
4. REM sleep having the same EEG pattern as while awake and alert has spawned the terms "paradoxical sleep" and "desynchronized sleep"
5. Benzodiazepines shorten stage 4 sleep; thus useful for night terrors and sleepwalking
6. Imipramine is used to treat enuresis since it decreases stage 4 sleep

REM sleep

Increased and variable pulse, rapid eye movements (REM), increased and variable blood pressure, penile/clitoral tumescence. 25% of total sleep. Occurs every 90 minutes; duration increases through the night. REM sleep decreases with age. Acetylcholine is the principal neurotransmitter involved in REM sleep.

REM rebound

Body compensates for missed REM sleep. Drugs that decrease the amount of REM sleep (e.g., barbiturates, alcohol, phenothiazines, and MAO inhibitors) cause an increased amount of REM sleep after the specific drug is discontinued.	Benzodiazepines decrease the amount of REM sleep without causing REM rebound.

Sleep apnea

Central sleep apnea: no respiratory effort.

Obstructive sleep apnea: respiratory effort against airway obstruction.

Person stops breathing for at least 10 sec during sleep.

Associated with obesity, loud snoring, systemic/pulmonary hypertension, arrhythmias, and possibly sudden death.

Individuals may become chronically tired.

HIGH-YIELD FACTS

Behavioral Science

Narcolepsy	Person falls asleep suddenly. May include hypnagogic (just before sleep) or hypnopompic (with awakening) hallucinations. The person's nocturnal and narcoleptic sleep episodes start off with REM sleep. Cataplexy (sudden collapse when awake) in some patients. Strong genetic component. Treat with stimulants (e.g., amphetamines).

Sleep patterns of depressed patients	Patients with depression typically have the following changes in their sleep stages: 1. Reduced slow-wave sleep 2. Decreased REM latency 3. Early morning waking (important screening question)

Sensory deprivation effects	1. Suppression of EEG 2. Decreased galvanic skin response 3. Decreased respiration 4. Increased urinary epinephrine	Seen in the ICU setting or after excessive studying.

Stress effects	Stress induces production of free fatty acids, 17-OH corticosteroids, lipids, cholesterol, catecholamines; affects water absorption, muscular tonicity, gastrocolic reflex, and mucosal circulation.

BEHAVIORAL SCIENCE—PSYCHIATRY

Forensic psychiatry	Confidentiality: breachable in child abuse, emergencies, communicable diseases. Good samaritan law protects roadside MD from malpractice liability. Involuntary hold: danger to self, others, unable to provide food/clothing/shelter.

Cultural/ethnic psychiatry	Specific diseases: Amok = killing rampage (seen in southeast Asia). Latah = echolalia, coprolalia (Malaysia). Koro = fear of penile regression, death (seen in Chinese men).	The origin of "running amok." Echolalia = repetition of another person's words or phrases. Coprolalia = "filthy" language.

Orientation as to person	Is the patient aware of him- or herself as a person? Does the patient know his or her own name? Anosognosia = unaware that one is ill. Autopagnosia = unable to locate one's own body parts. Depersonalization = body seems unreal or dissociated.	Generally, the last thing to go (first = time, second = place, last = person).

Orientation as to place	Deficiency in orientation as to place, including jamais vu (person is in a familiar surrounding but feels he or she has never been there before) and déjà vu (person is in an unfamiliar situation and feels he or she has been there before).

Amnesia types	*Antero*grade amnesia is being unable to remember things that occurred after a CNS insult (no new memory).	*Antero* = after
	Korsakoff's amnesia is a classic anterograde amnesia that is caused by thiamine deficiency (bilateral destruction of the mamillary bodies), is seen in alcoholics, and is associated with confabulations.	
	*Retro*grade amnesia is being unable to remember things that occurred before a CNS insult.	*Retro* = before

Substance dependence	Maladaptive pattern of substance use.
	Defined as 3 or more of the following signs in 1 year:
	1. Tolerance
	2. Withdrawal
	3. Substance taken in larger amounts than intended
	4. Persistent desire or attempts to cut down
	5. Lots of energy spent trying to obtain substance
	6. Important social, occupational, or recreational activities given up or reduced because of substance use
	7. Use continued in spite of knowing the problems that it causes

Substance abuse	Maladaptive pattern leading to clinically significant impairment or distress. Symptoms have not met criteria for substance dependence. One or more of the following in 1 year:
	1. Recurrent use resulting in failure to fulfill major obligations at work, school, or home
	2. Recurrent use in physically hazardous situations
	3. Recurrent substance-related legal problems
	4. Continued use in spite of persistent problems caused by use

Substance withdrawal syndromes		
Alcohol	Tremor, tachycardia, hypertension, nausea, malaise, seizure, delirium tremens.	
Opioids	Fever, rhinorrhea, nausea, sweating, "goose bumps," anxiety, insomnia (many features look like the flu).	
Cocaine	Hypersomnolence, depression, craving (peaks at 2–4 d).	
Amphetamines	Lethargy, headache, anxiety, GI cramps, depression.	

| **Delirium tremens** | Severe alcohol withdrawal syndrome that peaks 2–5 d after last drink. |
| | Confusion, delusions, hallucinations, autonomic system hyperactivity, tremors. |

Delirium	Decreased attention span and level of arousal, disorganized thinking, hallucination, illusions, misperceptions, disturbance in sleep–wake cycle, cognitive dysfunction.	De**lirium** = changes in senso**rium**
	Key to diagnosis: waxing and waning level of consciousness, develops rapidly.	Most common psychiatric illness on medical and surgical floors. Often reversible.
	Often due to substance use/abuse or medical illness.	

Dementia

Development of multiple cognitive deficits: memory, aphasia, apraxia, agnosia, loss of abstract thought, behavioral/personality changes, impaired judgment. Key to diagnosis: rule out delirium—patient is alert, no change in level of consciousness. More often gradual onset.

De**mem**tia characterized by **mem**ory loss. Commonly irreversible.

Major depressive episode

Characterized by 5 of the following for 2 weeks, including (1) depressed mood or (2) anhedonia:

1. **S**leep disturbances
2. Loss of **I**nterest
3. **G**uilt
4. Loss of **E**nergy
5. Loss of **C**oncentration
6. Change in **A**ppetite
7. **P**sychomotor retardation
8. **S**uicidal ideations
9. Depressed mood

SIG: Energy **CAPS**ules

Major depressive disorder, recurrent—requires 2 or more episodes with a symptom-free interval of 2 months.

Manic episode

Distinct period of abnormally and persistently elevated, expansive or irritable mood lasting at least 1 week. During mood disturbance, 3 or more of the following:

1. **D**istractibility
2. **I**nsomnia: ↓ need for sleep
3. **G**randiosity: inflated self-esteem
4. **F**light of ideas
5. Increase in goal-directed **A**ctivity/psychomotor agitation
6. Pressured **S**peech
7. **T**houghtlessness: seeks pleasure without regard to consequences

DIG FAST

Hypomanic episode

Like manic episode except mood disturbance not severe enough to cause marked impairment in social and/or occupational functioning or to necessitate hospitalization, and there are no psychotic features.

Bipolar disorder

Six separate criteria sets exist for bipolar I disorders with combinations of manic, hypomanic, and depressed episodes. Lithium is drug of choice. Different studies have linked bipolar disorder to chromosomes X, 11, 18, and 23.

Cyclothymic disorder

A period of at least 2 years with hypomanic symptoms and depressive symptoms that do not meet criteria for major depressive episode.

Malingering

Patient fakes or claims to have a disorder in order to attain a specific gain (e.g., financial).

Factitious disorder	Consciously creates symptoms in order to assume "sick role" and to get medical ~~a~~ Also known as Münchausen syndrome.
Somatoform disorders	Several types: 1. Conversion—symptoms suggest neurologic or physical disorder but tests and physical exam are negative 2. Somatoform pain disorder—conversion disorder with pain as presenting complaint 3. Hypochondriasis—misinterpretation of normal physical findings, leading to preoccupation with and fear of having a serious illness in spite of medical reassurance 4. Somatization—variety of complaints in multiple organ systems 5. Body dysmorphic disorder—patient convinced that part of own anatomy is malformed 6. Pseudocyesis—false belief of being pregnant associated with objective signs of pregnancy
Gain: 1°, 2°, 3°	1° gain = what the symptom does for the patient's internal psychic economy. 2° gain = what the symptom gets the patient (sympathy, attention). 3° gain = what the caretaker gets (like an MD on an interesting case).
Panic disorder	Discrete periods of intense fear or discomfort peaking in 10 minutes with 4 of the following: 1. Palpitations, racing heart 2. Sweating 3. Trembling 4. Shortness of breath 5. Choking feeling 6. Chest pain/discomfort 7. Nausea/abdominal distress 8. Dizziness, faintness, lightheadedness 9. Derealization 10. Fear of losing control 11. Fear of dying 12. Paresthesias 13. Chills or hot flashes Panic disorder must be diagnosed in context of occurrence (e.g., panic disorder with agoraphobia). High prevalence during Step 1 exam.
Specific phobia	Fear that is excessive or unreasonable, cued by presence or anticipation of a specific object or entity. Exposure provokes anxiety response. Person (not necessarily children) recognizes fear is excessive. Fear interferes with normal routine. Treatment options include systematic desensitization.
Social phobia	Fear of one or more social performance situations. Person fears acting in a way that is embarrassing or humiliating.
Obsession	Recurrent, intrusive and persistent thoughts, impulses, or images that cannot be ignored or suppressed by logical effort. Associated with anxiety.

Repetitive behaviors or mental acts that person feels driven to perform. Committing act produces transient relief from anxiety.

Obsessions and compulsions. Patient may have poor insight. Treatment options include clomipramine, fluvoxamine, paroxetine, behavioral therapy, and insight-based psychotherapy.

stress ~~disorder~~

Person experienced or witnessed event that involved actual or threatened death or serious injury. Response involves intense fear, helplessness, or horror. Traumatic event is persistently reexperienced, and person persistently avoids stimuli associated with the trauma. Person experiences persistent symptoms of increased arousal. Disturbance lasts longer than 1 month and causes distress or social/occupational impairment.

Personality disorders	Personality trait is an enduring pattern of perceiving, relating to, and thinking about the environment and oneself that is exhibited in a wide range of important social and personal contexts. Personality disorder—when these patterns become inflexible and maladaptive, causing impairment in social or occupational functioning or subjective distress.
Cluster A personality disorder	Paranoid, schizoid, schizotypal Characteristics: paranoid, suspicious, social isolation, odd beliefs, shy, withdrawn, impoverished personal relationships. Clinical dilemma: patient is suspicious of and does not trust doctor.
Cluster B personality disorder	Borderline, histrionic, narcissistic, antisocial Characteristics: dramatic, self-indulgent, hostile, aggressive, exploitative relationships, attention seeking. Clinical dilemma: patient changes rules on doctor. Clingy and demands attention. Feels that he/she is VIP and special. Manipulates doctor. Narcissist demands "best specialist in the country."
Cluster C personality disorder	Obsessive-compulsive, avoidant, dependent, passive–aggressive Characteristics: fear of doing wrong thing, anxiety repressed, regulations, unable to express affect. Clinical dilemma: patient may subtly sabotage his/her own treatment. Person is very controlling.
Hallucination versus illusion versus delusion	Hallucinations are perceptions in the absence of external stimuli. Illusions are misinterpretations of actual external stimuli. Delusions are false beliefs not shared with other members of culture/subculture that are firmly maintained in spite of obvious proof to the contrary.
Delusion vs. loose association	A delusion is a disorder in the content of thought (the actual idea). A loose association is a disorder in the form of thought (the way ideas are tied together).

Hallucination types	Visual hallucination is common in acute organic brain syndrome.

Auditory hallucination is common in schizophrenia.

Olfactory hallucination often occurs as an aura of a psychomotor epilepsy.

Gustatory hallucination is rare.

Tactile hallucination (e.g., formications) is common in delirium tremens. Also seen in cocaine abusers ("cocaine bugs").

Hypnagogic hallucination occurs while going to sleep.

Hypnopompic hallucination occurs while waking from sleep.

Schizophrenia

Waxing and waning vulnerability to psychosis.

Positive symptoms: hallucinations, delusions, strange behavior, loose associations.

Negative symptoms: flat affect, social withdrawal, thought blocking, lack of motivation.

The **4 As** described by Bleuler:
1. **A**mbivalence (uncertainty)
2. **A**utism (self-preoccupation and lack of communication)
3. **A**ffect (blunted)
4. **A**ssociations (loose)

Fifth A should be **A**uditory hallucinations.

Genetic factors outweigh environmental factors in the etiology of schizophrenia.

Lifetime prevalence = 1.5% (males = females, blacks = whites).

Five subtypes:
1. Disorganized
2. Catatonic
3. Paranoid
4. Undifferentiated
5. Residual

Schizoaffective disorder: a combination of schizophrenia and a mood disorder.

Antipsychotic mechanism

Antipsychotics most commonly work by blocking dopamine (D_2 and probably D_4) receptors. Examples: haloperidol, chlorpromazine, thiothixene.

Phobias

More than 100, so use etymology to figure them out.
Examples include:
Gamophobia (*gam* = gamete) = fear of marriage.
Algophobia (*alg* = pain) = fear of pain.
Acrophobia (*acro* = height) = fear of heights.
Agoraphobia (*agora* = assembly) = fear of open places.

Systematic desensitization is a treatment used for phobias.

Electroconvulsive therapy

Treatment option for refractory depression.
ECT is painless and produces a seizure with transient memory loss and disorientation. Complications can result from anesthesia. The major adverse effect of ECT is retrograde amnesia.

Very controversial.

HIGH-YIELD FACTS

Behavioral Science

97

Structural theory of the mind	Freud's three structures of the mind:
Id	Primal urges, sex, and aggression. (I want it.)
Superego	Moral values, conscience. (You know you can't have it.)
Ego	Bridge and mediator between the unconscious mind and the external world. (Deals with the conflict.)

Ego defenses	All ego defenses are automatic and unconscious reactions to psychological stress.	
	Description	**Example**
Acting out	Unacceptable feelings and thoughts are expressed through actions.	Tantrums.
Denial	Avoidance of awareness of some painful reality.	A common reaction in newly diagnosed AIDS and cancer patients.
Displacement	Process whereby avoided ideas and feelings are transferred to some neutral person or object.	Seen in dreams (e.g., murderous wishes toward mother are redirected at crossing guard in dream).
Fixation	Partially remaining at a more childish level of development.	
Identification	Modeling behavior after another person.	Spouse develops symptoms that deceased patient had.
Isolation	Separation of feelings from ideas and events.	Describing murder in graphic detail with no emotional response.
Projection	An unacceptable internal impulse is attributed to an external source.	Common in paranoid states.
Rationalization	Proclaiming logical reasons for actions actually performed for other reasons, usually to avoid self-blame.	
Reaction formation	Process whereby a warded-off idea or feeling is replaced by an (unconsciously derived) emphasis on its opposite.	A patient with libidinous thoughts enters a monastery.
Regression	Turning back the maturational clock and going back to earlier modes of dealing with the world.	Seen in children under stress (e.g., bedwetting) and in patients on peritoneal dialysis.
Repression	Involuntary withholding of an idea or feeling from conscious awareness.	
Sublimation	Process whereby one replaces an unacceptable wish with a course of action that is similar to the wish but does not conflict with one's value system.	Aggressive impulses used to succeed in business ventures.
Suppression	Voluntary (unlike other defenses) withholding of an idea or feeling from conscious awareness.	
Dissociation	Temporary, drastic change in personality, memory, conciousness or motor behavior to avoid emotional stress.	Extreme forms can result in multiple personalities (dissociative identity disorder).

Oedipus complex	Repressed sexual feelings of a child for the opposite-sex parent, accompanied by rivalry with same-sex parent. First described by Freud.	
Sick role	Exempts sick person from duties, allows person to expect care and sympathy, and obligates sick person to try to get well (i.e., working toward being healthy, cooperation with health care personnel in getting well, and compliance with the treatment regimen).	
Dyad	A pair of people within an interactional situation (e.g., husband–wife, mother–child, therapist–patient).	
Factors in hopelessness	Four dynamic factors in the development of hopelessness: **IGAD!** 1. Sense of **I**mpotence (powerlessness) 2. Sense of **G**uilt 3. Sense of **A**nger 4. Sense of loss/**D**eprivation leading to depression	
Conditioners: fear	Moderate fear is better than severe or mild fear in changing behavior.	As in studying for big exams.
Classical conditioning	Learning in which a response (salivation) is elicited by a conditioned stimulus (bell) that previously was presented in conjunction with an unconditioned stimulus (food).	Programmed by habit, without any element of reward. As in Pavlov's **classical** experiments with dogs (ringing the bell provoked salivation).
Operant conditioning	Learning in which a particular action is elicited because it produces a reward.	Voluntary action and a reward.

Reinforcement schedules

Continuous	Shows the most rapid extinction when discontinued.	This explains why people can get addicted to slot machines at casinos and yet get upset when vending machines don't work.
Variable ratio	Shows the slowest extinction when discontinued.	

Gestalt therapy	Stresses treatment of the whole person, highlights sensory awareness of the here and now, uses role playing. Developed by Friedrich Perls.	
Psychoanalysis	A form of insight therapy—intensive, lengthy, costly, great demands on patient, developed by Freud. May be appropriate for changing chronic character problems.	
Topography (in psychoanalysis)	Conscious = what you are aware of. Preconscious = what you are able to make conscious with effort (like your phone number). Unconscious = what you are not aware of; the central goal of Freudian psychotherapy is to make the patient aware of what is hidden in his/her unconscious.	

Existential psychotherapy	Emphasis on confrontation and feeling experiences; each individual is responsible for his or her own existence.
Intelligence testing	Stanford–Binet and Wechsler are the most famous tests. Mean is defined at 100, with standard deviation of 15. IQ lower than 70 (or 2 standard deviations below the mean) is one of the criteria for diagnosis of mental retardation. IQ scores are correlated with genetic factors but are more highly correlated with school achievement. Intelligence tests are objective (not projective) tests.
Projective tests	Projective tests use ambiguous stimuli. Examples: Rorschach (ink blot), TAT, sentence completion, word association, draw-a-person. *The patient projects his or her personality into the test.*

Sexual dysfunction	Differential diagnosis includes:
	  1. Drugs (e.g., antihypertensives, neuroleptics, ethanol)
	  2. Diseases (e.g., depression, diabetes)
	  3. Psychological (e.g., performance anxiety)

Changes in the elderly	1. Sexual changes
	   Men: slower erection/ejaculation, longer refractory period
	   Women: vaginal shortening, thinning, and dryness; sexual interest does not decrease
	2. Sleep patterns: ↓ REM sleep, ↓ slow-wave sleep, ↑ sleep latency
	3. Common medical conditions: arthritis, hypertension, heart disease
	4. Suicide rate increases
	5. Psychiatric problems (e.g., depression) become more prevalent

Epidemiology/Biostatistics

1. Differences in the incidence of disease among various ethnic groups.
2. Leading causes and types of cancers in men versus women.
3. Prevalence of common psychiatric disorders (e.g., alcoholism, major depression, schizophrenia).
4. Differences in death rates among ethnic and racial groups.
5. Definitions of morbidity, mortality, and case fatality rate.
6. Epidemiology of cigarette smoking, including prevalence and success rates for quitting.
7. Modes of human immunodeficiency virus (HIV) transmission among different populations (e.g., perinatal, heterosexual, homosexual, intravenous).
8. Simple pedigree analysis for inheritance of genetic diseases (e.g., counseling, risk assessment).
9. Different types of studies (e.g., randomized clinical trial, cohort, case series).
10. Definition and use of standard deviation, p value, r value, mean, mode, and median.
11. Effects of changing a test's criteria on number of false positives and number of false negatives.

Neurophysiology

1. Physiologic changes (e.g., neurotransmitter levels) in common neuropsychiatric disorders (e.g., Alzheimer's disease, Huntington's disease, schizophrenia, bipolar disorder).
2. Changes in cerebrospinal fluid composition with common psychiatric diseases (e.g., depression).
3. Physiologic, physical, and psychologic changes associated with aging (e.g., memory, lung capacity, glomerular filtration rate, muscle mass, pharmacokinetics of drugs).
4. Differences between anterior and posterior lobes of the pituitary gland (e.g., embryology, innervation, hormones).

Psychiatry/Psychology

1. Diagnosis of common psychiatric disorders.
2. Indicators of prognosis in psychiatric disorders (e.g., schizophrenia, bipolar disorder).
3. Genetic components of common psychiatric disorders (e.g., schizophrenia, bipolar disorder).
4. Diseases associated with different personality types.
5. Clinical features and treatment of phobias.
6. Clinical features of child abuse.
7. Clinical features of common learning disorders (e.g., dyslexia, mental retardation).
8. Therapeutic application of learning theories (e.g., classical and operant conditioning) to psychiatric illnesses (e.g., disulfiram therapy for alcoholics).
9. Problems associated with the physician–patient relationship (e.g., reasons for patient noncompliance).
10. Management of the suicidal patient.
11. Addiction: risk factors, family history, behavior, factors contributing to relapse.
12. How physicians and medical students should help peers with substance abuse problems.

HIGH-YIELD FACTS

Behavioral Science

Biochemistry

This high-yield material includes molecular biology, genetics, cell biology, and principles of metabolism (especially vitamins, cofactors, minerals and single-enzyme diseases). The topics are especially high-yield and are worth learning in detail. When studying metabolic pathways, emphasize important regulatory steps and enzyme deficiencies that result in disease. Do not spend time on hard-core organic chemistry, mechanisms, and physical chemistry. Detailed chemical structures are infrequently tested. Familiarity with the latest biochemical techniques that have medical relevance—such as enzyme-linked immunosorbent assay, immunoelectrophoresis, Southern blotting, and PCR—is useful. Beware if you placed out of your medical school's biochemistry class, for the emphasis of the test differs from the emphasis of many undergraduate courses.

DNA and RNA
Genetic Errors
Metabolism
Protein/Cell
Vitamins
High-Yield Topics

Chromatin structure — Condensed by (–) charged DNA looped twice around (+) charged H2A, H2B, H3, and H4 histones (nucleosome bead). H1 ties nucleosomes together in a string (30-nm fiber). In mitosis, DNA condenses to form mitotic chromosomes.

Think of beads on a string.

Heterochromatin — Condensed, transcriptionally inactive.
Euchromatin — Less condensed, transcriptionally active.

Eu = true, "truly transcribed."

Nucleotides — Purines (A, G) have two rings. Pyrimidines (**C, T, U**) have one ring. Guanine has a ketone. Thymine has a methyl. Uracil found in RNA; thymine in DNA.
G-C bond (3 H-bonds) stronger than A-T bond (2 H-bonds).

CUT the **PY** (pie): pyrimidines.
PURe **A**s **G**old: purines.
THYmine has a me**THY**l.
Crypts (**C**ytosine) and **T**ombs (**T**hymine) are found **U**nder (**U**racil) the **P**yramids (**P**yrimidines).

AUG codon — AUG (or rarely GUG) is the mRNA initiation codon. AUG codes for methionine, which may be removed before translation is completed. In prokaryotes the initial AUG codes for a formyl-**met**hionine (**f-met**).

AUG in**AUG**urates protein synthesis.

Genetic code: features — Unambiguous = each codon specifies only one amino acid.
Degenerate = more than one codon may code for same amino acid.
Commaless, nonoverlapping (except some viruses).
Universal (exceptions include mitochondria, archaebacteria, *Mycoplasma,* and some yeasts).

Mutations in DNA — Silent = same aa, often base change in third position of codon.
Missense = changed aa. (Conservative = new aa is similar in chemical structure.)
Nonsense = change resulting in early stop codon.
Frameshift = change resulting in misreading of all nucleotides downstream usually resulting in a truncated protein.

Severity of damage: nonsense > missense > silent.

Transition versus transversion — Transition = substituting purine for purine or pyrimidine for pyrimidine.
Transversion = substituting purine for pyrimidine or vice versa.

Transversion = **Trans**conversion (one type to another).

DNA replication

Origin of replication: continuous DNA synthesis on leading strand and discontinuous (Okazaki fragments) on lagging strand. DNA polymerase reaches primer of preceding fragment; $5' \rightarrow 3'$ exonuclease activity of DNA polymerase degrades RNA; DNA ligase seals; $3' \rightarrow 5'$ exonuclease activity of DNA polymerase "proofreads" each added nucleotide.

Eukaryotic genome has multiple origins of replication. Bacteria, viruses, and plasmids have only one origin of replication.

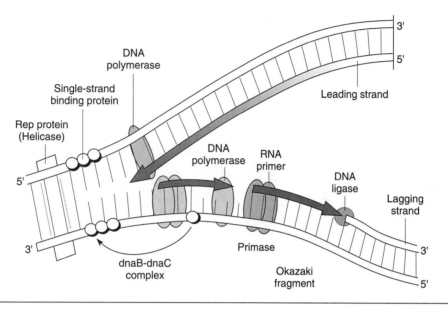

Polymerases: DNA

Functions in *E coli*:
DNA polymerase I removes RNA primers, fills gaps, and participates in repair.
DNA polymerase II function is unknown.
DNA polymerase III (holoenzyme) elongates most efficiently, makes bulk of DNA (high fidelity).

Enzymes that proofread cannot initiate (because initiation is a sloppy process). **Primase** makes an RNA primer on which DNA polymerase can initiate replication.

Polymerase chain reaction (PCR)

Molecular biology laboratory procedure that is used to synthesize many copies of a desired fragment of DNA.

Steps:

1. DNA is denatured by heating to generate 2 separate strands
2. During cooling, excess of premade primers anneal to a specific sequence on each strand to be amplified
3. Heat-stable DNA polymerase replicates the DNA sequence following each primer

These steps are repeated multiple times for DNA sequence amplification.

GENETIC DISEASES DETECTABLE BY PCR	
Disease	**Gene**
SCID	Adenosine deaminase
Lesch–Nyhan syndrome	HGPRT
Cystic fibrosis	CFTR
Familial hypercholesterolemia	LDL-R
Retinoblastoma	Rb
Sickle cell anemia and β-thalassemia	β-globin gene
Hemophilia A and B	Factor VIII (A) and IX (B)
Von Willebrand's disease	VWF
Lysosomal storage diseases	See "sphingolipidoses" on p. 112
Glycogen storage diseases	See p. 110

Molecular biology techniques

Southern blot — A DNA sample is electrophoresed on a gel and then transferred to a filter. The filter is then soaked in a denaturant and subsequently exposed to a labeled DNA probe that recognizes and anneals to its complementary strand. The resulting double-stranded labeled piece of DNA is visualized when the filter is exposed to film. — DNA–DNA hybridization

Northern blot — Similar technique, except that Northern blotting involves radioactive DNA probe binding to sample RNA. — DNA–RNA hybridization

Western blot — Sample protein is separated via gel electrophoresis and transferred to a filter. Labeled antibody is used to bind to relevant protein. — Antibody–protein hybridization

Southwestern blot — Protein sample is run on a gel, transferred to a filter, and exposed to labeled DNA. Used to detect DNA–protein interactions as with transcription factors (e.g., p53, *jun*). — DNA–protein interaction

DNA repair: single strand	Single-strand, excision-repair–specific glycosylase recognizes and removes damaged base. Endonuclease makes a break several bases to the 5′ side. Exonuclease removes short stretch of nucleotides. DNA polymerase fills gap. DNA ligase seals.	If both strands are damaged, repair may proceed via recombination with undamaged homologous chromosome.
DNA/RNA synthesis direction	DNA and RNA are both synthesized $5′ \rightarrow 3′$. Remember that the 5′ of the incoming nucleotide bears the triphosphate (energy source for bond). The 3′ hydroxyl of the nascent chain is the target.	Imagine the incoming nucleotide bringing a gift (triphosphate) to the 3′ host. **BYOP** (phosphate) from **5 to 3.**
Polymerases: RNA	**Eukaryotes:** RNA polymerase I makes **r**RNA. RNA polymerase II makes **m**RNA. RNA polymerase III makes **t**RNA. No proofreading function, but can initiate chains. RNA polymerase II opens DNA at promoter site (A-T-rich upstream sequence—TATA and CAAT). α-amanitin inhibits RNA polymerase II. **Prokaryotes:** RNA polymerase makes all three kinds of RNA.	I, II, and III are numbered as their products are used in protein synthesis. Or I, II, III ≈ **rem**o**t**e.
Regulation of gene expression		
Promoter	Site where RNA polymerase and multiple other transcription factors bind to DNA.	Promoter mutation commonly results in dramatic decrease in amount of gene transcribed.
Enhancer	Stretch of DNA that alters gene expression by binding transcription factors. May be located close to, far from, or even within (in an intron) the gene whose expression it regulates.	
Introns versus exons	Exons contain the actual genetic information coding for protein. Introns are intervening noncoding segments of DNA.	**INT**rons **INT**errupt (or **INT**ervene). **IN**trons stay **IN** the nucleus whereas **EX**ons **EX**it and are **EX**pressed.
Types of RNA	mRNA is the largest type of RNA. rRNA is the most abundant type of RNA. tRNA is the smallest type of RNA.	**Mr²**
Splicing of mRNA	Introns are precisely spliced out of primary mRNA transcripts. A lariat-shaped intermediate is formed. Small nuclear ribonucleoprotein particles (snRNP) facilitate splicing by binding to primary mRNA transcripts and forming spliceosomes.	*Lariat* = lasso.

HIGH-YIELD FACTS

Biochemistry

RNA processing (eukaryotes)

Occurs in nucleus. After transcription:
1. **Capping** on 5′ end (7-methyl-G)
2. **Polyadenylation** on 3′ end (≈200 A's)
3. **Splicing** out of introns occurs

Initial transcript is called heterogeneous nuclear RNA (hnRNA).

Capped and tailed transcript is called mRNA.

Only processed RNA is transported out of the nucleus. The cap goes on a head (the beginning of the strand) and the polyA tail goes at the end of the strand.

tRNA structure

75–90 nucleotides, cloverleaf form, anticodon end is opposite 3′ aminoacyl end. All tRNAs, both eukaryotic and prokaryotic, have CCA at 3′ end along with a high percentage of chemically modified bases. The amino acid is covalently bound to the 3′ end of the tRNA.

tRNA charging

Aminoacyl-tRNA synthetase (one per aa, uses ATP) scrutinizes aa before and after it binds to tRNA. If incorrect, bond is hydrolyzed by synthetase. The aa-tRNA bond has energy for formation of peptide bond. A mischarged tRNA reads usual codon but inserts wrong amino acid.

Aminoacyl-tRNA synthetase and binding of charged tRNA to the codon are responsible for accuracy of amino acid selection.

tRNA wobble

Third nucleotide of mRNA codon "wobble" pairs, allowing formation of non–Watson-Crick base pairs. A tRNA normally reads one to three specific codons— but each codon it reads designates the same one amino acid. Economizes number of tRNAs needed.

"G-U" is **wobble (gee, you wobble)**, rest is standard A-U and G-C. Inosine has three-way wobble: I-U, I-C, or I-A.

Modes of inheritance

Autosomal dominant

50% of offspring inherit disease. Often due to defects in structural genes. Many generations, both male and female, affected.

Often pleiotropic and, in many cases, present clinically after puberty. Family history crucial to diagnosis.

Autosomal recessive

25% of offspring from 2 carrier parents are affected. Often due to enzyme deficiencies. Usually seen in only one generation.

Commonly more severe than dominant disorders; patients often present in childhood.

X-linked recessive

Sons of heterozygous mothers have a 50% chance of being affected. No male-to male transmission.

Commonly more severe in males. Heterozygous females may be affected.

Mitochondrial inheritance

Transmitted only through mother. All offspring of affected females may show signs of disease.

Leber's hereditary optic neuropathy, mitochondrial myopathies.

Genetic terms

Variable expression	Nature and severity of the phenotype varies from one individual to another.
Incomplete penetrance	Not all individuals with a mutant genotype show the mutant phenotype.
Pleiotropy	One gene has more than one effect on an individual's phenotype.
Imprinting	Differences in phenotype depend on whether the mutation is of maternal or paternal origin (e.g., Angelman syndrome [paternal], Prader-Willi syndrome [maternal]).
Anticipation	Severity of disease worsens or age of onset of disease is earlier in succeeding generations (e.g., Huntington's disease).
Loss of heterozygosity	If a patient inherits or develops a mutation in a tumor suppressor gene, the complementary allele must be deleted/mutated before cancer develops. This is not true of oncogenes.

DNA repair defects

Xeroderma pigmentosum (skin sensitivity to UV light), ataxia-telangiectasia (x-rays), Bloom syndrome (radiation) and Fanconi's anemia (cross-linking agents).

Xeroderma pigmentosum

Defective excision repair such as uvr ABC exonuclease. Results in inability to repair thymidine dimers, which form in DNA when exposed to UV light.
Associated with dry skin and with melanoma and other cancers.

Fructose intolerance

Hereditary deficiency of aldolase B. Fructose-1-phosphate accumulates, causing a decrease in available phosphate, which results in inhibition of glycogenolysis and gluconeogenesis, thus causing severe hypoglycemia.

Must decrease intake of both fructose and sucrose (glucose + fructose).

Galactosemia

Absence of galactose-1-phosphate uridyltransferase. Autosomal recessive. Damage is caused by accumulation of toxic substances (including galactitol) rather than absence of an essential compound.
Symptoms: cataracts, hepatosplenomegaly, mental retardation.
Treatment: exclude galactose and lactose (glactose + glucose) from diet.

Lactase deficiency

Age-dependent and/or hereditary lactose intolerance (blacks, Asians).
Symptoms: bloating, cramps, osmotic diarrhea.
Treatment: avoid milk or add lactase pills to diet.

Pyruvate dehydrogenase deficiency

Causes backup of substrate (pyruvate and alanine), resulting in lactic acidosis.
Findings: neurologic defects.
Treatment: increased intake of ketogenic nutrients.

Lysine and leucine—the only purely ketogenic amino acids.

Glucose-6-phosphate dehydrogenase deficiency

G6PD is rate-limiting enzyme in HMP shunt (which yields NADPH). ↓ NADPH in RBCs leads to **hemolytic anemia** due to poor RBC defense against oxidizing agents (fava beans, aspirin, sulfonamides, antimalarial drugs) and anti-tuberculosis drugs. X-linked recessive disorder.

G6PD deficiency more prevalent among blacks. NADPH is necessary to keep glutathione reduced, which in turn keeps the heme iron reduced so that O_2 can bind.

HIGH-YIELD FACTS

Biochemistry

Glycolytic enzyme deficiency	Hexokinase, glucose-phosphate isomerase, aldolase, triose-phosphate isomerase, phosphate-glycerate kinase, and enolase deficiencies are associated with hemolytic anemia.	RBCs depend on glycolysis (energy and reducing equivalents).
Glycogen storage diseases	12 types, all resulting in abnormal glycogen metabolism and an accumulation of glycogen within cells.	
Type I	**Von Gierke's disease** = glucose-6-phosphatase deficiency. Findings: severe fasting hypoglycemia, ↑↑ glycogen in liver.	Von Gierke's: liver.
Type II	**Pompe's disease** = lysosomal α-1,4-glucosidase deficiency. Findings: cardiomegaly and systemic findings, leading to early death.	Pompe's: liver, heart, and muscle.
Type V	**McArdle's disease** = muscle glycogen phosphorylase deficiency. Findings: ↑ glycogen in muscle but cannot break it down, leading to painful cramps, myoglobinuria with strenuous exercise.	McArdle's: muscle.
Hartnup's disease	Defect in GI uptake of neutral amino acids. Symptoms mimic pellagra (diarrhea, dementia, dermatitis) because of malabsorption of tryptophan (precursor of niacin). Carcinoid syndrome may also cause pellagra.	**Hard-N-Up** = **Hard N**eutral **U**ptake
Homocystinuria	Defect in cystathionine synthase. Two forms: 1. Deficiency (treatment: ↓ Met and ↑ Cys in diet) 2. Decreased affinity of synthase for pyridoxal phosphate (treatment: ↑↑ vitamin B$_6$ in diet)	Results in excess homocystine in the urine. Cysteine becomes essential.
Maple syrup urine	Blocked degradation of **branched** amino acids (**I**le, **V**al, **L**eu). Causes severe CNS defects, mental retardation, and death.	Urine smells like maple syrup. Think of cutting (blocking) **branches** of a maple tree. **I** lo**V**e **L**ucy
Phenylketonuria	Normally, phenylalanine is converted into tyrosine (nonessential aa). In PKU, there is ↓ phenylalanine hydroxylase or ↓ tetrahydrobiopterin cofactor. Tyrosine becomes essential and phenylalanine builds up, leading to excess phenylketones. Findings: mental retardation, fair skin, eczema, musty body odor. Treatment: ↓ phenylalanine and ↑ tyrosine in diet (no Nutrasweet).	Screened for at birth. Phenylketones = phenylacetate, phenyllactate, and phenylpyruvate in urine.

Alkaptonuria	Congenital deficiency of homogentisic acid oxidase in the degradative pathway of tyrosine. Resulting alkapton bodies cause **dark urine.** Also, the connective tissue is dark. Benign disease.	*Alkapton* = alkali-hapten bodies (homogentisic acid) bind to alkali. These are in the urine.
Albinism	Congenital deficiency of tyrosinase. Results in an inability to synthesize melanin from tyrosine. Can result from a lack of migration of neural crest cells.	Lack of melanin results in an increased risk of skin cancer.
Adenosine deaminase deficiency	ADA deficiency can cause **SCID.** Excess ATP and dATP imbalances nucleotide pool via feedback inhibition of ribonucleotide reductase. This prevents DNA synthesis and thus lowers lymphocyte count. First disease to be treated by experimental human gene therapy.	**SCID** = **S**evere **C**ombined (T and B) **I**mmunodeficiency **D**isease. SCID happens to kids.
Lesch-Nyhan syndrome	Purine salvage problem owing to absence of HGPRTase, which converts hypoxanthine to inosine monophosphate (IMP) and guanine to guanosine monophosphate (GMP). X-linked recessive. Findings: retardation, self-mutilation, aggression, hyperuricemia, choreoathetosis.	**LNS** = **L**acks **N**ucleotide **S**alvage (purine).
Ehlers-Danlos syndrome	10 types, all resulting in faulty collagen synthesis. Skin is stretchy (hyperextensible) with poor wound healing, joints are hypermobile. Inheritance varies from autosomal dominant (type IV) to autosomal recessive (type VI) to X-linked recessive (type IX). Type I findings: Diaphragmatic hernia. Type IV findings: Ecchymoses, arterial rupture. Type VI findings: Retinal detachment, corneal rupture.	Sounds like "feller's damn loose" (loose joints).

Sphingolipidoses	Each is caused by a deficiency in one of the many lysosomal enzymes.	
Fabry's disease	Caused by deficiency of α-galactosidase A, resulting in accumulation of ceramide trihexoside. Finding: renal failure.	X-linked recessive.
Gaucher's disease	Caused by deficiency of β-glucocerebrosidase, leading to glucocerebroside accumulation in brain, liver, spleen, and bone marrow (Gaucher's cells with characteristic "crinkled paper" enlarged cytoplasm). Type I, the more common form, is compatible with a normal life span.	Autosomal recessive.
Niemann-Pick disease	Deficiency of sphingomyelinase causes buildup of sphingomyelin and cholesterol in reticuloendothelial and parenchymal cells and tissues. Patients die by age 3.	Autosomal recessive. No man picks (Nieman-Pick) his nose with his sphinger.
Tay-Sachs disease	Absence of hexosaminidase A results in GM_2-ganglioside accumulation. Death occurs by age 3. Cherry-red spot visible on macula. Carrier rate is 1 in 30 in Jews of European descent (1 in 300 for others).	Autosomal recessive. **Tay-saX** sounds like he**X**osaminidase.

BIOCHEMISTRY—METABOLISM

ATP	Base (adenine), ribose, 3 phosphoryls. 2 phosphoanhydride bonds, 7 kcal/mol each. Aerobic metabolism produces 38 ATP via malate shuttle, 36 ATP via G3P shuttle. Anaerobic glycolysis produces only 2 ATP per glucose molecule. ATP hydrolysis can be coupled to energetically unfavorable reactions.
Activated carriers	Phosphoryl (ATP) Electrons (NADH, NADPH, $FADH_2$) Acyl (coenzyme A, lipoamide) CO_2 (biotin) One-carbon units (tetrahydrofolates) CH_3 groups (SAM) Aldehydes (TPP) Glucose (UDP-glucose) Choline (CDP-choline)

Extracellular messengers	Examples	Mechanism
	Nicotinic receptor, norepinephrine receptor on K^+ channel in the heart	Open or close ion channels in cell membrane
	Thyroid hormones, retinoic acid, steroid hormones, vitamin D_3	Act via cytoplasmic or nuclear receptors to increase transcription of target genes
	Angiotensin II, α_1-receptor, ADH	Activate phospholipase C with intracellular production of DAG, IP_3, protein kinase C and Ca^{++}
	β_1-receptor, β_2-receptor ($\uparrow$ cAMP), α_2-receptor ($\downarrow$ cAMP)	Activate or inhibit adenylate cyclase
	ANP, nitric oxide (EDRF)	Increase cyclic GMP in the cell
	Insulin, EGF, PDGF, M-CSF	Increased tyrosine kinase activity
	TGF-β	Increased serine kinase activity

NAD$^+$/NADPH		
	NAD$^+$ is generally used in **catabolic** processes to carry reducing equivalents away as NADH. **NADPH** is used in **anabolic** processes as a supply of reducing equivalents.	NADPH is a product of the HMP shunt and the malate dehydrogenase reaction.

S-adenosyl-methionine		
	ATP + methionine $\rightarrow$ SAM. SAM transfers methyl units to a wide variety of acceptors (e.g., in synthesis of phosphocreatine, high-energy phosphate active in muscle ATP production). Regeneration of methionine (and thus SAM) is dependent on vitamin B_{12}.	SAM the methyl donor man.

Metabolism sites		
Mitochondria	Fatty acid **O**xidation, **A**cetyl-CoA production, **K**rebs cycle.	Mity **OAK**
Cytoplasm	Glycolysis, fatty acid synthesis, HMP shunt, protein synthesis (RER), steroid synthesis (SER).	
Both	Gluconeogenesis, urea cycle.	

Hexokinase versus glucokinase		
	Hexokinase is found throughout body. **Glucokinase** (lower affinity [$\uparrow K_m$] but higher capacity [$\uparrow V_{max}$]) is found only in the liver.	Only hexokinase is feedback inhibited by G6P.

HIGH-YIELD FACTS

Biochemistry

REGULATION OF METABOLIC PATHWAYS

Pathway	Major Regulatory Enzyme(s)	Activator	Inhibitor	Effector Hormone	Remarks
Citric acid cycle	Citrate synthase		ATP, long-chain acyl-CoA		Regulated mainly by the need for ATP and therefore by the supply of NAD^+
Glycolysis and pyruvate oxidation	Phosphofructokinase	AMP, fructose 2,6-bisphosphate in liver, fructose 1,6-bisphosphate in muscle	Citrate (fatty acids, ketone bodies), ATP, cAMP	Glucagon ↓	Induced by insulin
	Pyruvate dehydrogenase	CoA, NAD, ADP, pyruvate	Acetyl-CoA, NADH, ATP (fatty acids, ketone bodies)	Insulin ↑ (in adipose tissue)	Also important in regulating the citric acid cycle
Gluconeogenesis	Pyruvate carboxylase Phosphoenolpyruvate carboxykinase	Acetyl-CoA cAMP?	ADP	Glucagon?	Induced by glu-cocorticoids, glucagon, cAMP
	Fructose-1,6-bisphosphatase	cAMP	AMP, fructose 2,6-bisphosphate	Glucagon	Repressed by insulin
Glycogenesis	Glycogen synthase		Phosphorylase (in liver) cAMP, Ca^{2+} (muscle)	Insulin ↑ Glucagon ↓ (liver) Epinephrine ↓	Induced by insulin
Glycogenolysis	Phosphorylase	cAMP, Ca^{2+} (muscle)		Insulin ↓ Glucagon ↑ (liver) Epinephrine ↑	
Pentose phosphate pathway	Glucose-6-phosphate dehydrogenase	$NADP^+$	NADPH		Induced by insulin
Lipogenesis	Acetyl-CoA carboxylase	Citrate	Long-chain acyl-CoA, cAMP	Insulin ↑ Glucagon ↓ (liver)	Induced by insulin
Cholesterol synthesis	HMG-CoA reductase		Cholesterol, cAMP	Insulin ↑ Glucagon ↓ (liver)	Inhibited by certain drugs, eg, lovastatin

Organ	Major Function	Major Pathways	Main Substrates	Major Products	Specialist Enzymes
Liver	Service for the other organs and tissues	Most represented, including gluco-neogenesis; β-oxidation; keto-genesis; lipopro-tein formation; urea, uric acid & bile acid forma-tion; cholesterol synthesis	Free fatty acids, glucose (well fed), lactate, glycerol, fructose, amino acids (Ethanol)	Glucose, VLDL (triacylglycerol), HDL, ketone bodies, urea, uric acid, bile acids, plasma proteins (Acetate)	Glucokinase, glu-cose-6-phospha-tase, glycerol kinase, phospho-enolpyruvate carboxykinase, fructokinase, arginase, HMG-CoA synthase and lyase, 7 α-hydroxylase
Brain	Coordination of the nervous system	Glycolysis, amino acid metabolism	Glucose, amino acids, ketone bodies (in starva-tion) Polyunsaturated fatty acids in neonate	Lactate	
Heart	Pumping of blood	Aerobic pathways, eg, β-oxidation and citric acid cycle	Free fatty acids, lactate, ketone bodies, VLDL and chylomicron tria-cylglycerol, some glucose		Lipoprotein lipase Respiratory chain well developed
Adipose tissue	Storage and breakdown of triacylglycerol	Esterification of fatty acids and lipolysis	Glucose, lipopro-tein triacylgly-cerol	Free fatty acids, glycerol	Lipoprotein lipase, hormone-sensitive lipase
Muscle Fast twitch Slow twitch	Rapid movement Sustained move-ment	Glycolysis Aerobic pathways, eg, β-oxidation and citric acid cycle	Glucose Ketone bodies, triacylglycerol in VLDL and chylo-microns, free fatty acids	Lactate	Lipoprotein lipase Respiratory chain well developed

HIGH-YIELD FACTS

Biochemistry

Glycolysis regulation, irreversible enzymes

D-glucose ⟶ Glucose-6-phosphate
　　　　Hexokinase

Glucose-6-P ⊖

Fructose-6-P ⟶ Fructose-1,6-BP
　　　　Phosphofructokinase
　　　　(rate-limiting step)

ATP ⊖, AMP⊕, citrate ⊖, fructose 2, 6-BP⊕

Phosphoenolpyruvate ⟶ Pyruvate
　　　　Pyruvate kinase

ATP ⊖, alanine ⊖, fructose-1,6-BP⊕

Pyruvate ⟶ Acetyl-CoA
　　　　Pyruvate
　　　　dehydrogenase

ATP ⊖, NADH ⊖, acetyl-CoA ⊖

Gluconeogenesis, irreversible enzymes

Pyruvate carboxylase	In mitochondria. Pyruvate → oxaloacetate.	Requires biotin, ATP. Activated by acetyl-CoA.
PEP carboxykinase	In cytosol. Oxaloacetate → phosphoenolpyruvate.	Requires GTP.
Fructose-1,6-bisphosphatase	In cytosol. Fructose-1,6-bisphosphate → fructose-6-P	
Glucose-6-phosphatase	In cytosol. Glucose-6-P → glucose	

Above enzymes found only in liver, kidney, intestinal epithelium.

Hypoglycemia is caused by a deficiency of these key gluconeogenic enzymes listed above (e.g., von Gierke's disease, which is caused by a lack of glucose-6-phosphatase in the liver).

Pentose phosphate pathway

Produces ribose-5-P from G6P for nucleotide synthesis.
Produces NADPH from NADP⁺ for fatty acid and steroid biosynthesis and for maintaining reduced glutathione inside RBCs.
Part of HMP shunt.
All reactions of this pathway occur in the cytoplasm.
Sites: lactating mammary glands, liver, adrenal cortex—all sites of fatty acid or steroid synthesis.

Cori cycle

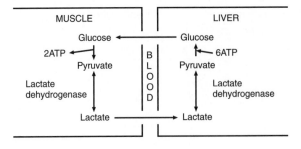

Transfers excess reducing equivalents from RBCs and muscle to liver, allowing muscle to function anaerobically (net 2 ATP).

Pyruvate dehydrogenase complex	The complex contains three enzymes that require five cofactors: pyrophosphate (from **T**hiamine, **L**ipoic acid, **C**oA (from pantothenate), **F**AD (riboflavin), **N**AD (niacin). Reaction: pyruvate + NAD$^+$ + CoA → acetyl-CoA + CO$_2$ + NADH.	Complex is similar to the α-ketoglutarate dehydrogenase complex (same cofactors, similar substrate and action). **T**ender **L**oving **C**are **F**or **N**obody

TCA cycle

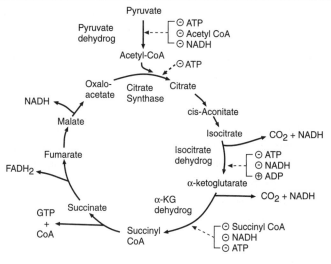

Produces 3NADH, 1FADH$_2$, 2CO$_2$, 1GTP per acetyl CoA = 12ATP/acetyl CoA (2x everything per glucose)

α-Ketoglutarate dehydrogenase complex cofactors:
1. Thiamine pyrophosphate
2. Lipoamide
3. CoA
4. FAD
5. NAD$^+$

Citric acid **i**s **K**rebs' **s**tarting substrate for **m**itochondrial **o**xidation.

Biochemistry

HIGH-YIELD FACTS

Biochemistry

Electron transport chain and oxidative phosphorylation

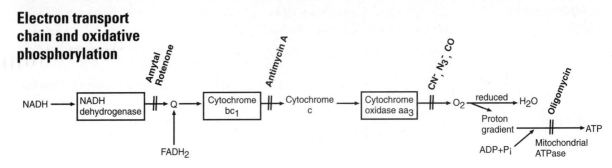

| Electron transport chain | 1 NADH → 3ATP; 1 FADH$_2$ → 2ATP |

Oxidative phosphorylation poisons

1. Electron transport inhibitors (rotenone, antimycin A, CN$^-$, CO) directly inhibit electron transport, causing ↓ of proton gradient and block of ATP synthesis.
2. ATPase inhibitor (oligomycin) directly inhibits mitochondrial ATPase, causing ↑ of proton gradient, but no ATP is produced because electron transport stops.
3. Uncoupling agents (2,4-DNP) increase permeability of membrane, causing ↓ of proton gradient and ↑ oxygen consumption. ATP synthesis stops. Electron transport continues.

Liver: fed state vs fasting state

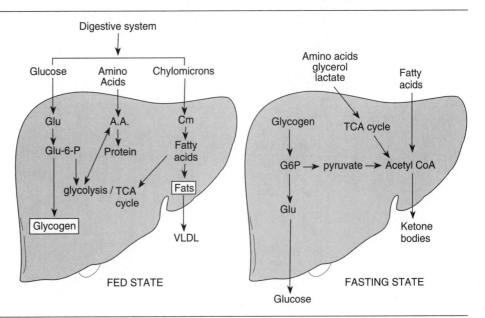

| **RBC energetics** | RBCs have no mitochondria (no TCA) and thus depend on glycolysis (ATP) for energy and HMP shunt (NADPH) for reducing equivalents. | Brain and RBCs rely on glucose for energy. (Brain can use ketone bodies in starvation.) |

| **Fatty acid metabolism sites** | Fatty acid synthesis = cytosol.
Fatty acid degradation = mitochondria.
Fatty acid entry into mitochondrion is via carnitine shuttle (inhibited by cytoplasmic malonyl-CoA). | Fatty acid degradation occurs where its products will be consumed—in the mitochondrion. |

Sphingolipid components	Sphingosine precursors are serine + palmitate.

Sphingolipid components

Sphingosine precursors are serine + palmitate.
Ceramide = sphingosine + fatty acid.
Sphingomyelin = ceramide + phosphoryl choline.
Cerebroside = ceramide + glucose/galactose.
Ganglioside = ceramide + oligosaccharide + sialic acid.

Cholesterol synthesis

Rate-limiting step is catalyzed by **HMG-CoA reductase,** which converts HMG-CoA to mevalonate. Two-thirds of plasma cholesterol is esterified by lecithin-cholesterol acyltransferase (LCAT), also known as phosphatidylcholine-cholesterol acyltransferase (PCAT).

Lovastatin inhibits HMG-CoA reductase.

Lipoproteins

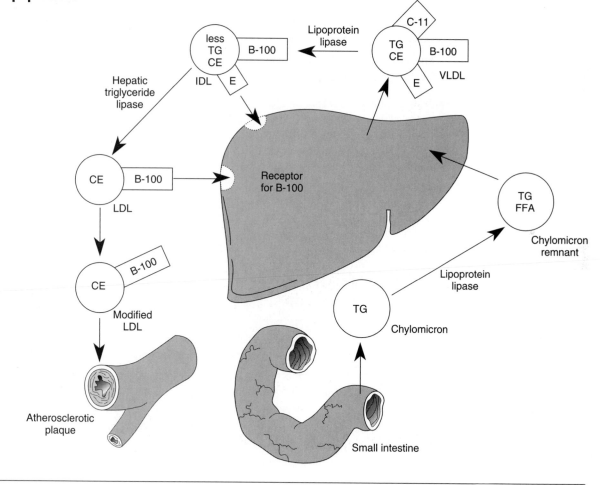

Lipoprotein functions

	Function and route	Apolipoproteins
Chylomicron	Delivers dietary triglycerides to peripheral tissues and dietary cholesterol to liver. Secreted by intestinal epithelial cells.	B-48 mediates secretion. A's are used for formation of new HDL. C-II activates lipoprotein lipase. E mediates remnant uptake by liver.
VLDL	Delivers hepatic triglycerides to peripheral tissues. Secreted by liver.	B-100 mediates secretion. C-II activates lipoprotein lipase. E mediates remnant uptake by liver.
LDL	Delivers hepatic cholesterol to peripheral tissues. Formed by lipoprotein lipase modification of VLDL in the peripheral tissue. Taken up by target cells via receptor-mediated endocytosis.	B-100 mediates binding to cell surface receptor for endocytosis.
HDL	Mediates centripetal transport of cholesterol (reverse cholesterol transport). Acts as a repository for apoC and apoE (which are needed for chylomicron and VLDL metabolism). Secreted from both liver and intestine.	A's help form HDL structure. A-I in particular activates LCAT (which catalyzes esterification of cholesterol). CETP mediates transfer of cholesteryl esters to other lipoprotein particles.

Major apolipoproteins

A-I: **A**ctivates LCAT.
B-100: **B**inds to LDL receptor.
C-II: **C**ofactor for lipoprotein lipase.
E: Mediates **E**xtra (remnant) uptake.

Aminolevulinate (ALA) synthase

Rate-limiting step for heme synthesis. The end product (heme) feedback inhibits this enzyme. Found in the mitochondria, where it converts succinyl CoA and glycine to ALA.

Heme synthesis

Occurs in the liver and bone marrow. Committed step is glycine + succinyl CoA → δ-aminolevulinate. Catalyzed by ALA synthase. Accumulation of intermediates causes porphyrias. Lead inhibits ALA dehydratase and ferrochelatase, preventing incorporation of iron and causing anemia and porphyria.

Under production of heme causes microcytic hypochromic anemia.

Heme catabolism

Heme is scavenged from RBCs and Fe^{2+} is reused. Heme → biliverdin → bilirubin (sparingly water soluble, toxic to CNS, transported by albumin). Bilirubin removed from blood by liver, conjugated with glucuronate and excreted in bile. In the intestine it is processed into its excreted form. Some urobilinogen, an intestinal intermediate, is reabsorbed into blood and excreted as urobilin into urine.

Hyperbilirubinemia	From conjugated (direct) and/or unconjugated (indirect) bilirubin. Causes: massive hemolysis, block in subsequent catabolism of heme, displacement from binding sites on albumin (e.g., liver damage or bile duct obstruction). Bilirubin is yellow, causing jaundice.	**UN**conjugated is **IN**direct and **IN**soluble. Conjugated bilirubin is excreted in the urine.
Essential amino acids	Ketogenic: **Leu, Lys.** Glucogenic/ketogenic: **Ile, Phe, Trp.** Glucogenic: **Met,** Thr, **Val, Arg, H**is.	Pri**VaTe TIM HALL.** Arg and His are required during periods of growth.
Acidic and basic amino acids	At body pH (7.4), acidic amino acids Asp and Glu are negatively charged; basic amino acids Arg and Lys are positively charged. Basic amino acid His at pH 7.4 has no net charge. Arginine is the most basic amino acid. Arg and Lys are found in high amounts in histones, which bind to negatively charged DNA.	Asp = aspartic ACID, Glu = glutamic ACID. Arg and Lys have an extra NH_3 group. The **ASP**iring **GLU**tton was **ACID**ic so others **BASIC**ally **ARG**ued with, **LY**ed to, and **HIS**sed at him.
Protein synthesis: ATP versus GTP	P site = peptidyl, A site = aminoacyl. ATP is used in tRNA charging, whereas GTP is used in binding of tRNA to ribosome and for translocation.	P = peptidyl, A = amino acid or acceptor site (on deck). Erythromycin inhibits the translocation step of protein synthesis.
Protein synthesis direction	Synthesis proceeds from N terminus to C terminus. mRNA is read $5' \rightarrow 3'$. Signal sequences are found on the N terminus of newly synthesized secretory and nuclear proteins.	The ami**N**o a**C**ids are tied together from **N** to **C**.
Urea cycle	$NH_4^+ + Asp + CO_2 + ATP$ Urea + Fumarate (Liver) Carbamoyl Phosphate, Mitoch., Cytoplasm, Citrulline, Aspartate +ATP, Ornithine, Urea, H_2O, Arginine, Fumarate, Argininosuccinate	**O**rdinarily, **C**areless **C**rappers **A**re **A**lso **F**rivolous **A**bout **U**rination.

Arachidonic acid products

Phospholipase A_2 liberates arachidonic acid from cell membrane. Lipoxygenase pathway yields leukotrienes. Cyclooxygenase pathway yields thromboxanes, prostaglandins, and prostacyclin. **L** for **L**ipoxygenase and **L**eukotriene.

Tx A_2 stimulates platelet aggregation.

PG I_2 inhibits platelet aggregation.

LT B_4 is a neutrophil chemoattractant.

LT C_4, D_4, and E_4 (SRS-A) function in bronchoconstriction, vasoconstriction, contraction of smooth muscle, and increased vascular permeability.

Platelet **G**athering **I**nhibitor

Insulin

Made in β cells of pancreas. No effect on glucose uptake by brain, RBCs, and hepatocytes. Required for adipose and skeletal muscle uptake of glucose. Inhibits glucagon release by α cells of pancreas.

Brain, liver, and RBCs take up glucose independent of insulin. **In**sulin moves glucose **In**to cells.

Ketone bodies

In liver: fatty acid and amino acids → acetoacetate + β-hydroxybutyrate (to be used in muscle and brain). Ketone bodies found in prolonged starvation and diabetic ketoacidosis. Excreted in urine. Made from HMG-CoA. Ketone bodies are metabolized by the brain to 2 molecules of acetyl CoA.

Breath smells like acetone (fruity odor). Urine test for ketones does not detect β-hydroxybutyrate (favored by high redox state).

Ethanol hypoglycemia

Ethanol metabolism increases NADH/NAD⁺ ratio in liver, causing diversion of pyruvate to lactate and OAA to malate, thereby inhibiting gluconeogenesis and leading to hypoglycemia.

Ethanol metabolism

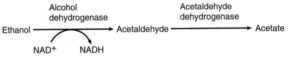

NAD⁺ is the limiting reagent.

Alcohol dehydrogenase operates via zero order kinetics.

Disulfiram (Antabuse) inhibits acetaldehyde dehydrogenase (acetaldehyde accumulates, contributing to hangover symptoms).

Kwashiorkor versus marasmus

Kwashiorkor = protein malnutrition resulting in skin lesions, edema, liver malfunction (fatty change). Clinical picture is small child with swollen belly. Marasmus = protein-calorie malnutrition resulting in tissue wasting.

Kwashiorkor results from a protein-deficient **MEAL**:
Malabsorption
Edema
Anemia
Liver (fatty)

Signal molecule precursors	ATP → cAMP via adenylate cyclase.
	GTP → cGMP via guanylate cyclase.
	Glutamate → GABA via glutamate decarboxylase (requires vit. B₆).
	Tyrosine → DOPA via tyrosine hydroxylase, the rate-limiting enzyme of catecholamine biosynthesis.
	Choline → ACh via choline acetyltransferase (ChAT).
	Arachidonate → prostaglandins, thromboxanes, leukotrienes via cyclooxygenase/lipoxygenase.
	Fructose-6-P → fructose-1,6-bis-P via phosphofructokinase (PFK), the rate-limiting enzyme of glycolysis.
	1,3-BPG → 2,3-BPG via bisphosphoglycerate mutase.

| **Tyrosine derivatives** | Tyrosine derivatives are thyroxine, dopamine, epinephrine, melanin. | Tire-sine ("tired without") substances that get you going: thyroxine, epinephrine, dopamine (as in Parkinson's), melanin (gets you outdoors). |

Enzyme kinetics

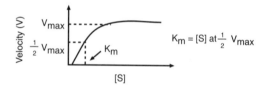

$$K_m = [S] \text{ at } \frac{1}{2} V_{max}$$

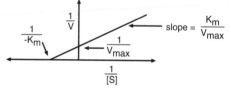

$$\text{slope} = \frac{K_m}{V_{max}}$$

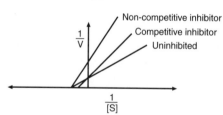

Competitive inhibitors:
Resemble substrates; bind reversibly to active sites of enzymes. High substrate concentration overcomes effect of inhibitor. V_{max} remains unchanged, K_m increases compared to uninhibited.

Noncompetitive inhibitors:
Do not resemble substrate; bind to enzyme but not at active site. Inhibition cannot be overcome by high substrate concentration. V_{max} decreases, K_m remains unchanged compared to uninhibited.

Cell cycle phases

M (mitosis: prophase–metaphase–
    anaphase–telophase)
G_1 (growth)
S (synthesis of DNA)
G_2 (growth)
G_0 (quiescent G_1 phase)
G_1 and G_0 are of variable duration. Mitosis is usually
    shortest phase. Most cells are in G_0.

G stands for **Gap** or **Growth**; **S** for **Synthesis**.

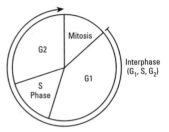

Plasma membrane composition

Plasma membranes contain cholesterol (≈50%, promotes membrane stability), phospholipids (≈50%), sphingolipids, glycolipids, and proteins. Only noncytoplasmic side of membrane contains glycosylated lipids or proteins (i.e., the plasma membrane is an asymmetric, fluid bilayer).

Phosphatidylcholine function

Phosphatidylcholine (lecithin) is a major component of RBC membranes, of myelin, of bile, and of surfactant (DPPC–dipalmitoyl phosphatidylcholine).

Keratin composition and function

Keratin is a protein with a high percentage of cysteine. It is found in intermediate filaments (nails and keratinized squamous epithelium).

Microtubule

Cylindrical structure 23 nm in diameter and of variable length. A helical array of polymerized dimers of α- and β-tubulin (13 per circumference). Each dimer has 2 GTP bound. Incorporated into flagella, cilia, mitotic spindles. Grows slowly, collapses quickly. Microtubules are also involved in slow axoplasmic transport in neurons.

Drugs that act on microtubules include colchicine (anti-gout), vinblastine/vincristine and taxol (anti-cancer), griseofulvin (anti-fungal), and mebendazole/thiabendazole (anti-helminthic). Colchicine inhibits microtubule polymerization. Vincristine and vinblastine interact with tubulin to block assembly of mitotic spindle.

Collagen synthesis

Preprocollagen is synthesized in the RER. Signal sequence is cleaved. Proline and lysine residues are hydroxylated by a reaction that requires vitamin C. Sugar residues are added to hydroxylysine residues. The procollagen fibrils arrange into a triple helix; the procollagen is secreted from the cell and cleaved to yield collagen. Lysine–hydroxylysine cross-links form and add stability to final structure.

Collagen structure

Collagen fibril = many staggered collagen molecules (linked by lysyl oxidase). Collagen molecule = 3 collagen α chains (usually X-Y-Gly, X and Y = proline, hydroxyproline, or hydroxylysine). Procollagen must be trimmed to collagen molecule.

Cholesterol lipoproteins

LDL and HDL carry most cholesterol. LDL transports cholesterol from liver to tissue; HDL tranports it from periphery to liver.

HDL is **H**ealthy.
LDL is **L**ousy.

Hemoglobin	Hemoglobin is composed of four polypeptide subunits (2α and 2β) and exists in two forms: 1. T (taut) form has low affinity for oxygen. 2. R (relaxed) form has high affinity for oxygen ($300\times$). Hemoglobin exhibits positive cooperativity and negative allostery (accounts for the sigmoid-shaped O_2 dissociation curve for hemoglobin), unlike myoglobin.	Carbon monoxide has a $200\times$ greater affinity for hemoglobin than oxygen.
Hb structure regulation	Increased Cl^-, H^+, CO_2, DPG, and temperature favor T form over **R** form (shifts dissociation curve to right, leading to $\uparrow O_2$ unloading). T form has low affinity for O_2.	When you're **R**elaxed, you do your job better (carry O_2).
CO_2 transport in blood	CO_2 binds to amino acids in globin chain (at N terminus) but not to heme. CO_2 binding favors T (taut) form of hemoglobin (and thus promotes O_2 unloading).	CO_2 must be transported from tissue to lungs, the reverse of O_2.
Hormonal effects on cAMP	Insulin reduces cAMP levels. Epinephrine, norepinephrine, and glucagon raise cAMP levels.	cAMP mobilizes resources (remember ATP → cAMP).
PIP_2 second messenger system	Involved in mast cell degranulation, α_1 receptor activation, and activation of some muscarinic receptors.	$PIP_2 \nearrow IP_3 \to \uparrow Ca^{2+}$ (from ER) $\searrow DAG \to$ protein kinase
Muscle activation: calcium	In skeletal muscle, calcium ions activate troponin, which moves tropomyosin, which exposes actin and allows actin-myosin interaction. In smooth muscle, Ca^{2+} activates contraction by binding to calmodulin (no troponins).	
Sodium pump	Na^+-K^+ATPase is located in the plasma membrane with ATP site on cytoplasmic side. For each ATP consumed, 3 Na^+ go out and 2 K^+ come in. During cycle, pump is phosphorylated (inhibited by vanadate). Ouabain inhibits by binding to K^+ site. Cardiac glycosides (digoxin, digitoxin) also inhibit the Na^+-K^+ATPase, causing increased cardiac contractility.	
Enzyme regulation methods	Enzyme concentration alteration (synthesis and/or destruction), covalent modification (e.g., phosphorylation), proteolytic modification (zymogen), allosteric regulation (e.g., feedback inhibition), and transcriptional regulation (e.g., steroid hormones).	

Vitamins

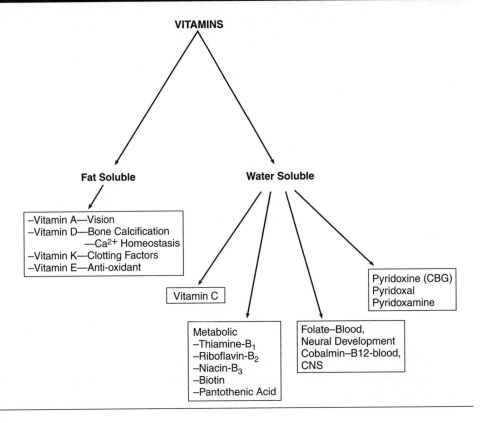

VITAMINS

Fat Soluble

–Vitamin A—Vision
–Vitamin D—Bone Calcification
  —Ca^{2+} Homeostasis
–Vitamin K—Clotting Factors
–Vitamin E—Anti-oxidant

Water Soluble

Vitamin C

Metabolic
–Thiamine-B_1
–Riboflavin-B_2
–Niacin-B_3
–Biotin
–Pantothenic Acid

Folate–Blood,
Neural Development
Cobalmin–B12-blood,
CNS

Pyridoxine (CBG)
Pyridoxal
Pyridoxamine

Vitamin A (retinol)

Deficiency	Night blindness and dry skin.	Retinol is vitamin A, so think Retin-A (used topically for wrinkles and acne).
Function	Constituent of visual pigments (retinal).	
Excess	Arthralgias, fatigue, headaches, skin changes, sore throat, alopecia	

Vitamin B_1 (thiamine)

Deficiency	Beriberi and Wernicke-Korsakoff syndrome. Seen in alcoholism and malnutrition.	Beriberi: characterized by polyneuritis, cardiac pathology, and edema. Spell beriberi as **Ber1Ber1**.
Function	In thiamine pyrophosphate, a cofactor for oxidative decarboxylation of α-keto acids (pyruvate, α-ketoglutarate) and a cofactor for transketolase.	Wet beriberi may lead to high output cardiac failure.

Vitamin B_2 (riboflavin)

Deficiency	Angular stomatitis.	**FAD** and **FMN** are derived from ribo**F**lavin (B_2 = 2 ATP).
Function	Cofactor in oxidation and reduction (e.g., $FADH_2$).	**N**AD derived from **N**iacin.

Niacin

Deficiency	Pellagra can be caused by Hartnup disease, malignant carcinoid syndrome and INH.	Pellagra's symptoms are the **3 Ds: D**iarrhea, **D**ermatitis, **D**ementia (also beefy glossitis).
Function	Constituent of NAD^+, $NADP^+$ (used in redox reactions). Derived from tryptophan.	

Vitamin B₅ (pantothenate)

Deficiency	Dermatitis, enteritis, alopecia, adrenal insufficiency.	
Function	Constituent of CoA, part of fatty acid synthase. Cofactor for acyl transfers.	Pantothen-**A** is in Co-**A**.

Vitamin B₆ (pyridoxine)

Deficiency	Convulsions, hyperirritability (deficiency inducible by INH).
Function	Converted to pyridoxal phosphate, a cofactor used in transamination (e.g., ALT and AST), decarboxylation, and transsulfuration.

Biotin

Deficiency	Dermatitis, enteritis. Caused by antibiotic use, ingestion of raw eggs.	Buy-a-tin of CO_2 for carboxylations.
Function	Cofactor for carboxylations but not decarboxylations.	

Folic acid

Deficiency	Macrocytic, megaloblastic anemia (often no neurologic symptoms), sprue.	Eat green leaves (because folic acid is not stored very long). PABA is the folic acid precursor in bacteria. Sulfa drugs and dapsone are PABA analogs.
Function	Coenzyme for one-carbon transfer; involved in methylation reactions. Important for the synthesis of nitrogenous bases in DNA and RNA.	

Vitamin B₁₂ (cobalamin)

Deficiency	Macrocytic, megaloblastic anemia, neurologic symptoms.	Vit. B₁₂ deficiency is usually caused by malabsorption (sprue, enteritis, *Diphyllobothrium latum*), no intrinsic factor (pernicious anemia), or no terminal ileum (Crohn's disease).
Function	Cofactor for homocysteine methylation and methyl-malonyl-CoA handling. Stored primarily in the liver. Synthesized only by microorganisms.	

Vitamin C (ascorbic acid)

Deficiency	Scurvy.
Function	Necessary for hydroxylation of proline and lysine in collagen synthesis.
	Scurvy findings: swollen gums, bruising, anemia, poor wound healing.

Vitamin **C** **C**ross-links **C**ollagen. British sailors carried limes to prevent scurvy (origin of the word "limey").

Vitamin D

	D_2 = ergocalciferol, consumed in milk.
	D_3 = cholecalciferol, formed in sun-exposed skin.
Deficiency	Rickets in children (bending bones), osteomalacia in adults (soft bones), and hypocalcemic tetany.
Function	Increases intestinal absorption of calcium and phosphate.
Excess	Hypercalcemia, loss of appetite, stupor. Seen in sarcoidosis, a disease where the epithelioid macrophages convert vit. D into its active form.

Remember that drinking milk (fortified with vitamin D) is good for bones.

Vitamin E

Deficiency	Increased fragility of erythrocytes.
Function	Antioxidant (protects erythrocytes from hemolysis).

Vitamin **E** is for **E**rythrocytes.

Vitamin K

Deficiency	Neonatal hemorrhage with ↑ PT, ↑ aPTT, but normal bleeding time.
Function	Catalyzes γ-carboxylation of glutamic acid residues on various proteins concerned with blood clotting. Synthesized by intestinal flora. Therefore, vit. K deficiency can occur after the prolonged use of broad-spectrum antibiotics.

K for **K**oagulation. Note that the vitamin K–dependent clotting factors are II, VII, IX, and X. Warfarin is a vitamin K antagonist.

Vitamins: fat soluble

A, D, E, K. Absorption dependent on gut (ileum) and pancreas. Toxicity more common than for water-soluble vitamins, because these accumulate in fat.

Malabsorption syndromes (steatorrhea) such as cystic fibrosis and sprue can cause fat-soluble vitamin deficiencies.

Mineral oil (laxative) can also cause malabsorption of fat-soluble vitamins.

Vitamins: water soluble

B_1 (thiamine: TPP)
B_2 (riboflavin: FAD, FMN)
B_5 (pantothenate: CoA)
B_6 (pyridoxine: PP)
B_{12} (cobalamin)
Niacin (nicotinate: NAD^+)
C (ascorbic acid)
Biotin
Folate

All wash out easily from body except B_{12} (stored in liver).

Electrolytes

Electrolyte	Functions	Causes and signs of deficiency	Causes and signs of toxicity
Ca^{2+}	• muscle contraction • neurotransmitter release • bones, teeth	• kids—rickets • adults—osteomalacia • contributes to osteoporosis	• excess vitamin D • hyperparathyroidism • sarcoid
Po_4^{3-}	• ATP • nucleic acids • phosphorylation • bones, teeth	• kids—rickets • adults—osteomalacia	• low serum Ca^{2+} • can cause bone loss
Na^+ K^+	• extracellular fluid • maintains plasma volume • nerve/muscle function • intracellular fluid • nerve/muscle function	• 2° to injury or illness • 2° to injury, illness, or diuretics • causes weakness, paralysis, confusion	• hypertension if salt sensitive • cardiac arrest • small bowel ulcers
Cl^-	• fluid/electrolyte balance • gastric acid • HCO_3^-/Cl^- shift in RBC	• 2° to emesis, diuretics, renal disease	• none that are clinically significant
Mg^{2+}	• bones, teeth • enzyme cofactor	• 2° to malabsorption diarrhea, alcoholism	↓ reflexes ↓ respiration

DNA/RNA/Protein

1. Molecular biology: tools and techniques (e.g., cloning, cDNA libraries, PCR, restriction fragment length polymorphism, restriction enzymes, sequencing).
2. Transcriptional regulation: the operon model (lac, trp operons) of transcription, eukaryotic transcription (e.g., TATA box, enhancers, effects of steroid hormones, transcription factors).
3. Protein synthesis: steps, regulation, energy (Which step requires ATP? GTP?), differences between prokaryotes and eukaryotes (N-formyl methionine), post-translational modification (targeting to organelles, secretion).
4. Acid base titration curve of amino acids, proteins.
5. SH2 domain: role.

Genetic Errors

1. Inherited hyperlipidemias: types, clinical manifestations, specific changes in serum lipids.
2. Glycogen and lysosomal storage diseases (e.g., type III glycogen storage disease), I cell disease.
3. Porphyrias: defects, clinical presentation, effect of barbiturates.
4. DNA repair defects (e.g., HNPCC, xeroderma pigmentosa).
5. Triplet repeat diseases (Huntington's chorea, Fragile X).
6. Inherited defects in amino acid metabolism.

Metabolism

1. Glycogen synthesis: regulation, inherited defects.
2. Oxygen consumption, carbon dioxide production, and ATP production for fats, proteins, and carbohydrates.
3. Amino acid degradation pathways (urea cycle, tricarboxylic acid cycle).
4. Effect of enzyme phosphorylation on metabolic pathways.
5. Rate limiting enzymes in different metabolic pathways (e.g., pyruvate decarboxylase).
6. Sites of different metabolic pathways (What organ? Where in the cell?).
7. Fed state versus fasting state: forms of energy used, direction of metabolic pathways.
8. Tyrosine kinases and their effects on metabolic pathways (insulin receptor, growth factor receptors).
9. Anti-insulin (gluconeogenic) hormones (e.g., glucagon, GH, cortisol).
10. Synthesis and metabolism of neurotransmitters (e.g., acetylcholine, epinephrine, norepinephrine, dopamine).
11. Purine/pyrimidine degradation.
12. Carnitine shuttle: function, inherited defects.
13. Cellular/organ effects of insulin secretion.
14. Effect of uncouplers on oxidative phosphorylation.

Microbiology

This high-yield material covers the basic concepts of microbiology and immunology. The emphasis in previous examinations has been approximately 40% bacteriology (20% basic, 20% quasi-clinical), 25% immunology, 25% virology (10% basic, 15% quasi-clinical), 5% parasitology, and 5% mycology. Learning the distinguishing characteristics, target organs, and method of spread of—as well as relevant laboratory tests for—major pathogens can improve your score substantially.

Many students preparing for this part of the boards make the mistake of studying bacteriology very well without devoting sufficient time to the other topics. For this reason, learning immunology and virology well is high yield. Learn the components of the immune response, including T cells, B cells, and the structure and functions of immunoglobulins as well as immunodeficiency diseases (e.g., agammaglobulinemia, DiGeorge's syndrome). Knowledge of viral structures and genomes is also very important.

Bugs

Viruses

Immunology

High-Yield Topics

Auxotroph, autotroph, heterotroph

Auxotroph	Nutritionally deficient species. Require nutrients not required by parental or prototype strain.	**Aux**otroph requires **Aux**iliary nourishment.
Heterotroph	Require carbon source, sugar, or amino acids.	All human pathogens are heterotrophs.
Autotroph	Require only CO_2 and energy source.	

Obligate aerobes

Examples include *Pseudomonas aeruginosa* and *Mycobacterium tuberculosis*.
Mycobacterium tuberculosis has a predilection for the apices of the lung, which have the highest Po_2.

*P **AER**uginosa* is an **AER**obe seen in burn wounds, nosocomial pneumonia, and pneumonias in cystic fibrosis patients.

Obligate anaerobes

Examples include *Clostridium* and *Bacteroides.* They lack catalase and/or superoxide dismutase and thus are susceptible to oxidative damage. They are generally foul-smelling (short-chain fatty acids), difficult to culture, and produce gas in tissue (CO_2 and H_2).

Anaerobes are normal flora in GI tract, pathogenic elsewhere. Aminoglycosides are ineffective against anaerobes because these antibiotics require O_2 to enter into bacterial cell.

Bacterial growth curve

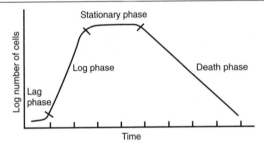

Bacterial structures

Structure	Function	Chemical composition
Peptidoglycan	Gives rigid support, protects against osmotic pressure	Sugar backbone with cross-linked peptide side chains
Cell wall/cell membrane (gram positives)	Major surface antigen	Teichoic acid induces TNF and IL-1
Outer membrane (gram negatives)	Site of endotoxin (lipopolysaccharide) Major surface antigen	Lipid A induces TNF and IL-1 Polysaccharide
Plasma membrane	Site of oxidative and transport enzymes	Lipoprotein bilayer
Ribosome	Protein synthesis	RNA and protein in 50S and 30S subunits
Nucleoid	Genetic material	DNA
Mesosome	Participates in cell division	Invagination of plasma membrane
Periplasm	Space between the cytoplasmic membrane and outer membrane	Contains many hydrolytic enzymes, including β-lactamases
Capsule	Protects against phagocytosis	Polysaccharide (except *Bacillus anthracis*)
Pilus/fimbria	Mediates adherence of bacteria to cell surface and attachment to bacteria during conjugation	Glycoprotein
Flagellum	Motility	Protein
Spore	Provides resistance to dehydration, heat, and chemicals	Keratin-like coat Dipicolinic acid
Plasmid	Contains a variety of genes for antibiotic resistance, enzymes, and toxins	DNA
Glycocalix	Mediates adherence to surfaces, especially foreign surfaces (e.g., indwelling catheters)	Polysaccharide

Cell walls

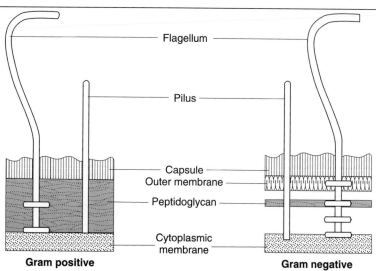

Gram positive   **Gram negative**

Component	Gram-positive Cells	Gram-negative Cells
Peptidoglycan	Thicker: multilayer	Thinner: single layer
Teichoic acids	Yes	No
Lipopolysaccharide (endotoxin)	No	Yes
Lipoprotein and phospholipid	No	Yes

Spores: bacterial	Only certain gram-positive rods form spores when nutrients are limited. Spores are highly resistant to destruction by heat and chemicals. Have dipicolinic acid in their core. Have no metabolic activity. Must autoclave to kill spores.	Gram-positive soil bugs ≈ spore formers (*Bacillus anthracis, Clostridium perfringens, C tetani*).
Spores: fungal	Most fungal spores are asexual. Both coccidioidomycosis and histoplasmosis are transmitted by inhalation of asexual spores. Ascospores from ascomycetes are sexual.	Conidia ≡ asexual fungal spores (e.g., blastoconidia, arthroconidia).
Antigenic variation	Classic examples: Bacteria: *Salmonella* (two flagellar variants), *Borrelia* (relapsing fever), *Neisseria gonorrhoeae* (pilus protein). Virus: influenza (major = shift, minor = drift). Parasites: trypanosomes (predictable sequence).	Some mechanisms for variation include DNA rearrangement and RNA segment rearrangement (e.g., influenza major shift).
Bacterial genetic transfer	Conjugation ≡ direct DNA transfer via sex (fertility, F) pilus. Transduction ≡ DNA transfer via bacteriophage vector. Transformation ≡ uptake of naked DNA from environment. Transposons ≡ "jumping genes," DNA sequences that jump from bacterium to bacterium or from bacterium to plasmid.	Conjugation = with joining. Transduction ≈ trans-**DUCK**-tion (imagine duck vector carrying DNA in bill). Transformation ≈ trans-**FROM**-ation (naked DNA **FROM** environment).
Exotoxins	Peptides that are excreted by both gram-positive and gram-negative bugs. They are highly antigenic and generally not associated with fever. They are relatively unstable to heat, are highly toxic, and have specific receptors. Usually encoded by lysogenic phage DNA.	**EX**otoxins are **EX**creted. Examples include tetanospasmin, botulinum toxin, and diphtheria toxin.

Bugs with exotoxins

Gram-positive bugs	Mode of action
Corynebacterium diphtheriae	Inactivates EF-2 by ADP ribosylation
Clostridium tetani	Blocks the release of the inhibitory neurotransmitter glycine
Clostridium botulinum	Blocks the release of acetylcholine: causes anticholinergic symptoms, CNS paralysis; spores found in canned food, honey (get floppy baby)
Clostridium perfringens	Alpha toxin is a lecithinase in gas gangrene. Get double zone of hemolysis on blood agar
Bacillus anthracis	One of the toxins is an adenylate cyclase
Staphylococcus aureus	Toxin is a superantigen that binds to class II MHC protein and T-cell receptor, inducing IL-1 and IL-2 synthesis in toxic shock syndrome
Streptococcus pyogenes	Erythrogenic toxin (causes rash of scarlet fever) and streptolysin O (antigen for ASO-antibody is found in rheumatic fever). Erythrogenic toxin is a superantigen; streptolysin O is a hemolysin

Gram-negative bugs	
Escherichia coli	Heat-labile toxin stimulates adenylate cyclase by ADP ribosylation of G protein Heat-stable toxin stimulates guanylate cyclase
Vibrio cholerae	Stimulates adenylate cyclase by ADP ribosylation of G protein; ↑ pumping of Cl⁻ and H_2O into gut
Bordetella pertussis	Stimulates adenylate cyclase by ADP ribosylation; causes whooping cough, lymphocytosis

Endotoxin

A lipopolysaccharide found only in cell wall of gram-negative bacteria. Lipid A is the toxic part. Can cause hemorrhagic tissue necrosis (via TNF), DIC, fever (via IL-1), shock, metabolic acidosis; also activates complement (via alternative pathway).

N-dotoxin in integral part of gram-**N**egative cell wall. Endotoxin is heat stable.

Endotoxins vs. exotoxins

	Exotoxin	Endotoxin
Source	Some gram-positive and gram-negative bacteria	Cell wall of most gram-negative bacteria
Secreted from cell	Yes	No
Composition	Polypeptide	Lipopolysaccharide (LPS)
Location of genes	Plasmid, bacteriophage, or bacterial chromosome	Bacterial chromosome
Clinical effects	Various effects	Fever, shock, DIC
Mode of action	Various modes	Induces TNF and IL-1 synthesis
Vaccines	Toxoids used as vaccines (highly antigenic)	No toxoids formed and no vaccine available (poorly antigenic)

Microbiology

HIGH-YIELD FACTS

Microbiology

Gram stain limitations	These bugs do not Gram stain well:	**T**hese **R**ascals **M**ay **M**icroscopically **L**ack **C**olor
	Treponema (too thin to be visualized)	Treponemes—darkfield microscopy and fluorescent antibody staining.
	Rickettsia (intracellular parasite)	
	Mycobacteria (high-lipid-content cell wall requires acid-fast stain)	Mycobacteria—acid fast.
	Mycoplasma (no cell wall)	
	Legionella pneumophila (primarily intracellular)	*Legionella*—silver stain.
	Chlamydia (intracellular parasite)	
Fermentation patterns of *Neisseria*	The pathogenic *Neisseria* species are differentiated on the basis of sugar fermentation.	**M**enin**G**ococci ferment **M**altose/**G**lucose; **G**onococci ferment **G**lucose.
Pigment-producing bacteria	*Staphylococcus aureus* produces a yellow pigment. *Pseudomonas aeruginosa* produces a blue-green pigment. *Serratia marcescens* produces a red pigment.	*Aureus* (Latin) = gold *Serratia marcescens* = maraschino cherries are red

| **IgA proteases** | IgA proteases allow these organisms to colonize mucosal surfaces: *Streptococcus pneumoniae, Neisseria meningitidis, Neisseria gonorrhoeae, Haemophilus influenzae.* |

Gram positive lab algorithm

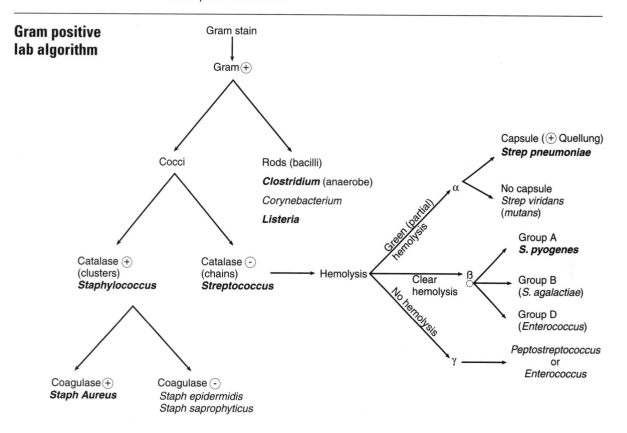

Important pathogens are in **Bold Type**

Note: Enterococcus is Group D but it is not β-hemolytic; it is α- or γ-hemolytic.

HIGH-YIELD FACTS

Microbiology

Gram negative lab algorithm

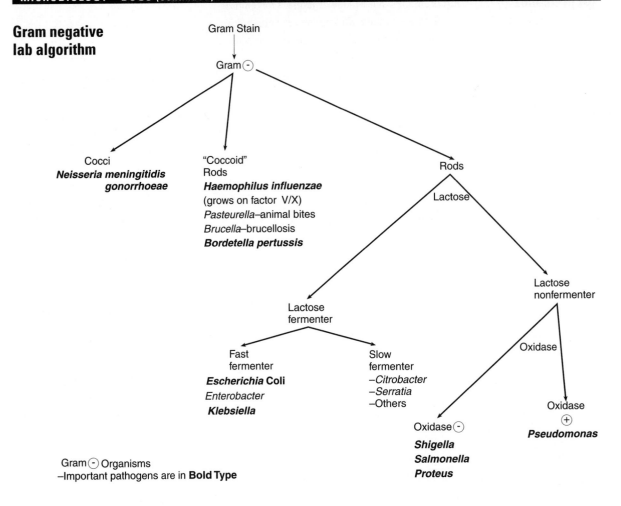

Gram Stain

Gram ⊖

Cocci
Neisseria meningitidis gonorrhoeae

"Coccoid" Rods
Haemophilus influenzae
(grows on factor V/X)
Pasteurella–animal bites
Brucella–brucellosis
Bordetella pertussis

Rods

Lactose

Lactose fermenter

Lactose nonfermenter

Fast fermenter
***Escherichia* Coli**
Enterobacter
Klebsiella

Slow fermenter
–*Citrobacter*
–*Serratia*
–Others

Oxidase

Oxidase ⊖
Shigella
Salmonella
Proteus

Oxidase ⊕
Pseudomonas

Gram ⊖ Organisms
–Important pathogens are in **Bold Type**

α-hemolytic bacteria

Include the following organisms:
1. *Streptococcus pneumoniae* (catalase-negative and optochin-sensitive)
2. Viridans streptococci (catalase-negative and optochin-resistant)

β-hemolytic bacteria

Include the following organisms:
1. *Staphylococcus aureus* (catalase- and coagulase-positive)
2. *Streptococcus pyogenes* (catalase-negative and bacitracin-sensitive)
3. *Streptococcus agalactiae* (catalase-negative and bacitracin-resistant)
4. *Listeria monocytogenes* (tumbling motility, meningitis in newborns, unpasteurized milk.)

Catalase/coagulase (gram-positive cocci)	Catalase degrades H_2O_2, an antimicrobial product of PMNs. Staphylococci make catalase, whereas streptococci do not. S aureus makes coagulase, whereas S epidermidis does not.	Staph make catalase because they have more "staff." Bad staph (*aureus,* because *epidermidis* is skin flora) make coagulase and toxins.
Staphylococcus aureus	Protein A (virulence factor) binds Fc-IgG, inhibiting complement fixation and phagocytosis. *Staphylococcus aureus* produces exfoliative toxin (scalded skin syndrome), TSST-1 (toxic shock syndrome: high fever, rash, shock), hemolysins, enterotoxins (rapid-onset/food poisoning), and coagulase.	TSST is a superantigen that binds to class II MHC and T-cell receptor, resulting in polyclonal T-cell activation. S aureus food poisoning is due to ingestion of preformed toxin.
Streptococcus pyogenes (Group A β-hemolytic streptococci sequelae)	Pharyngeal infection can lead to acute rheumatic fever (fever, polyarthritis, carditis, elevated ASO titer). Skin infection (also known as erysipelas or impetigo) can lead to acute glomerulonephritis (elevated ASO titer, low C3).	Pharyngitis gives you rheumatic "phever." Rheumatic fever = **PECCS**: **P**olyarthritis, **E**rythema marginatum, **C**horea, **C**arditis, **S**ubcutaneous nodules
M protein	An antiphagocytic virulence factor on cell wall of *Streptococcus pyogenes* (strep group **A**). Antibody to **M** protein enhances host defenses against S pyogenes.	**AM/PM**
Enterococci	Enterococci (*Streptococcus faecalis* and S faecium) are penicillin G-resistant and cause UTI and subacute endocarditis. Lancefield group D includes the enterococci and the nonenterococcal group D streptococci. Lancefield grouping is based on differences in the C-carbohydrate on the bacterial cell wall.	*Entero* = intestine, *faecalis* = feces, *strepto* = twisted (chains), *coccus* = berry. Enterococci, hardier than nonenterococcal group D, can thus grow in 6.5% NaCl (lab test).

Diarrhea

Species	Typical findings	Fever/leukocytosis
Escherichia coli	Ferments lactose	No
Vibrio cholerae	Comma-shaped organisms	No
Salmonella	Does not ferment lactose, motile	Yes
Shigella	Does not ferment lactose, nonmotile, very low ID_{50}	Yes
Campylobacter jejuni	Comma- or S-shaped organisms; growth at 42°C	Yes
Vibrio parahaemolyticus	Transmitted by seafood	Yes
Yersinia enterocolitica	Usually transmitted from pet feces (e.g., puppies)	Yes

Viridans group streptococci	Viridans streptococci are α-hemolytic. They are normal flora of the oropharynx and cause dental caries (*Streptococcus mutans*) and bacterial endocarditis (*S sanguis*). Resistant to optochin, differentiating them from *S pneumoniae*, which is α-hemolytic but is optochin sensitive.	*Sanguis* (Latin) = blood. There is lots of blood in the heart (endocarditis). Viridans group strep live in the mouth because they are not afraid of-the-chin (op-to-chin resistant).
Clostridia (with exotoxins)	All gram-positive, spore-forming, anaerobic bacilli. *Clostridium tetani* produces an exotoxin causing tetanus. *C botulinum* produces a preformed, heat-labile toxin that inhibits ACh release, causing botulism. *C perfringens* produces α toxin, a hemolytic lecithinase that causes myonecrosis or gas gangrene. *C difficile* produces a cytotoxin, an exotoxin that kills enterocytes, causing pseudomembranous colitis.	**Tet**anus is **tet**anic paralysis (blocks glycine, an inhibitory neurotransmitter). **Bot**ulinum is from bad **bot**tles of food (causes a flaccid paralysis), **Perf**ringens **perf**orates a gangrenous leg, **Diff**icile causes **di**arrhea.
Diphtheria (and exotoxin)	Caused by *Corynebacterium diphtheriae* via exotoxin encoded by β-prophage. Potent exotoxin inhibits protein synthesis via ADP-ribosylation of EF-2. Symptoms include pseudomembranous pharyngitis (grayish-white membrane) with lymphadenopathy. Lab diagnosis based on gram-positive rods with metachromatic granules.	*Coryne* = club shaped. Grows on tellurite agar. **ABCDEFG:** **A**denopathy **B**eta-prophage **C**orynebacterium **D**iphtheriae **E**longation Factor 2 **G**ranules
Actinomycetes	Actinomycetes are bacteria (prokaryotes) that form filaments resembling hyphae of fungi (eukaryotes).	*Actino* = ray, radiating (as in the filaments they form).
Actinomyces* versus *Nocardia	*Actinomyces israelii*, a gram-positive anaerobe, causes oral/facial abscesses with "sulfur granules" that may drain through sinus tracts in skin. *Nocardia asteroides*, a gram-positive and also a weakly acid-fast aerobe in soil, causes pulmonary infection in immunocompromised patients.	*A israelii* forms "sulfur" granules in sinus tracts. ***Nocardia*** has **no car,** so it walks fast on acid (acid fast) and on soil but gets out of breath (pulmonary infection).
Penicillin and gram-negative bugs	Gram-negative bugs are resistant to benzyl penicillin G but may be susceptible to penicillin derivatives like ampicillin. The gram-negative outer membrane layer inhibits entry of penicillin G and vancomycin.	

Periplasmic space	Space between outer membrane and cytoplasmic membrane in gram-negative bacteria. Periplasm contains enzymes (e.g., β-lactamases such as penicillinases).	Only gram-negatives have a periplasmic space.
Bugs causing food poisoning	*Vibrio parahaemolyticus* and *Vibrio vulnificus* contaminated seafood. *Bacillus cereus* in reheated rice. *Staphylococcus aureus* in meats, mayonnaise, custard. *Clostridium perfringens* in reheated meat dishes.	**V**omit **B**ig **S**melly **C**hunks. *Staphylococcus aureus* food poisoning starts quickly, ends quickly. "Food poisoning from reheated rice? Be serious!" (*B cereus*)
Enterobacteriaceae	All species have somatic (O) antigen (which is the polysaccharide of endotoxin). The capsular (K) antigen is related to the virulence of the bug. The flagellar (H) antigen is found in motile species. All ferment glucose and are oxidase negative.	Think **KOH**: **K**apsular s**O**matic flag**H**ellar (or think flagella spin like **H**elicopter blades).
Haemophilus influenzae	Causes meningitis, otitis media, pneumonia, epiglottitis. Small gram-negative (coccobacillary) rod. Aerosol transmission. Most invasive disease caused by capsular type b. Produces IgA protease. Culture on chocolate agar, requires factors V (NAD) and X (hemin) for growth. Treat meningitis with ceftriaxone. Rifampin prophylaxis in close contacts. Does not cause the flu (influenza virus does).	When a child has "flu," mom goes to five (V) and dime (X) store to buy some chocolate. Vaccine contains type b capsular polysaccharide conjugated to diphtheria toxoid or other protein. Given between 2 and 18 months of age.
Legionella pneumophila	Legionnaire's disease ("atypical" pneumonia). Gram-negative rod. Gram stains poorly—use silver stain. Grow on charcoal yeast extract culture buffered with iron and cysteine. Aerosol transmission from environmental water source habitat. No person-to-person transmission. Treat with erythromycin.	Think of a French legionnaire (soldier) with his **silver** helmet, sitting around a campfire (**charcoal**) with his **iron** dagger—he is no sissy (**cysteine**).
Pseudomonas aeruginosa	Causes wound and burn infections, UTI, pneumonia (especially in cystic fibrosis), sepsis (black lesions on skin), external otitis (swimmer's ear), hot tub folliculitis. Aerobic gram-negative rod. Non–lactose fermenting, oxidase positive. Produces pyocyanin (blue-green) pigment. Water source. Produces endotoxin (fever, shock) and exotoxin A (inactivates EF-2). Treat with aminoglycoside plus extended-spectrum penicillin (e.g., piperacillin, ticarcillin).	**AER**uginosa—**AER**obic Think water connection and blue-green pigment.

Helicobacter pylori	Causes gastritis. Risk factor for peptic ulcer and gastric carcinoma. Gram-negative rod. Urease positive. Creates alkaline environment. Treat with triple therapy: bismuth (Pepto-Bismol), metronidazole, and either tetracycline or amoxicillin.	Pylori—think pyloris of stomach. *Proteus* and *H pylori* are both urease positive (cleave urea to ammonia).
Lactose-fermenting enteric bacteria	These bacteria grow pink colonies on MacConkey's agar. Examples include ***C**itrobacter*, ***E** coli*, ***E**nterobacter*, and ***K**lebsiella*.	They **"CEEK"** (seek) lactose.
Salmonella* versus *Shigella	Both are non–lactose fermenters; both invade intestinal mucosa and cause bloody diarrhea. Only *Salmonella* is **m**otile and can invade further and disseminate hematogenously. Symptoms of salmonellosis may be prolonged with antibiotic treatments.	Salmon swim (motile and disseminate). *Salmonella* has an animal reservoir; *Shigella* does not and is transmitted via "food, fingers, feces, and flies."
Bugs causing watery diarrhea	Include *Vibrio cholerae* (associated with rice-water stools), enterotoxigenic *E coli*, viruses (e.g., rotaviruses), and protozoans (e.g., *Cryptosporidium* and *Giardia*).	
Bugs causing bloody diarrhea	Include *Salmonella, Shigella, Campylobacter jejuni*, enterohemorrhagic/enteroinvasive *E coli, Yersinia enterocolitica,* and *Entamoeba histolytica* (a protozoan).	
Cholera and pertussis toxins	*Vibrio cholerae* toxin permanently activates G_s, causing rice-water diarrhea. Pertussis toxin permanently disables G_i, causing whooping cough. Both toxins act via ADP ribosylation that permanently activates adenyl cyclase (resulting in ↑ cAMP).	Cholera turns the "on" on. Pertussis turns the "off" off. Pertussis toxin also promotes lymphocytosis.

Zoonotic bacteria

Species	Disease	Transmission and source	
Borrelia burgdorferi	Lyme disease	Tick bite; *Ixodes* ticks that live on deer and mice	**B**ugs
Francisella tularensis	Tularemia	Tick bite; rabbits, deer	**F**rom
Yersinia pestis	Plague	Flea bite; rodents, especially prairie dogs	**Y**our
Pasteurella multocida	Cellulitis	Animal bite; cats, dogs	**P**et

Undulant fever/ brucellosis	Caused by ingestion of unpasteurized dairy products contaminated with *Brucella abortus* (cattle) or *B melitensis* (goats) or contact with animals (goats, cattle, pigs). *Brucella* can replicate within macrophages. Undulant fever is an occupational hazard for butchers and meat handlers. Treat with tetracycline.	Picture ungulates (hoofed mammals) "hoofing it up" in your macrophages— **un**gulates give you **un**dulant fever.
Intracellular bugs Obligate intracellular Facultative intracellular	*R*ickettsia, *C*hlamydia *Mycobacterium, Brucella, Francisella, Listeria*	Stay inside (cells) when it is **R**eally **C**old.
Mycobacteria: atypical	*Mycobacterium tuberculosis* (TB) *M kansasii* (pulmonary TB-like symptoms). *M scrofulaceum* (cervical lymphadenitis in kids). *M avium–intracellulare* (often resistant to multiple drugs; causes disseminated disease in AIDS). All mycobacteria are acid-fast organisms.	TB symptoms include fever, night sweats, weight loss, hemoptysis.
Leprosy (Hansen's disease)	Caused by *Mycobacterium leprae,* an acid-fast bacillus that likes cool temperatures (infects skin and super-ficial nerves), and cannot be grown in vitro. Reservoir in US: armadillos. Treatment: long-term oral dapsone; toxicity is hemolysis and metHb. Alternate treatments include rifampin and combination of clofazimine and dapsone.	Hansen's disease has two forms: lepromatous and tuberculoid; lepromatous is worse (failed cell-mediated immunity), tuberculoid is self-limited. **LE**promatous = **LE**thal
Rickettsiae	Rickettsiae are obligate intracellular parasites (except *R quintana*) and need CoA and NAD. All except *Coxiella* are transmitted by an arthropod vector and cause headache, fever, and rash; *Coxiella* is an atypical rickettsia, because it is transmitted by aerosol. Tetracycline is the treatment of choice for most rickettsial infections.	Classic triad: headache, fever, rash (vasculitis)
Lyme disease	Classic symptom is erythema chronicum migrans, an expanding "bull's eye" red rash with central clearing. Also affects joints, CNS, and heart. Caused by *Borrelia burgdorferi,* which is transmitted by the tick *Ixodes.* Mice are important reservoirs. Deer required for tick life cycle. Treat with tetracycline. Named after Lyme, Connecticut; disease is common in northeastern U.S.	3 stages of Lyme disease: Stage 1: Erythema chronicum migrans, flu-like symptoms Stage 2: Neurologic and cardiac manifestations Stage 3: Autoimmune migratory polyarthritis

Rickettsial diseases and vectors

Rocky Mountain spotted fever (tick):
  Rickettsia rickettsii
Endemic typhus (fleas): *R typhi*
Epidemic typhus (human body louse): *R prowazekii*
Scrub typhus (mite): *R tsutsugamushi*
Q fever (inhaled aerosols): *Coxiella burnetii*
Treatment for all: tetracycline.

TyPHus has centriPHugal (outward) spread of rash, sPotted fever is centriPetal (inward). Q fever is Queer because it has no rash, has no vector, has negative Weil-Felix, and its causative organism can survive outside for a long time and does not have *Rickettsia* as its genus name.

Rocky Mountain spotted fever

Caused by *Rickettsia rickettsii*.
Symptoms: rash on palms and soles (migrating to wrists, ankles, then trunk), headache, fever.
Endemic to East Coast (in spite of name).

Palm and sole rash is seen in Rocky Mountain spotted fever, syphilis, and coxsackievirus infection (hand, foot, and mouth disease).

Chlamydiae

Chlamydiae are obligate intracellular parasites that cause mucosal infections. Two forms:
  1. Elementary body (small, dense), which Enters cell via endocytosis
  2. Initial or Reticular body, which Replicates in cell by fission
Chlamydiae cause arthritis, conjunctivitis, and nongonococcal urethritis. The peptidoglycan wall is unusual in that it lacks muramic acid.
Treatment: erythromycin or tetracycline.

Chlamys = cloak (intracellular).
Chlamydia psittaci notable for an avian reservoir.
C trachomatis infects only humans.
Lab diagnosis: cytoplasmic inclusions seen on Giemsa or fluorescent-antibody stained smear.

Chlamydia trachomatis serotypes

Types A, B, and C: chronic infection, causes blindness in Africa.
Types D–K: urethritis/PID, neonatal pneumonia, or neonatal conjunctivitis.
Types L1, L2, and L3: lymphogranuloma venereum (acute lymphadenitis: positive Frei test).
TWAR = new strain, pneumonia. Now called *C pneumoniae*.

ABC = **A**frica/**B**lindness/**C**hronic infection.
L1–3 = **L**ymphogranuloma venereum.
D–K = everything else.
Neonatal disease acquired by passage through infected birth canal.

Spirochetes

The spirochetes are spiral-shaped bacteria with axial filaments and include *Borrelia* (big size), *Leptospira*, and *Treponema*. Only *Borrelia* can be visualized using aniline dyes (Wright's stain or Giemsa stain).

BLT. B is **B**ig. **L** is **L**ean (thin spiral).
Leptospira = thin spiral.

Treponemal disease	Treponemes are spirochetes. *Treponema pallidum* causes syphilis. *T pertenue* causes yaws (a tropical infection that is not an STD although VDRL test is positive).	
Syphilis 1° syphilis 2° syphilis 3° syphilis	Caused by spirochete *Treponema pallidum.* Presents with painless chancre. Constitutional symptoms, maculopapular rash. Gummas, aortitis, neurosyphilis.	Treat with penicillin G.
VDRL versus FTA-ABS	FTA-ABS is specific for treponemes, turns positive earliest in disease, and remains positive longest during disease. VDRL is less specific.	**FTA-ABS** = **F**ind **T**he **A**ntibody-**ABS**olutely: 1. Most specific 2. Earliest positive 3. Remains positive the longest
VDRL false positives	VDRL detects nonspecific Ab that reacts with beef cardiolipin. Used for diagnosis of syphilis, but many biologic false positives, including viral infection (mononucleosis, hepatitis), some drugs, rheumatic fever, rheumatoid arthritis, SLE, and leprosy.	**VDRL** = **V**enereal **D**isease (also **V**ery **D**oubtful) **R**esearch **L**aboratory. The **3 As** of false positives: **A**ged, **A**ddiction, **A**utoimmune.
Mycoplasma pneumoniae	*Mycoplasma pneumoniae* is classic cause of atypical "walking" pneumonia (insidious onset, headache, nonproductive cough). X-ray looks worse than patient. High titer of cold agglutinins. Grown on Eaton's agar. Treatment: tetracycline or erythromycin (bugs are penicillin resistant because they have no cell wall).	No cell wall. Only bacterial membrane containing cholesterol. Mycoplasma pneumonia is less frequent in patients older than age 30. Frequent outbreaks in military recruits and prisons.
Candida albicans	Systemic or superficial fungal infection (budding yeast with pseudohyphae, germ tube formation at 37°C). Thrush in throat with immunocompromised patients (neonates, steroids, diabetes, AIDS), endocarditis in IV drug users, vaginitis (post-antibiotic), diaper rash. Treatment: nystatin for superficial infection; amphotericin B for serious systemic infection.	*Alba* = white.

Systemic mycoses

Disease	Endemic location	Notes
Coccidioidomycosis	Southwestern US, California.	San Joaquin Valley or desert (desert bumps)
Histoplasmosis	Mississippi and Ohio river valleys	Bird or bat droppings. Intracellular.
Blastomycosis	States east of Mississippi River and Central America	**B**ig, **B**road-**B**ased **B**udding
Paracoccidioidomy-cosis	Rural Latin America	"Captain's wheel" appearance
	All of the above are dimorphic fungi, which are mold in soil (at lower temperature) and yeast in tissue (at higher/body temperature: 37 ˚C) except coccidioidomycosis, which is a spherule in tissue.	**Cold = Mold** Culture on Sabouraud's agar.

Opportunistic fungal infections

Candida albicans	Thrush in immunocompromised (neonates, steroids, diabetes, AIDS), vulvovaginitis (high pH, diabetes, use of antibiotics), disseminated candidiasis (to any organ), chronic mucocutaneous candidiasis.
Aspergillus fumigatus	Ear fungus, lung cavity aspergilloma ("fungus ball"), invasive aspergillosis. **Mold** with septate hyphae that branch at a V-shaped (45°) angle. Not dimorphic.
Cryptococcus neoformans	Cryptococcal meningitis, cryptococcosis. Heavily encapsulated **yeast.** Not dimorphic. Found in soil, pigeon droppings. Culture of Sabouraud's agar. Stains with India ink. Latex agglutination test detects polysaccharide capsular antigen. Cryptographer uses India ink.
Mucor and *Rhizopus* species	Mucormycosis. **Mold** with irregular nonseptate hyphae branching at wide angles (≥ 90°). Disease mostly in ketoacidotic diabetic and leukemic patients.

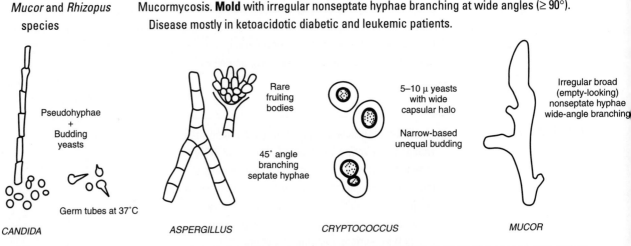

CANDIDA — Pseudohyphae + Budding yeasts — Germ tubes at 37˚C

ASPERGILLUS — Rare fruiting bodies — 45˚ angle branching septate hyphae

CRYPTOCOCCUS — 5–10 μ yeasts with wide capsular halo — Narrow-based unequal budding

MUCOR — Irregular broad (empty-looking) nonseptate hyphae wide-angle branching

Pneumocystis carinii	Causes pneumonia (PCP). Yeast (originally classified as protozoan). Inhaled. Most infections asymptomatic. Immunosuppression (e.g., AIDS) predisposes to disease. Silver stain of lung tissue. Treat with TMP-SMX, pentamidine.

Sporothrix schenckii

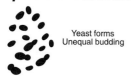

Yeast forms
Unequal budding

Sporotrichosis. Dimorphic fungus that lives on vegetation. When traumatically introduced into the skin, typically by a thorn ("rose gardener's" disease), causes local pustule or ulcer with nodules along draining lymphatics. Little systemic illness. Cigar-shaped budding cells visible in pus.

Encapsulated bacteria

Examples are *Streptococcus pneumoniae* (also known as pneumococcus), *Haemophilus influenzae* (especially b serotype), *Neisseria meningitidis* (also known as meningococcus), and *Klebsiella pneumoniae*.

Polysaccharide capsule is an antiphagocytic virulence factor.

Positive **Quellung** reaction: if encapsulated bug is present, capsule **swells** when specific anticapsular antisera are added.

IgG_2 necessary for immune response. Capsule serves as antigen in vaccines (Pneumovax, *H influenzae* b, meningococcal vaccines).

Quellung = capsular **"swellung."**

Pneumococcus associated with "rusty" sputum, sepsis in sickle cell anemia.

Normal flora: dominant

Skin–*S epidermidis*
Nose–*S aureus*
Oropharynx–Viridans streptococci
Dental plaque–*S mutans*
Colon–*B fragilis* > *E coli*
Vagina–*Lactobacillus, E coli,* group B strep

Neonates delivered by cesarean section have no flora, but are rapidly colonized after birth.

Common causes of pneumonia

Children (6 wk–18 yo) ──► Adults (18–40 yo) ──► Adults (40–65 yo) ──────► Elderly

Children (6 wk–18 yo)	Adults (18–40 yo)	Adults (40–65 yo)	Elderly
Viruses (RSV)	**Mycoplasma**	*S. pneumoniae*	***S. pneumoniae***
Mycoplasma	*C. pneumoniae*	*H. influenzae*	Anaerobes
Chlamydiae pneumonia	*S. pneumoniae*	Anaerobes	*H. influenzae*
S. pneumonia		*Viruses*	*Gram-negative rods*
		Mycoplasma	***Viruses***

Special Groups
—Nosocomial (hospital acquired)   —*Staphylococcus*
                                        —*Gram-negative rods*
—Immunocompromised   —*Staphylococcus*
                                        —*Gram-negative rods*
                                        —Fungi
                                        —*Viruses*
                                        —*Pneumocystis carinii*—with HIV
—Aspiration   —Anaerobes
—Alcoholic/IV drug user   —*S. pneumoniae*
                                        —*Klebsiella*
                                        —*Staphylococcus*
—Post-viral   —*Staphylococcus*
                                        —*H. influenzae*
—Neonate   —Group B *Streptococcus*
                                        —*E coli*

Causes of meningitis

Newborn (0–6 mo) →	Child (6 mo–6 y) →	6 y–60 y →	60 y +
Group B strep	*H influenzae* b	Enteroviruses	*S. pneumoniae*
E. coli	*S. pneumonia*	*N. meningitidis*	Gram-negative rods
Listeria	*N. meningitidis*	*S. pneumoniae*	Listeria
Klebsiella	Enteroviruses	HSV	

HIV—*Cryptococcus,* CMV, toxoplasmosis (abscess), JC virus (PML)

Note: Incidence of *H. influenzae* meningitis has ↓ greatly with introduction of *H. influenzae* vaccine in last 10–15 years.

CSF findings in meningitis

Bacterial: pressure ↑, polys ↑, proteins ↑, sugar ↓.

Viral: pressure normal/↑, lymphs ↑, proteins **normal,** sugar **normal.**

TB/fungal: pressure ↑, lymphs ↑, proteins ↑, sugar ↓.

Osteomyelitis

Most people: *S aureus*

Sexually active: *N gonorrhoeae* (also septic arthritis)

Drug addicts: *Pseudomonas aeruginosa*

Sickle cell: *Salmonella*

Hip replacement: *S aureus* and *S epidermidis*

Assume *S aureus* if no other information.

Most osteomyelitis occurs in children.

Elevated ESR.

Urinary tract infections

Ambulatory: *E coli* (50–80%), *Klebsiella* (8–10%).

Staphylococcus saprophyticus (10–30%) is the second most common cause of UTI in young ambulatory women.

Hospital: *E coli, Proteus, Klebsiella, Serratia, Pseudomonas.*

Epidemiology: women to men = 30 to 1 (short urethra colonized by fecal flora).

UTIs mostly caused by ascending infections. In males: babies with congenital defects; elderly with enlarged prostates.

UTI: dysuria, frequency, urgency, suprapubic pain.

Pyelonephritis: fever, chills and flank pain.

UTI bugs

Species	Features of the organism	Ferments lactose
Escherichia coli	Colonies show metallic sheen on EMB agar	Yes
Enterobacter cloacae	Often nosocomial and drug-resistant	Yes
Klebsiella pneumoniae	Large mucoid capsule and viscous colonies	Yes
Serratia marcescens	Some strains produce a red pigment; often nosocomial and drug-resistant	No
Proteus mirabilis	Motility causes "swarming" on agar; produces urease; associated with Struvite stones	No
Pseudomonas aeruginosa	Blue-green pigment and fruity odor; usually nosocomial and drug-resistant	No

Pelvic inflammatory disease	Top bugs: *Chlamydia trachomatis* (subacute, often undiagnosed), *N gonorrhoeae* (acute, high fever). *C trachomatis* is the most common STD in the US (3–4 million cases per year). Cervical motion tenderness, purulent cervical discharge. PID may include salpingitis, endometritis, hydrosalpinx, and tubo-ovarian abscess.	Salpingitis is a risk factor for ectopic pregnancy, infertility, chronic pelvic pain, and adhesions. Other STDs include *Gardnerella* (clue cells) and *Trichomonas* (motile on wet prep).
Nosocomial infections	By risk factor: Newborn nursery: CMV, RSV Urinary catheterization: *E coli*, *Proteus mirabilis* Respiratory therapy equipment: *P aeruginosa* Work in renal dialysis unit: HBV Hyperalimentation: *Candida albicans* Water aerosols: *Legionella*	The two most common causes of nosocomial infections are *E coli* (UTI) and *S aureus* (wound infection). Presume *Pseudomonas* **air**-*uginosa* when **air** or burns are involved. *Legionella* when water source is involved.
Bug hints (if all else fails)	Pus, empyema, abscess: *S aureus* Pediatric infection: *H influenzae* (including epiglottitis) Aerobic infection: *P aeruginosa* (pneumonia in CF, burn infections) Branching rods in oral infection: *Actinomyces israelii*	
Weil-Felix reaction	Weil-Felix reaction assays for antirickettsial antibodies, which cross-react with *Proteus* antigen. Weil-Felix is usually positive for typhus and Rocky Mountain spotted fever but negative for Q fever.	

Special culture requirements

Bug	Media used for isolation
H influenzae	Chocolate agar with factors V (NAD) and X (hematin)
N gonorrhoeae	Thayer–Martin media
B pertussis	Bordet–Gengou (potato) agar
C diphtheriae	Tellurite agar
M tuberculosis	Löwenstein–Jensen agar
S aureus	Mannitol–salt agar
M pneumoniae	Eaton's agar
Lactose-fermenting enterics (e.g., *Escherichia*, *Klebsiella*, and *Enterobacter*)	Pink colonies on MacConkey's agar
Legionella pneumophila	Charcoal yeast extract agar buffered with ↑ iron and cysteine
Fungi	Sabouraud's agar

HIGH-YIELD FACTS

Microbiology

DNA viral strands	All DNA viruses except the Parvoviridae are dsDNA. All are linear except papovaviruses and hepadnaviruses (circular).	All are dsDNA (like our cells) except "part-of-a-virus" (parvovirus) is ssDNA.
RNA viral strands	All RNA viruses except Reoviridae are ssRNA.	All are ssRNA (like our mRNA) except "**re**pe**a**t**o**-virus" (**Reo**virus) is dsRNA.
Naked viral genome infectivity	Naked nucleic acids of most dsDNA (except poxviruses and HBV) and (+) strand ssRNA (≈mRNA) viruses are infectious. Naked nucleic acids of (–) strand ssRNA and dsRNA viruses are not infectious. **Naked** (nonenveloped) RNA viruses include **C**alicivirus, **P**icornavirus, and **R**eovirus.	Viral nucleic acids with the same structure as host nucleic acids are infective alone; others require special enzymes (contained in intact virion). **Naked CPR.**
Enveloped viruses	Generally, enveloped viruses acquire their envelopes from plasma membrane when they exit from cell. Exceptions are herpesviruses, which acquire envelopes from nuclear membrane.	
Virus ploidy	All viruses are haploid (with one copy of DNA or RNA) except retroviruses, which have two identical ssRNA molecules (≈diploid).	
Viral vaccines	Live attenuated: measles, mumps, rubella, Sabin polio, VZV. Killed: rabies, influenza, hepatitis A, and Salk polio vaccines. Recombinant: HBV (antigen = recombinant HBsAg).	**MMR** = **M**easles, **M**umps, **R**ubella. sal**K** = **K**illed.

Viral replication

DNA viruses	All replicate in the nucleus (except poxvirus).
RNA viruses	All replicate in the cytoplasm (except influenza virus and retroviruses).

Viral genetics

Recombination	Exchange of genes between 2 chromosomes by crossing over within regions of significant base sequence homology.
Reassortment	When viruses with segmented genomes (e.g., influenza virus) exchange segments. High-frequency recombination.
Complementation	When one of 2 viruses that infects the cell has a mutation that results in a nonfunctional protein. The nonmutated virus "complements" the mutated one by making a functional protein that serves both viruses.
Phenotypic mixing	Genome of virus A can be coated with the surface proteins of virus B. Type B protein coat determines the infectivity of the phenotypically mixed virus. However, the progeny from this infection has a type A coat and is encoded by its type A genetic material.

Viral vaccines: dead or alive

Live attenuated vaccines induce humoral and cell-mediated immunity, but have reverted to virulence on rare occasion. Killed vaccines induce only humoral immunity but are stable.

Dangerous to give live vaccines to immunocompromised patients or their close contacts.

Viral pathogens

Structure	Viruses
DNA enveloped viruses	Herpesviruses (herpes simplex virus types 1 and 2, varicella-zoster virus, cytomegalovirus, Epstein-Barr virus), hepatitis B virus, smallpox virus
DNA nucleocapsid viruses	Adenovirus, papillomaviruses
RNA enveloped viruses	Influenza virus, parainfluenza virus, respiratory syncytial virus, measles virus, mumps virus, rubella virus, rabies virus, human T cell leukemia virus, human immunodeficiency virus
RNA nucleocapsid viruses	Enteroviruses (poliovirus, coxsackievirus, echovirus, hepatitis A virus), rhinovirus, reovirus

Prions

Infectious agents that do not contain RNA or DNA (consist only of proteins); diseases include Creutzfeldt-Jakob disease (CJD: rapid progressive dementia), kuru, scrapie (sheep), and "mad cow disease."

Latent virus infections

Virus exists in patient for months to years before it manifests as clinical disease. SSPE (late sequela of measles), PML (reactivation of JC virus) in immuno-compromised patients.

Hepatitis transmission

HAV (RNA virus) is transmitted primarily by fecal–oral route. Short incubation (3 wk). No carriers.

Hep **A: A**symptomatic (usually)

HBV (DNA virus) is transmitted primarily by parenteral, sexual, and maternal–fetal routes. Long incubation (3 mo). Carriers.

Hep **B: B**lood-borne

HCV is transmitted primarily via blood and resembles HBV in its course and severity. Carriers. Common cause of posttransfusion and IV drug use hepatitis in the United States.

Hep **C: C**hronic, **C**irrhosis, **C**arcinoma, **C**arriers

HDV (delta agent) is a defective virus that requires HBsAg as its envelope. Carriers.

Hep **D: D**efective, **D**ependent on HBV

HEV is transmitted enterically and causes water-borne epidemics. Resembles HAV in course, severity, incubation. High mortality rate in pregnant women.

Hep **E: E**nteric

Both HBV and HCV predispose a patient to hepato-cellular carcinoma.

Hepatitis serologic markers

	Description
IgM HAVAb	IgM antibody to HAV; best test to detect active hepatitis A.
HBsAg	Antigen found on surface of HBV; continued presence indicates carrier state.
HBsAb	Antibody to HBsAg; provides immunity to hepatitis B.
HBcAg	Antigen associated with core of HBV.
HBcAb	Antibody to HBcAg; positive during window phase. IgM HBcAb is an indicator of recent disease.
HBeAg	A second, different antigenic determinant in the HBV core. Important indicator of transmissibility.
HBeAb	Antibody to e antigen; indicates low transmissibility.

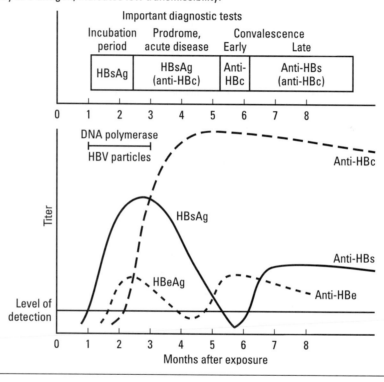

DNA viruses

Viral family	Envelope?	DNA structure	Medical importance
Parvovirus	No	SS-linear	B19 virus—aplastic crises in sickle cell disease —"slapped cheeks" rash—erythema infectiosum
Papovavirus	No	DS-circular	AAV—adeno-assisted virus HPV—warts, CIN, cervical cancer JC—progressive multifocal leukoencephalopathy in HIV BK—in kidney transplant patients
Adenovirus	No	DS-linear	Possible gene therapy vector Febrile pharyngitis—sore throat Pneumonia Conjunctivitis—"pink eye"

Hepadnavirus	Yes	DS-partial circular	Hepatitis B virus
			   Acute or chronic hepatitis
			   Vaccine available—use has ↑ tremendously

Herpesviruses	Yes	DS-linear	HSV 1—oral (and some genital) sores HSV 2—genital (and some oral) sores Varicella-zoster virus—chickenpox, zoster, shingles Epstein-Barr virus—Mononucleosis, Burkitt's lymphoma Cytomegalovirus—infection in immunosuppressed patients, esp. transplant recipients HHV 6 HHV 7—monkey bites (fatal in humans) KSAV—Kaposi's sarcoma-associated virus
Poxvirus	Yes	DS-linear	Smallpox eradication Vaccinia—cowpox ("milkmaid's blisters")

RNA viruses

Viral Family	Envelope?	RNA Structure	Capsid Symmetry	Medical Importance

Picornaviruses	No	SS + linear	Icosahedral	Poliovirus— polio-Salk/Sabin vaccines KPV/OPV
				Rhinovirus—"common cold"
				Coxsackievirus—aseptic meningitis
				  Herpangina—febrile pharyngitis
				  "Hand, foot, and mouth" disease
				  Myocarditis
				Hepatitis A—acute viral hepatitis

Caliciviruses	No	SS + linear	Icosahedral	Hepatitis E Norwalk virus—viral gastroenteritis
Reoviruses	No	DS linear	Icosahedral	Reovirus—Colorado tick fever Rotavirus—#1 cause of fatal diarrhea in humans
Flaviviruses	Yes	SS + linear	Icosahedral	Yellow fever Dengue
Togaviruses	Yes	SS + linear	Icosahedral	Rubella—German measles Congenital heart defects
Retroviruses	Yes	SS + linear	Icosahedral	Have reverse transcriptase HIV—AIDS HTLV—T cell leukemia
Orthomyxoviruses	Yes	SS – linear Segmented	Helical	Influenza virus
Paramyxoviruses	Yes	SS – linear Non-segmented	Helical	Measles Mumps Parainfluenza—croup RSV—bronchiolitis in babies
Rhabdoviruses	Yes	SS – linear	Helical	Rabies
Filoviruses	Yes	SS – linear	Helical Marburg	Ebola/Marburg Hemorrhagic fever—often fatal!
Coronaviruses	Yes	SS + linear	Helical	Coronavirus— "common cold"
Arenaviruses	Yes	SS – circular	Helical	LCV—lymphocytic choriomeningitis Meningitis—spread by mice
Bunyaviruses	Yes	SS – circular	Helical	California encephalitis Sandfly/Rift Valley fevers Crimea-Congo hemorrhagic fever Hantavirus—hemorrhagic fever, pneumonia

SS, single-stranded; DS, double-stranded; +, + polarity; –, – polarity

Segmented viruses	All are RNA viruses. They include arenaviruses, reoviruses, bunyaviruses, and orthomyxoviruses (influenza viruses). Influenza virus consists of 8 segments of negative-stranded RNA. These segments can undergo reassortment, causing worldwide epidemics of the flu.	Arena = "grains of sand" (due to ribosomes in the viral capsid as seen on electron microscopy). **Reo** = **re**peat**o** = segmented.
Picornavirus	Includes poliovirus, rhinovirus, coxsackievirus, echovirus, hepatitis A virus. RNA is translated into one large polypeptide that is cleaved by proteases into many small proteins. Can cause aseptic meningitis (except rhinovirus and hep A virus).	The discovery of **polio**, on a **rhino** in **Coxsackie**, NY, was **echo**ed around the world. picoRNAvirus = small RNA virus.
Rhinovirus	Nonenveloped RNA virus. Cause of common cold: more than 100 serologic types.	**Rhino** has a runny nose.
Rotavirus	Rotavirus, the most important global cause of infantile gastroenteritis, is a segmented dsRNA virus (a reovirus). Major cause of acute diarrhea in US during winter.	**ROTA** = **R**ight **O**ut **T**he **A**nus.
Paramyxoviruses	Paramyxoviruses include those that cause parainfluenza (croup), mumps, and measles as well as RSV, which causes respiratory tract infection (bronchiolitis, pneumonia) in infants. Paramyxoviruses cause disease in children. All paramyxoviruses have 1 serotype.	
Mumps virus	A paramyxovirus with one serotype. Symptoms: parotitis, orchitis (inflammation of testes), and aseptic meningitis. Can cause sterility (especially after puberty).	**M**umps gives you **b**umps (parotitis).
Measles virus	A paramyxovirus that causes measles. Koplik spots (bluish-gray spots on buccal mucosa) are diagnostic. SSPE, encephalitis (1 in 2000), or giant cell pneumonia (rarely, in immunosuppressed) are possible sequelae.	**3 C**s of measles: **C**ough **C**oryza **C**onjunctivitis Also look for Koplik spots.
Influenza viruses	Enveloped, single-stranded RNA viruses with segmented genome. Contain hemagglutinin and neuraminidase antigens. Responsible for worldwide influenza epidemics; patients at risk for fatal bacterial superinfection. Rapid genetic changes.	Killed viral vaccine is major mode of protection; reformulated vaccine offered each fall to elderly, health-care workers, etc.
Genetic shift	Reassortment of viral genome (such as when human flu virus recombines with swine flu virus).	Amantadine and rimantadine are approved for use against
Genetic drift	Minor changes based on random mutation.	influenza A (especially prophylaxis), but are not useful against influenza B or C.

Rabies virus	Negri bodies are characteristic cytoplasmic inclusions in neurons infected by rabies virus. Has bullet-shaped capsid. Rabies has long incubation period (weeks to 3 mo). Causes fatal encephalitis with seizures and hydrophobia. More commonly from bat, raccoon, and skunk bites than from dog bites.	Travels to the CNS by migrating in a retrograde fashion up nerve axons.
Arboviruses	Transmitted by arthropods (mosquitoes, ticks). Classic examples are dengue fever (also known as break-bone fever) and yellow fever. A variant of dengue fever in Southeast Asia is hemorrhagic shock syndrome.	**Arbo** virus = **Ar**thropod = **bo**rne virus
Yellow fever	Caused by flavivirus, an arbovirus transmitted by *Aedes* mosquitos. Virus has a monkey or human reservoir. Symptoms: high fever, black vomitus, and jaundice. Councilman bodies (acidophilic inclusions) may be seen in liver.	*Flavi* = yellow.

Herpesviruses	**Diseases**	**Route of transmission**
HSV-1	Gingivostomatitis, temporal lobe encephalitis, herpes labialis	Respiratory secretions, saliva
HSV-2	Herpes genitalis, neonatal herpes	Sexual contact, perinatal
VZV	Varicella zoster (shingles), encephalitis, pneumonia	Respiratory secretions
EBV	Infectious mononucleosis, Burkitt's lymphoma	Respiratory secretions, saliva
CMV	Congenital infection, mononucleosis, pneumonia	Congenital, transfusion, sexual contact, saliva, urine, transplant
KSAV	Kaposi's sarcoma (HIV patients)	Sexual contact

Mononucleosis	Caused by EBV, a herpesvirus. Characterized by fever, hepatosplenomegaly, pharyngitis, and lymphadenopathy (especially posterior auricular nodes). Peak incidence 15–20 y old. Positive heterophil Ab test. Abnormal circulating cytotoxic T cells (atypical lymphocytes).	Most common during peak kissing years ("kissing disease").
Tzanck test	A smear of an opened skin vesicle to detect multi-nucleated giant cells. Used to assay for herpesvirus.	Tzanck heavens I do not have herpes.
HIV diagnosis	Presumptive diagnosis made with ELISA; positive results are then confirmed with Western blot assay. HIV PCR/viral load tests are increasing in popularity; they allow physician to monitor the effect of drug therapy on viral load.	ELISA/Western blot tests look for antibodies to viral proteins; these tests are often falsely negative in the first 1–2 months of HIV infection.

Complement

Complement defends against gram-negative bacteria. Activated by Ig**G** or Ig**M** in the **classic** pathway, and activated by toxins (including endotoxin), aggregated IgA, or other conditions in the alternate pathway.

GM makes **classic** cars.
C1, C2, C3, C4: viral neutralization.
C3b: opsonization.
C3a, C5a: anaphylaxis.
C5a: neutrophil chemotaxis.
C5b-9: cytolysis by **M**embrane **A**ttack **C**omplex (**MAC**) (deficiency in *Neisseria* sepsis).
Deficiency of C1 esterase inhibitor leads to angioedema (overactive complement).

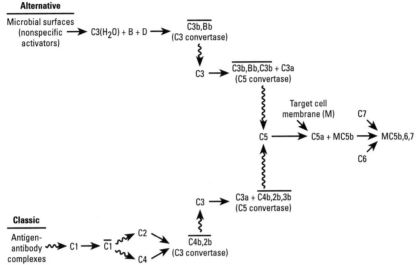

Interferon mechanism

Interferons are proteins that place uninfected cells in an antiviral state. Interferons induce the production of a second protein that inhibits viral protein synthesis by degrading viral mRNA (but not host mRNA).

Interferes with viral protein synthesis.

Hypersensitivity

Type I	**Anaphylactic and atopic:** Ag cross-links IgE on presensitized mast cells and basophils, triggering release of vasoactive amines. Reaction develops rapidly after Ag exposure due to preformed Ab. Possible manifestations include anaphylaxis, asthma, or local wheal and flare.	**F**irst and **F**ast (anaphylaxis). I, II, and III are all antibody mediated.
Type II	**Cytotoxic:** IgM, IgG bind to Ag on "enemy" cell, leading to lysis (by complement) or phagocytosis. Examples include autoimmune hemolytic anemia, Rh disease (erythroblastosis fetalis), Goodpasture's syndrome.	Cy-**2**-toxic. Antibody and complement mediated.
Type III	**Immune complex:** Ag-Ab complexes activate complement, which attracts neutrophils; neutrophils release lysosomal enzymes (e.g., PAN, immune complex GN).	Imagine an immune complex as **three** things stuck together: Ag–Ab–complement.
	Serum sickness: an immune complex disease (type III) in which Abs to the foreign proteins are produced (takes 5 days). Immune complexes form and are deposited in membranes, where they fix complement (leads to tissue damage). More common than Arthus reaction.	Most serum sickness is now caused by drugs (not serum). Fever, urticaria, arthralgias, proteinuria lymphadenopathy 5–10 days after Ag exposure.
	Arthus reaction: a local subacute Ab-mediated hypersensitivity (type III) reaction. Intradermal injection of Ag induces antibodies, which form Ag-Ab complexes in the skin. Characterized by edema, necrosis, and activation of complement.	Ag-Ab complexes cause the Arthus reaction.
Type IV	**Delayed (cell-mediated) type:** Sensitized T lymphocytes encounter antigen and then release lymphokines (leads to macrophage activation). Examples include TB skin test, transplant rejection, contact dermatitis.	**4th** and last = delayed. Cell mediated; therefore, it is not transferable by serum. **ACID** = **A**naphylactic and **A**topic (type I) **C**ytotoxic (type II) **I**mmune complex (type III) **D**elayed (cell-mediated) (type IV)

Passive versus active immunity

Passive	Based on receiving preformed antibodies from another host. Rapid onset. Short life span of antibodies.	After exposure to tetanus toxin, botulinum toxin, rabies, or HBV patients are given preformed antibodies (passive) for rapid availability of protection.
Active	Induced after exposure with foreign antigens. Slow onset. Long-lasting protection.	

Immune deficiencies

Thymic aplasia (DiGeorge's syndrome)	**T**-cell deficiency. Thymus and parathyroids fail to develop owing to failure of development of the 3rd and 4th pharyngeal pouches. Presents with tetany owing to hypocalcemia.
Severe combined immunodeficiency	B- and T-cell deficiency. Defect in early stem-cell differentiation. Presents with recurrent viral, bacterial, fungal, and protozoal infections. May have multiple causes (e.g., failure to synthesize class II MHC antigens, defective IL-2 receptors, or adenosine deaminase deficiency).
Wiskott–Aldrich syndrome	B- and T-cell deficiency. Defect in the ability to mount an IgM response to capsular poly-saccharides of bacteria. Associated with elevated IgA levels, normal IgE levels, and low IgM levels. Triad of symptoms includes recurrent pyogenic infections, eczema, and thrombocytopenia.
Chronic granulomatous disease	Phagocyte deficiency. Defect in phagocytosis of neutrophils owing to lack of NADPH oxidase activity or similar enzymes. Presents with marked susceptibility to opportunistic infections with bacteria, especially *S aureus* and *Aspergillus*.
Chédiak–Higashi disease	Autosomal recessive defect in phagocytosis that results from microtubular and lysosomal defects of phagocytic cells. Presents with recurrent pyogenic infections by staphylococci and streptococci.
Job's syndrome	Neutrophils fail to respond to chemotactic stimuli. Associated with high levels of IgE. Presents with recurrent cold staphylococcal abscesses.
Bruton's agammaglobulinemia	B-cell deficiency. X-linked recessive defect associated with low levels of all classes of immunoglobulins. Associated with recurrent bacterial infections after 6 months of age, when levels of maternal IgG antibody decline.
Selective immunoglobulin deficiency	Deficiency in a specific class of immunoglobulins. Possibly due to a defect in isotype switching. Selective IgA deficiency is the most common selective immunoglobulin deficiency.
Ataxia–telangiectasia	B- and T-cell deficiency, with associated IgA deficiency. Presents with cerebellar problems (ataxia) and spider angiomas (telangiectasia).
Chronic mucocutaneous candidiasis	T-cell dysfunction specifically against *Candida albicans*.

Transplant rejection

Hyperacute rejection—Antibody mediated due to the presence of preformed anti-donor antibodies in the transplant recipient. Occurs within minutes after transplantation.

Acute rejection—Cell mediated due to cytotoxic T lymphocytes reacting against foreign MHCs. Occurs weeks after transplantation. Reversible with immunosuppressants such as cyclosporin and OKT3.

Chronic rejection—Antibody-mediated vascular damage (fibrinoid necrosis); occurs months to years after transplantation. Irreversible.

Microbiology

1. Principles and interpretation of bacteriologic lab tests (culture, incubation time, drug sensitivity, specific growth requirements).
2. Dermatologic manifestations of bacterial and viral infections (e.g., syphilis, Rocky Mountain spotted fever, meningococcemia, herpes zoster, coxsackievirus infection).
3. Common sexually transmitted diseases (e.g., syphilis, AIDS, HSV, gonorrhea, chlamydia).
4. Viral gastroenteritis in the pediatric and adult populations.
5. Common causes of community acquired and nosocomial pneumonia.
6. Infections that cause congenital/neonatal complications (ToRCHeS: toxoplasmosis, rubella, CMV, HSV, syphilis).
7. Common nosocomial pathogens (e.g., *Pseudomonas, Klebsiella*).
8. Protozoa that frequently cause disease in the U.S. (e.g., Entamoeba histolytica, Giardia).
9. Parasites (protozoa, helminthes) that more commonly cause disease outside the U.S. (e.g., malaria, Chagas' disease, elephantiasis).
10. Mononucleosis (EBV or other pathogens that cause mono-like syndromes).
11. Herpes simplex virus encephalitis (medial temporal lobe lesion, mental status changes, treat with acyclovir).
12. Virulence factors and specific sites of bacterial infection (e.g., pili, capsules).
13. Salmonella infection: typhoid fever (rare in U.S.) versus enteric fever (seen in U.S.).
14. Tests available for diagnosis of viral infections (e.g., plaque assay, PCR).

Immunology

1. Principles and interpretation of immunologic tests (e.g., ELISA, complement-fixation tests, direct and indirect Coombs' test, Ouchterlony reactions).
2. Immune complex diseases (e.g., Goodpasture's syndrome, systemic lupus erythematosus, serum sickness).
3. Genetics of immunoglobulin variety and specificity (class switching, VDJ recombination, affinity maturation).
4. Mechanisms of antigenic variation and immune system evasion employed by bacteria, fungi, protozoa, and viruses.
5. How different types of immune deficiencies lead to different susceptibilities to infection (e.g., T-cell defects and viral/fungal infection; splenectomy and encapsulated organisms).
6. Helper T-cell pathways (Th1 versus Th2).
7. MHC/HLA serotypes: transplant compatibility, disease associations, familial inheritance.
8. Allergies: common antigens, antigen-IgE-mast cell complex, presumed mechanism of immunotherapy (blocking antibodies).
9. Granulomas: role of macrophages, foreign body versus immune granulomas, caseating (TB) versus noncaseating (sarcoid) granulomas, common causes (e.g., TB, sarcoid, fungi).

Pathology

Questions dealing with this discipline are difficult to prepare for because of the sheer volume of material. Review the basic principles and hallmark characteristics of each key disease. Given the clinical orientation of the Step 1, it is no longer enough to know the "trigger words" or key associations of certain diseases (e.g., café au lait macules and neurofibromatosis); you must also know the clinical descriptions of these trigger words. With the clinical slant of the USMLE Step 1, it is also important to review the classic presenting signs and symptoms of diseases as well as their associated laboratory findings. The examination includes a number of color photomicrographs and photographs of gross specimens, which are presented in the setting of a brief clinical history. However, read the question and the choices carefully before looking at the illustration, because the history will help you identify the pathologic process. Flip through your illustrated pathology textbook and look at the pictures for a few hours in the days before the exam. Pay attention to potential clues such as age, sex, ethnicity, and activity.

Congenital

Neoplastic

Gastrointestinal

Neurologic

Rheumatic/ Autoimmune

Vascular/Cardiac

Other

Findings

Photomicrographs

High-Yield Topics

Common congenital malformations

1. Heart defects (congenital rubella)
2. Hypospadias
3. Cleft lip with or without cleft palate
4. Congenital hip dislocation
5. Spina bifida
6. Anencephaly
7. Pyloric stenosis (associated with polyhydramnios); projectile vomiting

Neural tube defects (spina bifida and anencephaly) are associated with increased levels of AFP (in the amniotic fluid and maternal serum). Their incidence is decreased with maternal folate ingestion during pregnancy.

Congenital heart disease

R-to-L shunts (early cyanosis) "blue babies"

1. Tetralogy of Fallot (most common cause of early cyanosis)
2. Transposition of great arteries
3. Truncus arteriosus
4. Tricuspid atresia
5. Total anomalous pulmonary return

The **5 Ts:**
Tetralogy
Transposition
Truncus
Tricuspid
Total

L-to-R shunts (late cyanosis) "blue kids"

1. VSD (most common congenital cardiac anomaly)
2. ASD
3. PDA (close with indomethacin)

Frequency: VSD > ASD > PDA.
↑ pulmonary resistance due to arteriolar thickening
→ progressive pulmonary hypertension

Tetralogy of Fallot

1. Pulmonary stenosis
2. VSD
3. RVH
4. Large aorta overriding the VSD

This leads to early cyanosis from a R-to-L shunt across the VSD. On x-ray, boot-shaped heart due to RVH. Patients suffer "cyanotic spells."

The cause of tetralogy of Fallot is anterosuperior displacement of the infundibular septum.

Tetra = **4**
Think of pulmonary outflow stenosis/atresia as primary event with VSD and RVH as immediate consequences and with right-sided aorta as chronic compensation.

Transposition of great vessels

Aorta leaves RV (anterior) and pulmonary trunk leaves LV (posterior) → separation of systemic and pulmonary circulations. Not compatible with life unless a shunt is present to allow adequate mixing of blood (e.g., VSD, PDA, or patent foramen ovale).

Without surgical correction, most infants die within the first months of life. Common in offspring of diabetic mothers.

Coarctation of aorta

Infantile type: aortic stenosis proximal to insertion of ductus arteriosus (preductal).

Adult type: stenosis is distal to ductus arteriosus (postductal). Associated with notching of the ribs, hypertension in upper extremities, weak pulses in lower extremities.

Affects males:females 3:1.
Check femoral pulses on physical exam.
INfantile: **IN** close to the heart. (associated with Turner's syndrome.) A**D**ult: **D**istal to **D**uctus.

Patent ductus arteriosus	In fetal period, shunt is R-to-L (normal). In neonatal period, lung resistance decreases and shunt becomes L-to-R with subsequent RV hypertrophy and failure (abnormal). Associated with a continuous, "machine-like" murmur. Patency is maintained by PGE synthesis and low oxygen tension.	Indomethacin is used to close a PDA. PGE is used to keep a PDA open, which may be necessary to sustain life in conditions such as transposition of the great vessels.
Eisenmenger's syndrome	Uncorrected VSD, ASD, or PDA leads to progressive pulmonary hypertension. As pulmonary resistance increases, the shunt changes from L → R to R → L, which causes late cyanosis (clubbing and polycythemia).	

Autosomal trisomies

Down's syndrome (trisomy 21), 1:700	Most common chromosomal disorder and cause of congenital mental retardation. Findings: mental retardation, flat facial profile, prominent epicanthal folds, simian crease, **duodenal atresia** (double bubble sign on x-ray), congenital heart disease (most common malformation is **endocardial cushion defect**), **Alzheimer's disease** in affected individuals > 35 years old, associated with an increased risk of ALL. Ninety-five percent of cases are due to meiotic nondisjunction of homologous chromosomes, 4% of cases are due to Robertsonian translocation, and 1% of cases are due to Down mosaicism. Associated with advanced maternal age.
Edwards' syndrome (trisomy 18), 1:8000	Findings: severe mental retardation, **rocker bottom feet,** low-set ears, **micrognathia,** congenital heart disease, clenched hands (flexion of fingers), prominent occiput. Death usually occurs within 1 year of birth.
Patau's syndrome (trisomy 13), 1:6000	Findings: severe mental retardation, **microphthalmia,** microcephaly, cleft lip/palate, abnormal forebrain structures, polydactyly, congenital heart disease. Death usually occurs within 1 year of birth.

Genetic gender disorders

Klinefelter's syndrome [male] (XXY), 1:850	Testicular atrophy, eunuchoid body shape, tall, long extremities, gynecomastia, female hair distribution.	One of the most common causes of hypogonadism in males.
Turner's syndrome [female] (XO), 1:3000	Short stature, ovarian dysgenesis, webbing of neck secondary to cystic hygroma, coarctation of the aorta.	Imagine **turn**ing into a circle (XO).
Double Y males [male] (XYY), 1:1000	Phenotypically normal, very tall, severe acne, antisocial behavior (seen in 1–2% of XYY males).	Observed with increased frequency among inmates of penal institutions.

Pseudohermaphrodite

	Disagreement between the phenotypic (external genitalia) and gonadal (testes versus ovaries) sex.
Female pseudo-hermaphrodite (XX)	Ovaries present, but external genitalia are virilized or ambiguous. Due to excessive and inappropriate exposure to androgenic steroids during early gestation (i.e., congenital adrenal hyperplasia or exogenous administration of androgens during pregnancy).
Male pseudo-hermaphrodite (XY)	Testes present, but external genitalia are female or ambiguous. Most common form is testicular feminization (androgen insensitivity), which results from a mutation in the androgen receptor gene (X-linked recessive).

Cri-du-chat syndrome	Congenital deletion of short arm of chromosome 5 (46 XX or XY, 5p–). Findings: microcephaly, severe mental retardation, **high-pitched crying/mewing,** epicanthal folds, cardiac abnormalities.	*Cri-du-chat* = cry of the cat.
Fragile X syndrome	X-linked recessive defect. It is the second most common cause of genetic mental retardation (the most common cause is Down's syndrome). Associated with macro-orchidism (enlarged testes), long face with a large jaw, large everted ears, and autism.	Triplet repeat disorder that may show anticipation.
DiGeorge's syndrome	Due to failure of development of 3rd + 4th pharyngeal pouches and associated with: 1. Total absence of cell-mediated immune responses (lack of thymus) 2. Tetany (lack of parathyroids and hence hypocalcemia) 3. Congenital defects of heart and great vessels	Think "deep gorge" where thymus should have been. Recurrent viral and fungal infections because of defect in cellular immunity.
Duchenne's muscular dystrophy	An X-linked recessive muscular disease featuring a deleted dystrophin gene, leading to accelerated muscle breakdown. Onset before 5 years of age. Weakness begins in pelvic girdle muscles and progresses superiorly. Pseudohypertrophy of calf muscles due to fibro-fatty replacement of muscle; cardiac myopathy. The use of Gower's maneuver, requiring assistance of the upper extremities to stand up, is characteristic but not specific (indicates proximal lower limb weakness). Becker's muscular dystrophy is due to dystrophin gene mutations (not deletions) and is less severe.	
Cystic fibrosis	Autosomal recessive defect in CFTR gene on chromosome 7. Defective Cl^- channel → secretion of abnormally thick mucus that plugs lungs, pancreas, salivary glands, and liver → recurrent pulmonary infections (*Pseudomonas aeruginosa* and *Staphylococcus aureus*), chronic bronchitis, bronchiectasis, pancreatic insufficiency (malabsorption and steatorrhea), meconium ileus in newborns. Increased concentration of Cl^- ions in sweat test is diagnostic.	Infertility in males. Fat-soluble vitamin deficiencies (A, D, K). Can present as failure to thrive in infancy.
Juvenile polycystic kidney disease	Autosomal recessive bilateral enlargement of kidneys, with numerous small cysts of collecting ducts at right angles to the cortical surface. Associated with multiple liver cysts, congenital hepatic fibrosis, and proliferation of bile ducts.	

Autosomal dominant diseases

Adult polycystic kidney disease	Bilateral massive enlargement of kidneys due to multiple large cysts. Patients present with pain, hematuria, hypertension, progressive renal failure. Ninety percent of cases are due to mutation in APKD1 (chromosome 16). Associated with polycystic liver disease, berry aneurysms, mitral valve prolapse.
Familial hypercholesterolemia	Elevated LDL owing to defective or absent LDL receptor. Heterozygotes (1 in 500) have cholesterol ≈ 300 mg/dL. Homozygotes (very rare) have cholesterol ≈ 700+ mg/dL, severe atherosclerotic disease early in life and tendon xanthomas (classically in the Achilles tendon). Myocardial infarction may develop before age 20.
Marfan's syndrome	Fibrillin gene mutation → connective tissue disorders. Skeletal abnormalities: tall with long extremities, hyperextensive joints, and long, tapering fingers and toes Cardiovascular: cystic medial necrosis of aorta → aortic incompetence and dissecting aortic aneurysms. Floppy mitral valve. Ocular: subluxation of lenses.
Von Recklinghausen's disease (NFT1)	Findings: café au lait spots, neural tumors, Lisch nodules (pigmented iris hamartomas). On long arm of chromosome 17; 17 letters in von Recklinghausen.
Von Hippel-Lindau disease	Findings: hemangioblastomas of retina/cerebellum/medulla; about half of affected individuals develop multiple bilateral renal cell carcinomas and other tumors. Associated with deletion of VHL gene (tumor suppressor) on chromosome 3 (3p).
Huntington's disease	Findings: depression, progressive dementia, choreiform movements, caudate atrophy and decreased levels of GABA and acetylcholine in the brain. Symptoms manifest in affected individuals between the ages of 20 and 50. Gene located on chromosome 4; triplet repeat disorder.
Familial adenomatous polyposis	Colon becomes covered with adenomatous polyps after puberty; unless the colon is removed, the risk of cancer is 100%. Deletion of APC (tumor suppressor) gene on chromosome 5.

Neural tube defects

Associated with low folic acid intake during pregnancy. Spina bifida occulta: failure of bony spinal canal to close but no structural herniation. Usually seen at lower vertebral levels.
Meningocele: meninges herniate through spinal canal defect.
Meningomyelocele: meninges and spinal cord herniate through spinal canal defect.

Teratogens

Examples include actinomycin D (preimplantation), x-rays, iodine, thalidomide, aminopterin, DES, alcohol, warfarin, phenytoin, retinoic acid (Accutane). Most susceptible in 3rd–8th week of pregnancy. Alcohol is the number 1 known cause of congenital malformations in U.S.	Note that teratogens can act before pregnancy is discovered. Fetal infections can also cause congenital malformations.

Blood dyscrasias

Sickle cell anemia	Hb^S mutation is a single amino acid replacement in β-chain (substitution of normal glutamic acid with valine). Low O_2 precipitates sickling. Heterozygotes are relatively malaria resistant (balanced polymorphism). Complications in homozygotes (Hb^{SS}) include aplastic crisis (due to B19 parvovirus infection), autosplenectomy, ↑ risk of encapsulated organism infection, *Salmonella* osteomyelitis, painful crisis (vaso-occlusive), and splenic sequestration crisis. Hb^c defect is a different β chain mutation; patients with Hb^{cc} or Hb^{sc} (1 of each mutant gene) have milder disease than Hb^{ss} patients. New therapies for sickle cell anemia include hydroxyurea (↑ Hb^F) and bone marrow transplantation.	Eight percent of African-Americans carry the Hb^S trait. 0.2% have the disease. Sickled cells are crescent-shaped RBCs.
α-thalassemia	There are four α-globin genes. In α-thalassemia, the α-globin chain is underproduced (as a function of number of bad genes, one to four). There is no compensatory increase of any other chains. Hb Barts (γ_4-tetramers) or hydrops fetalis = non-functional α-globin chains and intrauterine fetal death.	Thalassemia is prevalent in Mediterranean populations (*thalassa* = sea). Think of thala**SEA**mia.
β-thalassemia	In β-minor thalassemia (heterozygote), the β-chain is underproduced; in β-major (homozygote), the β-chain is absent. In both cases, fetal hemoglobin production is compensatorily increased but is inadequate. Hb^s/β-thalassemia heterozygote has mild to moderate disease.	β-thalassemia major results in severe anemia requiring blood transfusions. Cardiac failure due to secondary hemochromatosis.

HLA associations

	Disease	
HLA-B27	**P**soriasis, **A**nkylosing spondylitis, **I**nflammatory bowel disease, **R**eiter's syndrome	**PAIR**
HLA-DR4	Rheumatoid arthritis	
HLA-DR3	Sjögren's syndrome; chronic active hepatitis	
HLA-DR2, HLA-DR3	Systemic lupus erythematosus	
HLA-A3	Primary hemochromatosis	
HLA-DR3, HLA-DR4	Type I diabetes mellitus (IDDM).	

Plasia definitions

Hyperplasia = Increase in number of cells (reversible).

Metaplasia = One adult cell type is replaced by another (reversible). Often secondary to irritation and/or environmental exposure (e.g., squamous metaplasia in trachea and bronchi of smokers).

Dysplasia = Abnormal growth with loss of cellular orientation, shape, and size in comparison to normal tissue maturation, commonly preneoplastic (reversible).

Anaplasia = Abnormal cells lacking differentiation; like primitive cells of same tissue, often equated with undifferentiated malignant neoplasms. Tumor giant cells may be formed.

Neoplasia = A clonal proliferation of cells that is uncontrolled and excessive.

Neoplastic progression

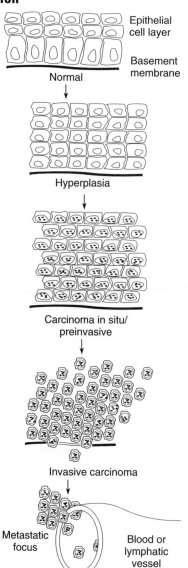

- normal cells with basal → apical differentiation

- cells have ↑ in number **HYPERPLASIA**
- no difference between cells at base and those at apex **ANAPLASIA**

- **IN SITU CARCINOMA**
- cells **LOOK LIKE CANCER CELLS** but **HAVE NOT INVADED BASEMENT MEMBRANE**
- **PYKNOSIS** - dark nuclei

- cells have invaded basement membrane using **COLLAGENASES** and **HYDROLASES**
- will metastasize if they reach a blood or lymphatic vessel

METASTASIS - spread to distant organ
- must survive immune attack
- "seed and soil" theory of metastasis
    - seed - tumor embolus
    - soil - target organ - liver, lungs, bone, brain...

Tumor nomenclature

Cell type	Benign	Malignant
Epithelium	Adenoma, papilloma	Adenocarcinoma, papillary carcinoma
Mesenchyme		
Blood Cells		Leukemia, lymphoma
Blood vessels	Hemangioma	Angiosarcoma
Smooth muscle	Leiomyoma	Leiomyosarcoma
Skeletal muscle	Rhabdomyoma	Rhabdomyosarcoma
More than one cell type	Mature teratoma	Immature teratoma

Precancerous conditions and associated neoplasms

Condition	Neoplasm
1. Down's syndrome	1. Acute lymphoblastic leukemia
2. Xeroderma pigmentosum	2. Squamous cell and basal cell carcinomas of skin
3. Chronic atrophic gastritis, pernicious anemia, postsurgical gastric remnants	3. Gastric adenocarcinoma
4. Tuberous sclerosis (facial angiofibroma, seizures, mental retardation)	4. Astrocytoma and cardiac rhabdomyoma
5. Café au lait skin patches	5. Neurofibromatosis I
6. Actinic keratosis	6. Squamous cell carcinoma of skin
7. Barrett's esophagus (chronic GI reflux)	7. Esophageal adenocarcinoma
8. Plummer–Vinson syndrome (atrophic glossitis, esophageal webs, plus anemia; all due to iron deficiency)	8. Squamous cell carcinoma of esophagus
9. Cirrhosis (alcoholic, hepatitis B/C)	9. Hepatocellular carcinoma
10. Ulcerative colitis	10. Colonic adenocarcinoma
11. Paget's disease of bone	11. Secondary osteosarcoma and fibrosarcoma
12. Immunodeficiency states	12. Malignant lymphomas
13. AIDS	13. Aggressive B-cell lymphomas and Kaposi's sarcoma
14. Autoimmune diseases (e.g., Hashimoto's thyroiditis, myasthenia gravis)	14. Malignant thymomas, benign thymomas, thymic hyperplasia

Oncogenes

Oncogenes	Associated tumor
myc	Burkitt's lymphoma
N-*myc*	Neuroblastoma
L-*myc*	Small cell carcinoma of lung
bcl-2	Follicular and undifferentiated lymphomas (inhibits apoptosis)
erb-B2	Breast, ovarian, and gastric carcinomas
ret	Multiple endocrine neoplasia (II, III)

Oncogenes act as dominant genes; one mutant copy of an oncogene is sufficient. Mutations in oncogenes "activate" the gene.

Tumor suppressor genes

Gene	Chromosome	Associated tumor
VHL	3p	Renal cell carcinoma, von Hippel-Lindau disease
APC	5q	Colorectal carcinoma, familial adenomatous polyposis coli
WT-1	11p	Wilms' tumor
Rb	13q	Retinoblastoma, osteosarcoma
BRCA-2	13q	Breast cancer
p53	17p	Most human cancers, Li-Fraumeni syndrome
NF-1	17q	Neurofibromatosis type I
BRCA-1	17q	Breast cancer, ovarian cancer
DCC	18q	Carcinomas of colon and stomach
DPC	18q	Pancreatic cancer
NF-**2**	**22**q	Neurofibromatosis type **II** (**bi**lateral acoustic neuroma)

Tumor suppressor genes act as recessive genes; both copies of gene must be "inactivated." If patient inherits or acquires one copy of a mutant tumor suppressor gene, the second copy must be mutated/deleted as well ("two-hit hypothesis").

Tumor markers

Marker	
PSA, prostatic specific acid phosphatase	Prostatic carcinoma
CEA	Carcinoembryonic antigen. Very nonspecific but produced by ~70% of colorectal and pancreatic cancers; also by gastric and breast carcinomas.
α-fetoprotein	Normally made by fetus. Hepatocellular carcinomas. Nonseminomatous germ cell tumors of the testis (e.g., yolk sac tumor).
β-hCG	Gestational trophoblastic tumors, hydatidiform moles, and choriocarcinomas.
α_1-antitrypsin	Liver and yolk sac tumors.
CA-125	Ovarian tumors.
S-100	Melanoma, neural tumors, astrocytomas.
Bombesin	Neuroblastoma, small cell carcinomas, gastric and pancreatic carcinomas.

Tumor markers should not be used as the primary tool for cancer diagnosis. They may be used to confirm diagnosis, to monitor for tumor recurrence, and to monitor response to therapy.

Oncogenic viruses

Virus	Associated cancer
HTLV-1	Adult T-cell leukemia
HBV	Hepatocellular carcinoma
EBV	Burkitt's lymphoma, nasopharyngeal carcinoma
HPV	Cervical carcinoma, penile/anal carcinoma
Kaposi's sarcoma–associated herpesvirus (KSAV)	Kaposi's sarcoma

Tumor grade versus stage

Grade	Histologic appearance of tumor. Usually graded I–IV based on degree of differentiation and number of mitoses per high-power field.	Stage has more prognostic value than grade. TNM staging system:
Stage	Based on site of primary lesion, spread to regional lymph nodes, presence of metastases.	**T** = size of **T**umor **N** = regional **N**ode involvement **M** = **M**etastases

Brain tumors

Adult	Seventy percent above tentorium (e.g., cerebral hemispheres). Incidence: metastases > astrocytoma (including glioblastoma) > meningioma > pituitary tumor.	Adults are taller than kids; therefore their tumors are supratentorial. Glioblastoma multiforme: necrosis, hemorrhage, and pseudo-palisading; "butterfly" glioma; very poor prognosis.
Childhood	Seventy percent below tentorium (e.g., cerebellum). Second most common childhood neoplasm after leukemia. Incidence: medulloblastoma > astrocytoma > ependymoma.	

Cardiac tumors

Myxomas are the most common 1° cardiac tumor in adults. Ninety percent occur in the atria (mostly LA). Myxomas are usually described as a "ball-valve" obstruction in the LA. Rhabdomyomas are the most frequent 1° cardiac tumor in children.

Skin cancer

Squamous cell carcinoma	Very common. Associated with excessive exposure to sunlight. Commonly appear on hands and face. Locally invasive but rarely metastasizes.	Actinic keratosis is a precursor to squamous cell carcinoma. Keratin "pearls." Arsenic exposure.
Basal cell carcinoma	Most common in sun-exposed areas of body. Locally invasive but almost never metastasizes.	Basal cell tumors have "palisading" nuclei.
Melanoma	Common tumor with significant risk of metastasis. Associated with sunlight exposure. Incidence increasing. Depth of tumor correlates with risk of metastasis.	Increased risk in fair-skinned persons. Dysplastic nevus is a precursor to melanoma.

Colorectal cancer risk factors	Risk factors for carcinoma of colon: colorectal villous adenomas, chronic inflammatory bowel disease, low-fiber diet, increasing age, familial adenomatous polyposis (FAP), hereditary nonpolyposis colorectal cancer (HNPCC), personal and family history of colon cancer. Screen patients > 50 years old with stool occult blood test.	
Barrett's esophagus	Glandular (columnar epithelial) metaplasia—replacement of stratified squamous epithelium with gastric (columnar) epithelium in the distal esophagus. Predisposes to esophageal adenocarcinoma; usually secondary to gastroesophageal reflux.	
Multiple endocrine neoplasias (MEN)	MEN type I (Werner's syndrome)—pancreas (e.g., ZE syndrome, insulinomas, VIPomas), parathyroid and pituitary tumors. MEN type IIa (Sipple's syndrome)—medullary carcinoma of the thyroid, pheochromocytoma, parathyroid tumor or adenoma. MEN type III (formerly MEN IIb)—medullary carcinoma of the thyroid, pheochromocytoma, and oral and intestinal ganglioneuromatosis (mucosal neuromas).	All MEN syndromes are autosomal dominantly inherited. MEN I = 3 "P" organs (**P**ancreas, **P**ituitary, and **P**arathyroid).

Most common leukemias by age group	Age	< 15	15–39	40–59	60+
		ALL (acute lymphocytic leukemia)	AML (acute myelocytic leukemia)	AML and CML (chronic myelocytic leukemia)	CLL (chronic lymphocytic leukemia)

Chromosomal translocations	t(9, 22), or the Philadelphia chromosome, is associated with CML (*abl-bcr* hybrid). t(8, 14) is associated with Burkitt's lymphoma (c-*myc* activation). t(14, 18) is associated with follicular lymphomas (*bcl*-2 activation).
Zollinger–Ellison syndrome	Gastrin-secreting tumor that is usually located in the pancreas. Causes recurrent ulcers. May be associated with MEN syndrome type I.
Multiple myeloma	Monoclonal plasma cell ("fried-egg" appearance) cancer that arises in the marrow and produces large amounts of IgG (55%) or IgA (25%). Most common 1° tumor arising within bone in adults. Destructive bone lesions and consequent hypercalcemia. Renal insufficiency, ↑ susceptibility to infection, and anemia. Ig light chains in urine (Bence Jones protein). Associated with primary amyloidosis and punched-out lytic bone lesions on x-ray. Characterized by monoclonal immunoglobulin spike (M protein) on serum protein electrophoresis.

Tumors of the adrenal medulla

Pheochromocytoma is the most common tumor of the adrenal medulla in adults.

Neuroblastoma is the most common tumor of the adrenal medulla in children, but it can occur anywhere along the sympathetic chain.

Pheochromocytomas may be associated with neurofibromatosis, MEN type II and MEN type III.

Pheochromocytoma

Most of these neoplasms secrete a combination of norepinephrine and epinephrine. Urinary VMA levels and plasma catecholamines are elevated. Associated with MEN type II and type III. Have a dusky color on gross pathology. Treated with α antagonists, especially phenoxybenzamine, a nonselective, **irreversible** α blocker.

Episodic hypercholinergic symptoms **(5 Ps):**

Pressure (elevated blood pressure)

Pain (headache)

Perspiration

Palpitations

Pallor/diaphoresis

Rule of 10s:

10% malignant

10% bilateral

10% extraadrenal

10% calcify

10% kids

10% familial

Also discussed **10**-fold more often than actually seen!

Lung cancer

Bronchogenic carcinoma

Tumors that arise **c**entrally:

1. **S**quamous cell carcinoma—clear link to smoking
2. **S**mall cell carcinoma—clear link to smoking. Associated with ectopic hormone production.

Tumors that arise peripherally:

1. Adenocarcinoma
2. Bronchioalveolar carcinoma (thought not to be related to smoking)
3. Large cell carcinoma—undifferentiated

Carcinoid tumor — Can cause carcinoid syndrome

Metastases — Very common

Lung cancer is the leading cause of cancer death.

Presentation: cough, hemoptysis, bronchial obstruction, "coin" lesion on x-ray.

Other clinical features:

1. Hoarseness
2. SVC syndrome
3. Pleural effusion
4. Paraneoplastic syndromes

Pancoast's tumor

Carcinoma that occurs in apex of lung and may affect cervical sympathetic plexus, causing Horner's syndrome.

Horner's syndrome: ptosis, miosis, anhydrosis.

Carcinoid syndrome

Rare syndrome caused by carcinoid tumors, especially those of the small bowel; the tumors secrete high levels of serotonin (5HT) that does not get metabolized by the liver due to liver metastases. Results in recurrent diarrhea, cutaneous flushing, asthmatic wheezing, and carcinoid heart disease. ↑ 5-HIAA in urine.

Rule of 1/3s:

1/3 metastasize

1/3 present with second malignancy

1/3 multiple

Treat with methysergide (5HT antagonist)

Metastasis to bone	These primary tumors metastasize to bone: **B**reast, **L**ung, **T**hyroid, **T**estes, **K**idney, **P**rostate. Metastasis from breast and prostate are most common. Metastatic bone tumors are far more common than 1° bone tumors.	**BLT**[2] with a **K**osher **P**ickle **L**ung = **L**ytic Prostate = blastic **B**reast = **B**oth lytic and blastic
Metastasis to brain	Primary tumors that metastasize to brain: lung (bronchogenic carcinoma) > breast > skin (melanoma) > kidney (renal cell carcinoma) > GI tract. Overall, approximately 50% of brain tumors are from metastases.	
Metastasis to liver	The liver is the second most common site of metastasis after the regional lymph nodes. Primary tumors that metastasize to the liver: colon (42%), stomach (23%), pancreas (21%), breast (14%), and lung (13%).	Metastatic liver tumors are far more common than primary liver tumors.
Hepatocellular carcinoma	Also called hepatoma. Most common primary malignant tumor of the liver in adults. Increased incidence of hepatocellular carcinoma is associated with hepatitis B/C, Wilson's disease, hemochromatosis, α_1-antitrypsin deficiency, alcoholic cirrhosis, and carcinogens (e.g., aflatoxin B1).	Hepatocellular carcinoma, like renal cell carcinoma, commonly spread by hematogenous dissemination.

Paraneoplastic syndromes

Cushing's syndrome	Mediated by ACTH or ACTH-like peptide. Causes include small cell lung carcinoma.
SIADH	Mediated by ADH or ANP. Causes include small cell lung carcinoma and intracranial neoplasms.
Hypercalcemia	Mediated by PTH-related peptide, TGFα, TNFα, IL-2. Causes include squamous cell lung carcinoma, renal carcinoma, breast carcinoma, and multiple myeloma.
Polycythemia	Mediated by erythropoietin. Causes include renal cell carcinoma (hypernephroma).
Myasthenia	Mechanism unclear. Causes include bronchogenic carcinoma.

Cancer epidemiology

	Male	Female	
Incidence	Prostate (32%) Lung (16%) Colon and rectum (12%)	Breast (32%) Lung (13%) Colon and rectum (13%)	Deaths from lung cancer have plateaued in males, but deaths continue to increase in females.
Mortality	Lung (33%) Prostate (13%)	Lung (23%) Breast (18%)	Cancer is the second leading cause of death in the U.S. (heart disease is first).

HIGH-YIELD FACTS

Pathology

Achalasia	Failure of relaxation of lower esophageal sphincter due to loss of myenteric (Auerbach's) plexus. Causes progressive dysphagia. Barium swallow shows dilated esophagus with an area of distal stenosis. Associated with an increased risk of esophageal carcinoma.	*A-chalasia* = absence of relaxation. 2° achalasia may arise from Chagas' disease. "Bird beak" on barium swallow.
Hirschsprung's disease	Congenital megacolon characterized by absence of parasympathetic ganglion cells (Auerbach's and Meissner's plexuses) on intestinal biopsy. Due to failure of neural crest cell migration. Presents as chronic constipation, early in life. Dilated portion of the colon proximal to the aganglionic segment resulting in a "transition zone."	Think of a giant spring that **sprung** in the colon.
Whipple's disease	Caused by *Tropheryma whippelli* and treated with antibiotics. Multisystem, affects mainly small bowel. Can also affect skin, joints, CNS, heart, liver, spleen. Small intestine infiltrated by PAS-positive macrophages containing rod-shaped bacilli. Symptoms: diarrhea, weight loss, polyarthritis, and lymphadenopathy. Affects mostly white adult males.	Mr. Whipple has diarrhea and can't squeeze the Charmin (arthritis). Surgical resection of terminal ileum can lead to vitamin B_{12} deficiency.

Gastritis

Type A	**A**utoimmune disorder characterized by **A**utoantibodies to parietal cells, pernicious **A**nemia, and **A**chlorhydria.	Type **A** = 4 **A**s
Type B	Caused by *H pylori* infection	Type **B** = a **B**ug, *H pylori*

Peptic ulcer disease

Gastric ulcer
Pain worse with meals
Weight loss
H pylori infection in 70%; NSAID use also implicated
Due to ↓ mucosal protection against gastric acid
↑ risk of malignancy

Duodenal ulcer
Pain lessens with meals
Almost 100% have *H pylori* infection
Due to ↑ gastric acid secretion or ↓ mucosal protection
No ↑ risk of malignancy

Potential complications include bleeding, perforation, and obstruction. *H pylori* infection can be treated with "triple therapy" (metronidazole, bismuth salicylate, and either amoxicillin or tetracycline) or new "double therapy" (omeprazole plus clarithromycin).

Crohn's disease	Inflammation mainly in the terminal ileum and cecum but can be anywhere along GI tract. Segmental involvement (skip lesions); transmural involvement; cobblestone mucosa; bowel wall thickening ("string sign" on x-ray); lymphoid infiltrates; noncaseating granulomas; linear ulcers, fissures, fistulas. Migratory arthritis, erythema nodosum.	Also called regional enteritis or ileitis. **Transmural** and **skip lesions** are key. Surgical resection of terminal ileum can lead to vitamin B_{12} deficiency.
Ulcerative colitis	Begins in rectum and extends proximally. Continuous involvement; microabscesses (crypt abscesses) and ulcers; pseudopolyps (inflamed mucosal tags). Inflammatory cell infiltration confined to mucosa and submucosa, not transmural. Pyoderma gangrenosum, sclerosing cholangitis.	*Colitis* = colon inflammation. Key is continuous cephalad progression; not transmural. Associated with increased risk of colorectal carcinoma and toxic megacolon.
Cirrhosis	Diffuse fibrosis of liver, destroys normal architecture. Nodular regeneration. Micronodular: nodules < 3 mm, uniform size. Macronodular: nodules > 3 mm, varied size. Causes portal hypertension, varices, ascites, splenomegaly, jaundice, and encephalopathy and is associated with an increased risk of hepatocellular carcinoma. Hematemesis, asterixis ("liver flap").	*Cirrho* (Greek) = tawny yellow. Micronodular cirrhosis is due to chronic insult (e.g., alcohol), whereas macronodular is usually due to an acute insult (e.g., postinfectious or drug-induced hepatitis).
Alcoholic hepatitis	Swollen and necrotic hepatocytes, neutrophil infiltration, Mallory bodies (hyaline), fatty change, and fibrosis around central vein. SGOT (AST) to SGPT (ALT) ratio is usually greater than 1.5.	
Wilson's disease	Due to failure of copper to enter circulation in the form of ceruloplasmin. Leads to copper accumulation, especially in liver, brain, cornea. Cirrhosis (micronodular to macronodular), Mallory bodies in liver. Neuronal degeneration in basal ganglia (especially putamen). Associated with dementia, asterixis (flapping tremor), and an increased risk of hepatocellular carcinoma.	↓ serum ceruloplasmin. Kayser–Fleischer rings (copper deposits in Descemet's membrane of the cornea). Treat with penicillamine.
Hemochromatosis	Increased iron deposition in many organs. Classic triad of micronodular pigment cirrhosis, "bronze" diabetes, skin pigmentation. Results in CHF and an increased risk of hepatocellular carcinoma. Disease may be a primary (autosomal recessive) disorder or secondary to chronic transfusion therapy. ↑ ferritin, ↑ transferrin saturation.	Total body iron may reach 50 g, enough to set off the metal detectors at airports. Treat with repeated phlebotomy, deferoxamine.

Hereditary hyperbilirubinemias

Crigler–Najjar syndrome, type I	Absent UDP-glucuronyl transferase. Presents early in life; patients die within a few years. Findings: jaundice, kernicterus (bilirubin deposition in brain), ↑ unconjugated bilirubin. Treatment: plasmapheresis and phototherapy.	Crigler-Najjar type I is a severe disease.
Gilbert's syndrome	Mildly ↓ UDP-glucuronyl transferase. Asymptomatic, but unconjugated bilirubin is elevated without overt hemolysis.	Gilbert's may represent a milder form.
Dubin–Johnson syndrome	Conjugated hyperbilirubinemia due to defective liver excretion. Grossly black liver.	Rotor's syndrome is similar, but less severe and does not cause black liver.

Gallstones

Gallstones	Form when solubilizing bile acids and lecithin are over-whelmed by increased cholesterol and/or bilirubin. Three types of stones: 1. Cholesterol stones: Associated with obesity, Crohn's disease, cystic fibrosis, advanced age, clofibrate, estrogens, multiparity, rapid weight loss, and Native American origin. 2. Mixed stones: Have both cholesterol and pigment components. 3. Pigment stones: Seen in patients with chronic RBC hemolysis, alcoholic cirrhosis, advanced age, and biliary infection. Diagnose with ultrasound. Treat with cholecystectomy.	Risk factors (5 Fs): 1. Female 2. Fat 3. Fertile 4. Forty 5. Flatulent Epigastric/RUQ pain, fever, nausea/emesis.

Acute pancreatitis

Acute pancreatitis	Abdominal pain: epigastric, radiates to the back. Elevated amylase, lipase. Can lead to DIC, ARDS, diffuse fat necrosis, and hypocalcemia.	Alcoholism Gallstones Trauma (children) Chronic pancreatitis is strongly associated with alcoholism.

Degenerative diseases

Cerebral cortex	**Alzheimer's disease:** Most common cause of dementia in the elderly. Associated with senile plaques (β amyloid core) and neurofibrillary tangles (abnormally phosphorylated tau protein). Familial form (10%) associated with genes on chromosomes 1, 11, 19 (Apo-E4 allele), and 21 (p-App gene).	Multi-infarct dementia is the second most common cause of dementia in the elderly.
	Pick's disease: Associated with Pick bodies and is specific for the frontal and temporal lobes.	
Basal ganglia and brainstem	**Huntington's disease:** Autosomal dominant inheritance, chorea, dementia. Lesion in caudate nucleus.	
	Parkinson's disease: Associated with Lewy bodies and depigmentation of the substantia nigra. Rare cases have been linked to exposure to MPTP, a contaminant in illicit street drugs.	Parkinsonian symptoms (**RAFT**): Cogwheel **R**igidity, **A**kinesia, **F**lat facies, and **T**remor (at rest).
Spinocerebellar	**Olivopontocerebellar atrophy**	
	Friedreich's ataxia	
Motor neuron	**Amyotrophic lateral sclerosis (ALS)**	ALS is associated with both lower and upper motor neuron signs. Commonly known as Lou Gehrig's disease (for famous New York Yankee baseball player who died of ALS).
	Werdnig–Hoffmann disease: Presents at birth as a "floppy baby"; tongue fasciculations.	
	Polio: Lower motor neuron signs.	

Demyelinating and dysmyelinating diseases

1. Multiple sclerosis (MS)—Higher prevalence in northern latitudes; periventricular plaques, preservation of axons, loss of oligodendrocytes, reactive astrocytic gliosis; ↑ protein (IgG) in CSF. Many patients have a relapsing–remitting course. Patients can present with optic neuritis (loss of vision), MLF syndrome (internuclear ophthalmoplegia), hemiparesis, hemisensory symptoms, or bladder/bowel incontinence.
2. Progressive multifocal leukoencephalopathy (PML)—Associated with JC virus and seen in 2–4% of AIDS patients (reactivation of latent viral infection).
3. Postinfectious encephalomyelitis
4. Metachromatic leukodystrophy (a sphingolipidosis)
5. Guillain-Barré syndrome—Inflammation and demyelination of peripheral nerves; ascending muscle weakness and paralysis beginning in distal lower extremities. In some cases it follows herpesvirus or *C jejuni* infection.

Seizures

Partial seizures: one area of the brain.
1. Simple partial (awareness intact): motor, sensory, autonomic, psychic.
2. Complex partial (impaired awareness).

Generalized seizures: diffuse.
1. Absence: blank stare (petit mal).
2. Myoclonic: quick, repetitive jerks.
3. Tonic-clonic: alternating stiffening and movement (grand mal).
4. Tonic: stiffening.
5. Atonic: "drop" seizures.

Epilepsy is a disorder of recurrent seizures.
Partial seizures can secondarily generalize.
Causes of seizures by age:
Children: genetic, infection, trauma, congenital, metabolic.
Adults: tumors, trauma, stroke, infection.
Elderly: stroke, tumor, trauma, metabolic, infection.
Febrile seizures are not epilepsy.

Wernicke–Korsakoff syndrome

Caused by vitamin B_1 (thiamine) deficiency in alcoholics. Classically may present with triad of psychosis, ophthalmoplegia, and ataxia (Wernicke's encephalopathy). May progress to memory loss, confabulation, confusion (Korsakoff's syndrome; irreversible). Associated with periventricular hemorrhage/necrosis, especially in mamillary bodies. Treatment: IV vitamin B_1 (thiamine).

Broca's versus Wernicke's aphasia

Broca's is nonfluent aphasia with intact comprehension (expressive aphasia). Wernicke's is fluent aphasia with impaired comprehension (receptive aphasia).
Broca's area = inferior frontal gyrus
Wernicke's area = superior temporal gyrus

BROca's is **BRO**ken speech; Wernicke's is **W**ordy but makes no sense.

Horner's syndrome

Sympathectomy of face:
1. Ptosis (slight drooping of eyelid)
2. Miosis (pupil constriction)
3. Anhidrosis (absence of sweating) and flushing (rubor) of affected side of face

Associated with Pancoast's tumor.

Arnold–Chiari malformation

Congenital protrusion of cerebellum and medulla through foramen magnum. Associated with lumbar meningomyelocele and obstructive hydrocephalus.

Syringomyelia

Softening and cavitation around central canal of spinal cord. Crossing fibers of spinothalamic tract are damaged. Bilateral loss of pain and temperature sensation in upper extremities with preservation of touch sensation.

Syrinx (Greek) = tube as in syringe.
Often presents in patients with Arnold-Chiari malformation.

Tabes dorsalis

Degeneration of dorsal columns and dorsal roots due to 3° syphilis, resulting in impaired proprioception and locomotor ataxia. Associated with Charcot joints, shooting (lightning) pain, Argyll-Robertson pupils, and absence of deep tendon reflexes.

Tabes (Latin) = wasting away.

Osteoarthritis

Destruction of articular cartilage (primarily weight-bearing joints), Heberden's nodes, eburnation, subchondral bone formation, sclerosis, osteophytes. Caused by wear and tear of joints. Classically hurts in evening after joint use, improves with rest. Commonly in older patients. No systemic symptoms.

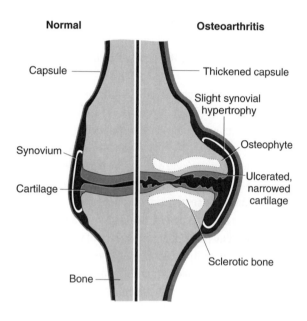

Rheumatoid arthritis

Pannus formation in joints (metacarpophalangeal, proximal interphalangeal); ulnar deviation, subluxation; subcutaneous rheumatoid nodules at pressure points (e.g., elbows); morning stiffness (decreased pain with use); symmetric involvement; 80% have positive rheumatoid factor (anti-IgG antibody). More common in females and is associated with HLA-DR4. Associated with systemic symptoms: fever, fatigue, pleuritis, pericarditis.

Gout

Precipitation of monosodium urate crystals into joints due to hyperuricemia. Asymmetric joint distribution. Favored manifestation is painful MTP joint in big toe joint (podagra). Crystals are needle-shaped and negatively birefringent. Tophus formation. Hyperuricemia can be caused by Lesch-Nyhan disease, PRPP excess, decreased excretion of uric acid, or G6P deficiency. Treatment is allopurinol, probenecid, colchicine, and NSAIDs. Gout is associated with the use of thiazide diuretics, because they competitively inhibit the secretion of uric acid. More common in men.

HIGH-YIELD FACTS

Pathology

Systemic lupus erythematosus

90% are female, most between ages 14 and 45. Fever, fatigue, weight loss. Joint pain, malar rash, pleuritis, pericarditis, nonbacterial verrucous endocarditis, Raynaud's phenomenon. **Wire loop** lesions in kidney with immune complex deposition (with nephrotic syndrome); death from renal failure and infections. False positives on syphilis tests (RPR/VDRL). Lab tests detect presence of:

1. Antinuclear antibodies (ANA): sensitive, but not specific for SLE
2. Antibodies to double-stranded DNA (anti-ds DNA): very specific
3. Anti-Smith antibodies (anti-Sm): very specific

Lupus (Latin) = wolf, a reference to the malar rash (on cheeks) causing wolflike facies. Also, **wire loopus** erythematosus.

Most common and severe in black females.

Drugs (procainamide, INH, hydralazine) can produce an SLE-like syndrome that is commonly reversible.

Sarcoidosis

Associated with restrictive lung disease, bilateral hilar lymphadenopathy, erythema nodosum, Bell's palsy, epithelial granulomas containing microscopic Schaumann and asteroid bodies, uveoparotitis, and hypercalcemia (due to elevated conversion of vit. D to its active form in epithelioid macrophages). Also associated with immune-mediated, widespread non-caseating granulomas and elevated serum ACE levels. Common in black females.

Sarko (Greek) = flesh, describing exuberant noncaseating granulomas.

GRUELING:
Granulomas
Rheumatoid arthritis
Uveitis
Erythema nodosum
Lymphadenopathy
Interstitial fibrosis
Negative TB test
Gammaglobulinemia

Scleroderma (progressive systemic sclerosis—PSS)

Excessive fibrosis and collagen deposition throughout the body. 75% female. Commonly sclerosis of skin but also of cardiovascular and GI systems, kidney. Two major categories:

1. Diffuse scleroderma: widespread skin involvement, rapid progression, early visceral involvement. Associated with anti-Scl-70 antibody.
2. **CREST** syndrome: **C**alcinosis, **R**aynaud's phenomenon, **E**sophageal dysmotility, **S**clerodactyly, and **T**elangiectasia. Limited skin involvement, often confined to fingers and face. More benign clinical course. Associated with anticentromere antibody.

Goodpasture's syndrome

Findings: pulmonary hemorrhages, renal lesions, hemoptysis, hematuria, anemia, proliferative glomerulonephritis, crescents.

Anti-glomerular basement membrane antibodies produce linear staining on immunofluorescence.

There are two **G**ood **P**astures for this disease: **G**lomerulus and **P**ulmonary. Also, a type **II** hypersensitivity disease.

Most common in men 20–40 yo.

HIGH-YIELD FACTS

Pathology

Reiter's syndrome	A seronegative spondyloarthropathy. Strong HLA-B27 link. Classic triad:
	   1. Urethritis
	   2. Conjunctivitis and anterior uveitis
	   3. Arthritis
	 Has a strong predilection for males.
		"Can't see (anterior uveitis/ conjunctivitis), can't pee (urethritis), can't climb a tree (arthritis)."

Sjögren's syndrome	Classic triad: dry eyes (conjunctivitis, xerophthalmia), dry mouth (dysphagia, xerostomia), arthritis. Parotid enlargement, ↑ risk of B-cell lymphoma. Predominantly affects females between 40 and 60 years of age.	Associated with rheumatoid arthritis. Sicca: dry eyes, dry mouth, nasal and vaginal dryness, chronic bronchitis, reflux esophagitis.
Reye's syndrome	Rare, often fatal childhood hepatoencephalopathy. Findings: fatty liver (microvesicular fatty change), hypoglycemia, coma. Associated with viral infection (especially VZV and influenza B) and salicylates; thus aspirin is no longer recommended for children (use acetaminophen).	Encephalopathy and liver failure. "Don't give your baby a baby aspirin."

PATHOLOGY—VASCULAR/CARDIAC

Intracranial hemorrhage

Epidural hematoma	Rupture of middle meningeal artery, often 2° to fracture of temporal bone.
Subdural hematoma	Rupture of bridging veins. Venous bleeding (less pressure) with delayed onset of symptoms. Seen in elderly individuals, alcoholics, blunt trauma.
Subarachnoid hemorrhage	Rupture of an aneurysm (usually berry aneurysm) or an AVM. Patients complain of "worst headache ever." Bloody or xanthochromic spinal tap.
Parenchymal hematoma	Caused by hypertension, amyloid angiopathy, and tumor.

Berry aneurysms	Berry aneurysms occur at the bifurcations in the circle of Willis. Most common site is bifurcation of the anterior communicating artery. Rupture (most common complication) leads to hemorrhagic stroke. Associated with adult polycystic kidney disease.	Red **b**erries at **b**ifurcations **b**ulge and **b**low out.
Infarcts: red versus pale	Red (hemorrhagic) infarcts occur in loose tissues with collaterals, such as lungs, intestine, or brain, or following reperfusion. Pale infarcts occur in solid tissues with single blood supply, such as heart, kidney, and spleen.	**RE**d = **RE**perfusion.

Atherosclerosis

Disease of elastic arteries and large and medium-sized muscular arteries.

Risk factors: smoking, hypertension, diabetes mellitus, hyperlipidemia.

Progression: fatty streaks → fibrous plaque → complex atheromas.

Complications: aneurysms, ischemia, infarcts, peripheral vascular disease, thrombus, emboli.

Location: abdominal aorta > coronary artery > popliteal artery > carotid artery.

Symptoms: angina, claudication, but can be asymptomatic.

Ischemic heart disease

Possible manifestations:

1. Angina: Stable: mostly 2° to atherosclerosis (retrosternal chest pain with exertion)

   Prinzmetal's variant: occurs at rest, 2° to coronary artery spasm

   Unstable/crescendo: thrombosis in a branch (worsening chest pain)

2. Myocardial infarction—most often occurs in CAD involving the left anterior descending artery

3. Sudden cardiac death—death from cardiac causes within 1 hour of onset of symptoms, most commonly due to a lethal arrhythmia

4. Chronic ischemic heart disease—progressive onset of congestive heart failure over many years due to chronic ischemic myocardial damage

Evolution of MI

Coronary artery occlusion: LAD > RCA > circumflex.

Symptoms: severe retrosternal pain, pain in left arm and/or jaw, shortness of breath, fatigue, adrenergic symptoms.

A. First day

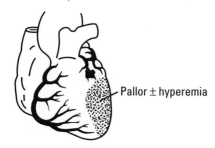

Occluded artery

Infarct

Pallor

Coagulative necrosis leads to release of contents of necrotic cells into bloodstream

Muscle shows minimal changes

B. 2 to 4 days

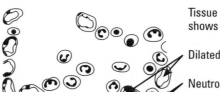

Pallor ± hyperemia

Tissue surrounding infarct shows acute inflammation

Dilated vessels (hyperemia)

Neutrophil emigration

Muscle shows microscopic changes of coagulative necrosis

C. 5 to 10 days

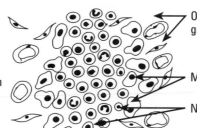

Hyperemic border; central yellow-brown softening— maximally yellow and soft by 10 days

Outer zone (ingrowth of granulation tissue)

Macrophage zone

Neutrophil zone

D. 7 weeks

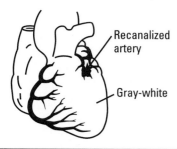

Recanalized artery

Gray-white

Contracted scar complete

Diagnosis of MI

CK-MB is test of choice in the first 24 hours post-MI.

LDH_1 is test of choice from 2 to 7 days post-MI.

AST is nonspecific and can be found in cardiac, liver, and skeletal muscle cells. EKG changes can include ST elevation (transmural ischemia) and Q waves (transmural infarct).

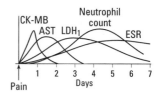

CK-MB AST LDH_1 Neutrophil count ESR

1 2 3 4 5 6 7

Pain

Days

MI complications

1. Cardiac arrhythmia (90%)
2. LV failure and pulmonary edema (60%)
3. Thromboembolism: mural thrombus
4. Cardiogenic shock (large infarct: high risk of mortality)
5. Rupture of ventricular free wall, interventricular septum, papillary muscle (4–7 days post-MI)
6. Fibrinous pericarditis: friction rub (3–5 days post-MI)
7. Dressler's syndrome: autoimmune phenomenon resulting in fibrinous pericarditis (several weeks post-MI)

Cardiomyopathies

Dilated (congestive) cardiomyopathy	Most common cardiomyopathy (90% of cases). Etiologies include EtOH toxicity, postviral myocarditis by coxsackievirus B, doxorubicin toxicity, beriberi, peripartum cardiomyopathy, chronic cocaine use. Heart dilates and looks like a balloon on chest x-ray.	Systolic dysfunction ensues.
Hypertrophic cardiomyopathy	Hypertrophy often asymmetric and involving the intraventricular septum. 50% of cases are familial and are inherited as an AD trait. Cause of sudden death in young athletes. Walls of LV are thickened and chamber becomes banana-shaped on echocardiogram.	Also referred to as IHSS, or idiopathic hypertrophic subaortic stenosis. Diastolic dysfunction ensues.
Restrictive/obliterative cardiomyopathy	Major causes include sarcoidosis, amyloidosis, endocardial fibroelastosis, and endomyocardial fibrosis (Löffler's).	

CHF

Abnormality	Cause
Ankle, sacral edema	RV failure → increased venous pressure → fluid transudation.
Hepatomegaly	Increased central venous pressure → increased resistance to portal flow. Rarely leads to "cardiac cirrhosis."
Pulmonary congestion	LV failure → increased pulmonary venous pressure → pulmonary venous distention and transudation of fluid.
Dyspnea on exertion	Failure of left ventricular output to increase during exercise.
Paroxysmal nocturnal dyspnea, pulmonary edema	Failure of left heart output to keep up with right heart output → acute rise in pulmonary venous and capillary pressure → transudation of fluid.
Orthopnea (shortness of breath when supine)	Pooling of blood in lungs in supine position adds volume to congested pulmonary vascular system; increased venous return not put out by left ventricle.
Cardiac dilation	Greater ventricular end-diastolic volume.

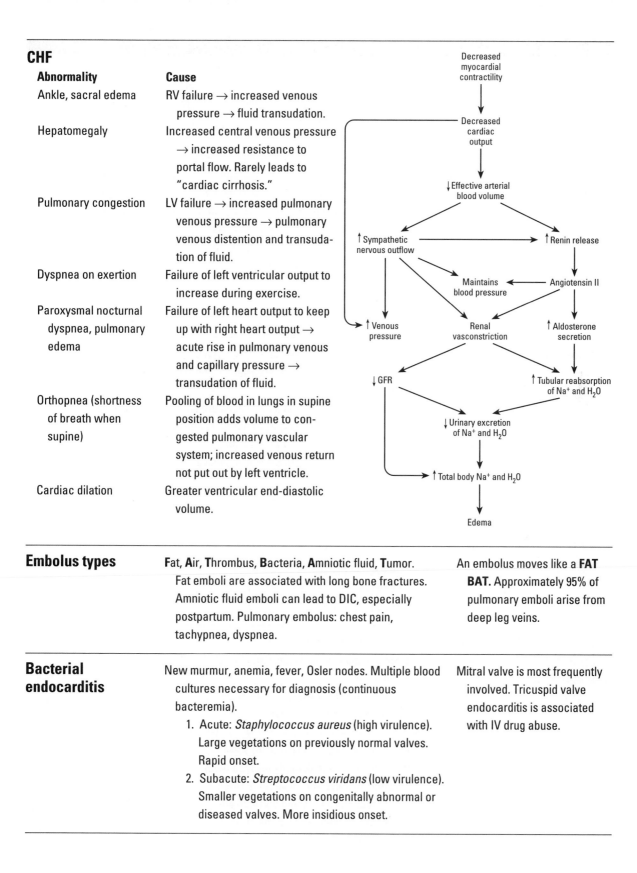

Embolus types	Fat, **A**ir, **T**hrombus, **B**acteria, **A**mniotic fluid, **T**umor. Fat emboli are associated with long bone fractures. Amniotic fluid emboli can lead to DIC, especially postpartum. Pulmonary embolus: chest pain, tachypnea, dyspnea.	An embolus moves like a **FAT BAT.** Approximately 95% of pulmonary emboli arise from deep leg veins.
Bacterial endocarditis	New murmur, anemia, fever, Osler nodes. Multiple blood cultures necessary for diagnosis (continuous bacteremia). 1. Acute: *Staphylococcus aureus* (high virulence). Large vegetations on previously normal valves. Rapid onset. 2. Subacute: *Streptococcus viridans* (low virulence). Smaller vegetations on congenitally abnormal or diseased valves. More insidious onset.	Mitral valve is most frequently involved. Tricuspid valve endocarditis is associated with IV drug abuse.

Marantic/ thrombotic endocarditis (nonbacterial)

Fibrin precipitation on valve leaflets, 2° to metastasis, renal failure, or sepsis. Vegetations are small and sterile but can produce emboli and infarctions. Often occurs in patients with deep venous thromboses and/or pulmonary emboli.

Rheumatic fever/ rheumatic heart disease

Rheumatic fever is a consequence of pharyngeal infection with group A, β-hemolytic streptococci. Multiple episodes can cause rheumatic heart disease, which affects heart valves: mitral > aortic >> tricuspid. Associated with Aschoff bodies, migratory polyarthritis, erythema marginatum, elevated ASO titers.

PHever follows **PH**aryngeal infection. High-pressure valves are affected most.
PECCS:
    Polyarthritis (migratory)
    Erythema marginatum
    Carditis
    Chorea
    Subcutaneous nodules

Pericarditis

Causes: infection (viruses, TB, pyogenic bacteria, often by direct spread from lung or mediastinal lymph nodes), ischemic heart disease, chronic renal failure → uremia, and connective tissue disease.

Effusions are usually serous; hemorrhagic effusions are associated with TB and malignancy. Renal failure causes serous or fibrinous effusions.

Findings: pericardial pain, friction rub, EKG changes.

Can resolve without scarring or lead to chronic adhesive or chronic constrictive pericarditis.

Pancytopenia

Pancytopenia is associated with the following pathologic conditions:
1. AML
2. Recurrent ovarian cancer
3. Aplastic anemia
4. Drug reactions

Diagnosis of congenital hematologic defects

Heinz bodies are seen in G6PD deficiency.

Ham's test is used to diagnose paroxysmal nocturnal hemoglobinuria (PNH).

Osmotic fragility test is used to diagnose hereditary spherocytosis (treat with splenectomy).

Syphilitic heart disease

Tertiary syphilis disrupts the vasa vasorum of aorta via endarteritis obliterans and disrupts elastica (with consequent dilation of aorta and valve ring). Often affects the aortic root and ascending aorta. Associated with a tree-bark appearance of the aorta.

Can result in aneurysm of ascending aorta or aortic arch and aortic valve incompetence.

Buerger's disease	Known as smoker's disease and thromboangiitis obliterans; idiopathic, segmental, thrombosing vasculitis of intermediate and small peripheral arteries and veins. Findings: intermittent claudication, superficial nodular phlebitis, cold sensitivity (Raynaud's phenomenon), severe pain in affected part; may lead to gangrene. Treatment: quit smoking.	
Takayasu's arteritis	Known as "pulseless disease": thickening of aortic arch and/or proximal great vessels, causing weak pulses in upper extremities and ocular disturbances. Associated with an elevated ESR. Primarily affects young Asian females. Fever, night sweats, myalgia, arthritis, skin nodules.	Affects medium and large arteries.
Temporal arteritis	Most common vasculitis that affects medium and small arteries, usually branches of carotid artery. Findings include unilateral headache, jaw claudication, impaired vision (occlusion of ophthalmic artery, which can lead to blindness). Half of patients have systemic involvement and syndrome of polymyalgia rheumatica. Associated with elevated ESR.	**Tem**poral = signs near **Tem**ples. ESR is markedly elevated. Also known as giant cell arteritis. Affects elderly females.
Budd–Chiari syndrome	Occlusion of IVC or hepatic veins with centrilobular congestion and necrosis, leading to congestive liver disease (hepatomegaly, ascites, abdominal pain, and eventual liver failure). Associated with polycythemia vera, pregnancy, hepatocellular carcinoma.	

Glomerular pathology

Nephritic syndrome: Hematuria, hypertension, oliguria.

1. Acute poststreptococcal glomerulonephritis
   LM: glomeruli enlarged and hypercellular; neutrophils.
   EM: subepithelial humps. IF: granular pattern.

   Most frequently seen in children. Peripheral, periorbital edema. Resolves spontaneously.

2. Rapidly progressive (crescentic) glomerulonephritis
   LM and IF: crescent-moon shape.

   Rapid course to renal failure from one of many causes.

3. Goodpasture's syndrome
   IF: linear pattern.

   Hemoptysis, hematuria.

4. Membranoproliferative glomerulonephritis
   EM: subendothelial humps.

   Slowly progresses to renal failure.

5. IgA nephropathy (Berger's disease)
   IF and EM: mesangial deposits of IgA.

   Mild disease.

Nephrotic syndrome: Massive proteinuria, hypoalbuminemia, generalized edema, hyperlipidemia.

1. Membranous glomerulonephritis
   LM: diffuse capillary thickening. IF: granular pattern.

   Most common cause of adult nephrotic syndrome.

2. Minimal change disease (lipoid nephrosis)
   LM: normal glomeruli. EM: foot process effacement (fusion).

   Most common cause of childhood nephrotic syndrome.

3. Focal segmental glomerular sclerosis with hyalinosis
   LM: segmental sclerosis and hyalinosis.

   More severe disease in HIV patients.

4. Diabetic nephropathy
   LM: Kimmelstiel-Wilson lesions.

(**LM** = light microscopy; **EM** = electron microscopy; **IF** = immunofluorescence)

Acidosis/alkalosis

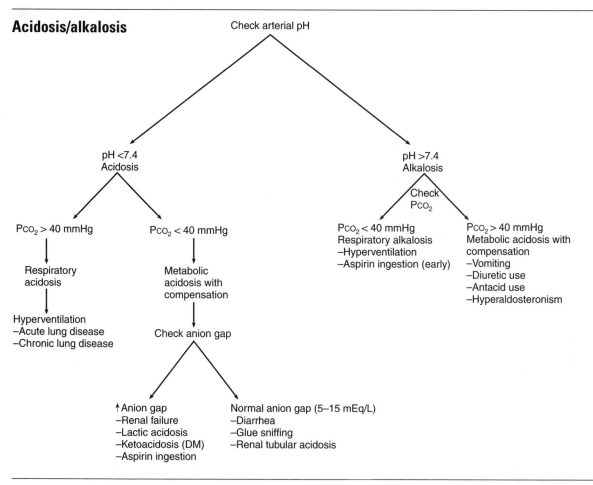

Check arterial pH

pH <7.4
Acidosis

pH >7.4
Alkalosis

Check Pco₂

Pco_2 > 40 mmHg

Pco_2 < 40 mmHg

Pco_2 < 40 mmHg
Respiratory alkalosis
–Hyperventilation
–Aspirin ingestion (early)

Pco_2 > 40 mmHg
Metabolic acidosis with compensation
–Vomiting
–Diuretic use
–Antacid use
–Hyperaldosteronism

Respiratory acidosis

Metabolic acidosis with compensation

Hyperventilation
–Acute lung disease
–Chronic lung disease

Check anion gap

↑Anion gap
–Renal failure
–Lactic acidosis
–Ketoacidosis (DM)
–Aspirin ingestion

Normal anion gap (5–15 mEq/L)
–Diarrhea
–Glue sniffing
–Renal tubular acidosis

Cretinism

Endemic cretinism occurs wherever endemic goiter is prevalent (lack of dietary iodine); sporadic cretinism is caused by defect in T4 formation or developmental failure in thyroid formation.

Findings: pot-bellied, pale, puffy-faced child with protruding umbilicus and protuberant tongue.

Cretin means Christ-like (French *chrétien*). Those affected were considered so mentally retarded as to be incapable of sinning. Still common in China.

Hydatidiform mole

A pathologic ovum ("empty egg"—ovum with no DNA) resulting in cystic swelling of chorionic villi and proliferation of chorionic epithelium (trophoblast). Most common precursor of choriocarcinoma. High β-**HCG**. "Honeycombed uterus," **"cluster of grapes"** appearance. Genotype of a complete mole is 46,XX and is purely paternal in origin (no maternal chromosomes). Partial mole is commonly triploid or tetraploid.

Asbestosis

Diffuse pulmonary interstitial fibrosis caused by inhaled asbestos fibers. Increased risk of pleural mesothelioma and bronchogenic carcinoma. Long latency. Ferruginous bodies in lung (asbestos fibers coated with hemosiderin). Ivory-white pleural plaques.

Smokers have synergistically higher risk of cancer.
Seen in ship builders and plumbers.

Neonatal respiratory distress syndrome

Surfactant deficiency leading to ↑ surface tension, resulting in alveolar collapse. Surfactant is made by type II cells most abundantly after 35th wk gestation. The lecithin-to-sphingomyelin ratio in the amniotic fluid, a measure of lung maturity, is usually less than 1.5 in neonatal respiratory distress syndrome.

Surfactant: dipalmitoyl phosphatidylcholine lecithin.

Prevention: maternal steroids before birth; artificial surfactant for infant.

Bleeding disorders

Platelet abnormalities	Mucous membrane bleeding Petechiae Purpura Prolonged bleeding time	Causes include ITP, TTP, drugs, and DIC (↑ fibrin split products)
Coagulation factor defects	Hemarthroses (bleeding into joints) Easy bruising Prolonged PT and/or aPTT	Coagulopathies include hemophilia A (factor VIII deficiency), hemophilia B (factor IX deficiency), and von Willebrand's disease (nasal, sinus, GI bleeds).

Hypothyroidism and hyperthyroidism

Hypothyroidism	Cold intolerance, hyperactivity, weight gain, fatigue, lethargy, ↓ appetite, constipation, amenorrhea, weakness, ↓ reflexes, myxedema (facial/periorbital), and dry, cool skin.	↑ TSH (sensitive test for 1° hypothyroidism), ↓ total T4, ↓ free T4, ↓ T3 uptake
Hyperthyroidism	Heat intolerance, hyperactivity, weight loss, chest pain/palpitations, arrhythmias, diarrhea, ↑ reflexes, and warm, dry skin.	↓ TSH (if 1°), ↑ total T4, ↑ free T4, ↑ T3 uptake
Graves' disease	Ophthalmopathy (proptosis, EOM swelling), pretibial myxedema.	An autoimmune hyperthyroidism with thyroid stimulating/TSH receptor antibodies

Osteoporosis

	Reduction of bone mass in spite of normal bone mineralization.	Blacks are affected more often than Asians, who are affected more often than whites.
Type I	Postmenopausal (10–15 years after menopause); ↑ bone resorption due to ↓ estrogen levels.	Vertebal crush fractures: acute back pain, loss of height, kyphosis.
Type II	Senile osteoporosis—affects men and women > 70 years.	Distal wrist (Colles') fractures, vertebral wedge fractures.

SIADH	Syndrome of inappropriate antidiuretic hormone secretion:	Causes include:
	Excessive water retention	Ectopic ADH (small cell lung cancer)
	Hyponatremia	CNS disorders
	Serum hypo-osmolarity with urine osmolarity > serum osmolarity	Pulmonary disease
	Very low serum sodium levels can lead to seizures.	Drugs

PATHOLOGY—FINDINGS

Aortic insufficiency	Pistol shot sound heard over femoral vessels (Traube sign). Water hammer pulse over carotid artery (Corrigan pulse). Quincke's capillary pulsations (pressure on fingernail results in visible pulsations).	
Argyll–Robertson pupil	Argyll–Robertson pupil constricts with accommodation but not reactive to light. Pathognomonic for 3° syphilis.	**A**rgyll–**R**obertson **P**upil. **ARP: A**ccommodation **R**esponse **P**resent. **PRA: P**upillary (light) **R**eflex **A**bsent.
Aschoff body	Aschoff bodies (granuloma with giant cells) and Anitschkow's cells (activated histiocytes) are found in rheumatic heart disease.	Think of two **RH**ussians with **RH**eumatic heart disease (Aschoff and Anitschkow).
Auer bodies (rods)	Auer rods are cytoplasmic inclusions in granulocytes and myeloblasts. Primarily seen in acute promyelocytic leukemia.	
Casts	Casts of nephron: RBC casts = glomerular inflammation, ischemia, or malignant hypertension. WBC casts = inflammation in renal interstitium, tubules, and glomeruli. Hyaline casts often seen in normal urine.	Presence of casts indicates that hematuria/pyuria is of renal origin.
Erythrocyte sedimentation rate	Very nonspecific test that measures acute-phase reactants. Dramatically increased with infection, malignancy, connective tissue disease. Also increased with pregnancy, inflammatory disease, anemia. Decreased with sickle cell anemia, polycythemia, congestive heart failure.	Simple, cheap, but nonspecific. Should not be used for asymptomatic screening; can be used to diagnose and monitor temporal arteritis and polymyalgia rheumatica.
Ghon complex	TB granulomas with lobar or perihilar lymph node involvement (Ghon focus and lymph node involvement). Reflects primary infection or exposure.	Ghon complex is the lung and the node; Ghon focus is just the focus of lung involvement.

Hyperlipidemia signs

Atheromata = plaques in blood vessel walls.

Xanthelasma = Plaques or nodules composed of lipid-laden histiocytes in the skin, especially the eyelids.

Tendinous xanthoma = lipid deposit in tendon, especially Achilles.

Corneal arcus = lipid deposit in cornea, nonspecific (arcus senilis).

Psammoma bodies

Laminated, concentric, calcific spherules seen in:

1. Papillary adenocarcinoma of thyroid   **P**apillary (thyroid)
2. Serous papillary cystadenocarcinoma of ovary   **S**erous (ovary)

       a

3. Meningioma   **M**eningioma
4. Malignant mesothelioma   **M**esotheli**oma**

RBC forms

Biconcave = normal.

Spherocytes = hereditary spherocytosis, autoimmune hemolysis.

Elliptocyte = hereditary elliptocytosis.

Macro-ovalocyte = megaloblastic anemia, marrow failure.

Helmet cell, schistocyte = DIC, traumatic hemolysis.

Sickle cell = sickle cell anemia.

Reed-Sternberg cells

Distinctive tumor giant cell seen in Hodgkin's disease; large cell that is binucleate or bilobed with the 2 halves as mirror images ("owl's eyes"). Necessary but not sufficient for a diagnosis of Hodgkin's disease.

There are 4 types of Hodgkin's disease; nodular sclerosis variant is the only one seen in women > men (excellent prognosis).

Target cell

Most commonly indicates hemolytic anemia, thalassemia, hemoglobinopathies, sickle cell anemia, or liver disease.

Looks like a shooting target (bull's-eye).

Roth's spots

White spots of coagulated fibrin in retina seen on funduscopic exam. Associated with bacterial endocarditis.

Sentinel loop (x-ray)

Represents a distended bowel loop suggestive of a localized ileus secondary to an inflamed abdominal viscus, as in pancreatitis, appendicitis, cholecystitis.

Virchow's (sentinel) node

A firm supraclavicular lymph node, often on left side, easily palpable (can be detected by medical students), also known as "jugular gland." Presumptive evidence of malignant visceral neoplasm (classically stomach).

Anemia

Type	Etiology
Microcytic, hypochromic	Iron deficiency: ↑ transferrin, ↓ ferritin, ↓ serum iron
	Anemia of chronic disease: ↓ transferrin, ↑ ferritin, ↓ serum iron, ↑ storage iron in marrow macrophages
	Thalassemias
	Lead poisoning
Macrocytic	Megaloblastic: Vitamin B_{12}/folate deficiency
	Drugs that block DNA synthesis (e.g., sulfa drugs, AZT)
	Marked reticulocytosis
Normocytic, normochromic	Hemorrhage
	Enzyme defects (e.g., G6PD deficiency, PK deficiency)
	RBC membrane defects (e.g., hereditary spherocytosis)
	Bone marrow disorders (e.g., aplastic anemia, leukemia)
	Hemoglobinopathies (e.g., sickle cell disease)
	Autoimmune hemolytic anemia

Vit. B_{12} and folate deficiencies are associated with hypersegmented PMNs. Unlike folate deficiency, vit. B_{12} deficiency is associated with neurologic problems.

Serum haptoglobin and serum LDH are used to determine RBC hemolysis. Direct Coombs' test is used to distinguish between immune vs. nonimmune mediated RBC hemolysis.

Peripheral blood smears

Normal

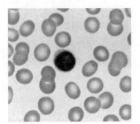

—normal

Microcytic hypochromic anemia

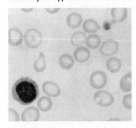

—normally 2° to **IRON DEFICIENCY**
—low serum ferritin
—elevated serum iron binding capacity

Megaloblastic anemia

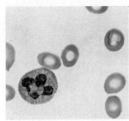

—2° to **FOLATE or B$_{12}$ deficiency**
—hypersegmented (5–7 lobes) PMN's
—large red blood cells (MCV > 100)
—**never** give folate to a patient who is deficient in B$_{12}$
—**PERNICIOUS ANEMIA**—autoimmune disease which causes B$_{12}$ deficiency by depleting
    INTRINSIC FACTOR, which is needed to absorb B$_{12}$ in **terminal ileum**

Target cells

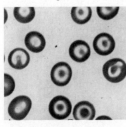

—thalassemia
—hemoglobin C disease
—liver disease

Hemoglobin SS with sickle cells

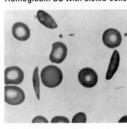

—**Hb^s**—β-globin GLU → VAL at #6; 8% of US blacks are Hb^s carriers
—cells will sickle 2° to hypoxia, dehydration, and ↑ blood viscosity
—anemia
—vaso-occlusive crises +/– chest pain
—aplastic crises (B19 virus)
—splenic sequestration crises
—strokes

Enzyme markers

Serum enzyme	Major diagnostic use
Aminotransferases (AST and ALT)	Myocardial infarction (AST only)
	Viral hepatitis (ALT > AST)
	Alcoholic hepatitis (AST > ALT)
Amylase	Acute pancreatitis, mumps
Ceruloplasmin (decreased)	Wilson's disease
CPK (creatine phosphokinase)	Muscle disorders (e.g., DMD) and myocardial infarction (CPK-MB)
γ-glutamyl transpeptidase	Various liver diseases
LDH-1 (lactate dehydrogenase fraction 1)	Myocardial infarction (LDH1 > LDH2)
Lipase	Acute pancreatitis

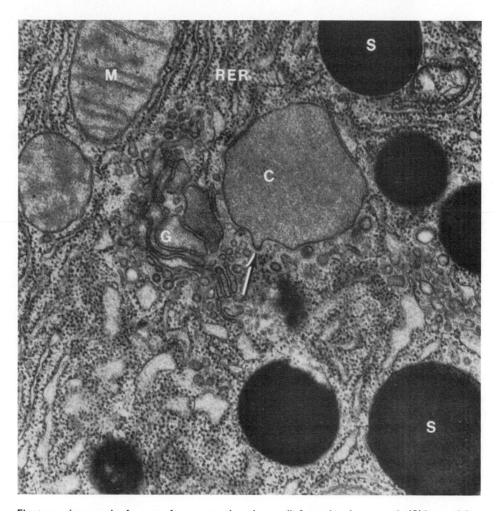

Electron micrograph of a part of a pancreatic acinar cell. A condensing vacuole (C) is receiving secretory product (arrow) from the Golgi complex (G). M, mitochondrion; RER, rough endoplasmic reticulum; S, mature condensed secretory (zymogen) granule.

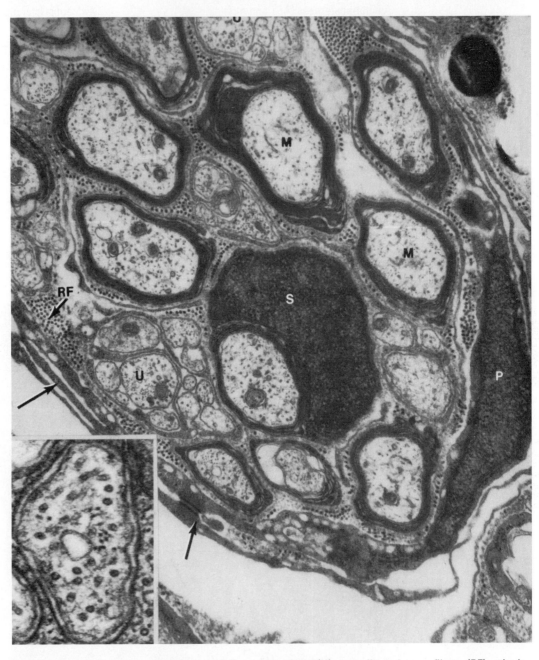

Electron micrograph of a peripheral nerve. (M) myelinated and (U) unmyelinated nerve fibers. (RF) reticular fibers (part of the endoneurium), (S) Schwann cell nucleus, (P, arrows) perineurial cells. Inset shows part of an axon with numerous neurofilaments.

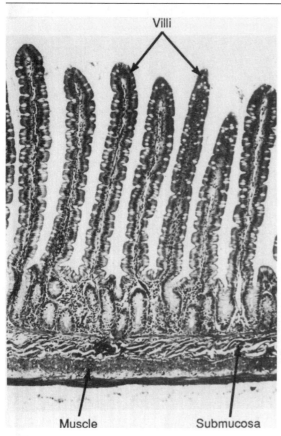

Photomicrograph of the small intestine.

An example of acute inflammatory response, with many polymorphonuclear cells mixed with strands of fibrin. Some macrophages are also present.

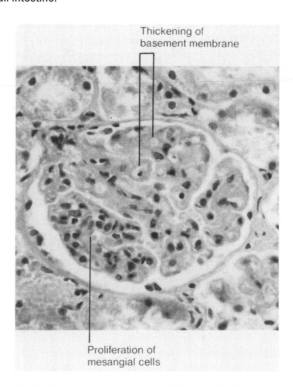

Systemic lupus erythematosus; kidney pathology.

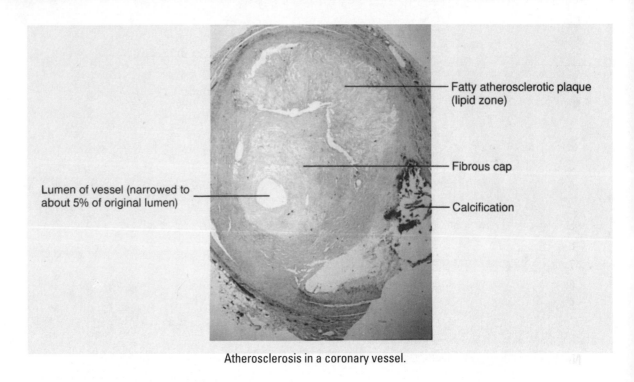

Fatty atherosclerotic plaque (lipid zone)

Fibrous cap

Calcification

Lumen of vessel (narrowed to about 5% of original lumen)

Atherosclerosis in a coronary vessel.

Congenital
1. Maternal complications of birth (e.g., Sheehan's syndrome, puerperal infection).
2. Failure to thrive: common causes.

Neoplasia
1. Bone and cartilage tumors (e.g., osteosarcoma, giant cell tumor, Ewing's sarcoma).
2. Clinical features of lymphomas (Burkitt's and other non-Hodgkin's lymphomas).
3. Risk factors for common carcinomas (e.g., lung, breast).
4. Prostate cancer: epidemiology, presentation (most commonly in peripheral region/posterior lobe), screening, treatment.
5. Chemical carcinogens (e.g., vinyl chloride, nitrosamines, aflatoxin).
6. Malignancies associated with pulmonary pneumoconiosis (e.g., asbestos, silicosis).
7. AIDS-associated neoplasms (Kaposi's sarcoma, B-cell lymphoma).
8. Pituitary tumors (e.g., prolactinomas) and other sellar lesions (e.g., craniopharyngioma).
9. Tumors of the mouth, pharynx, and larynx (e.g., vocal cord tumors in smokers).

Nervous System
1. Hydrocephalus: types (e.g., communicating, obstructive), sequelae.
2. CNS manifestations of viral infections (e.g., HIV, HSV).
3. Spinal muscular atrophies (e.g., Werdnig-Hoffmann disease, ALS).

Rheumatic/Autoimmune
1. Polyarteritis nodosa, Wegener's granulomatosis.
2. Transplant rejection (hyperacute, acute, graft versus host disease).
3. Differences between rheumatoid arthritis and graft versus host disease.
4. Psoriasis: skin/joint involvement.

Vascular/Hematology
1. Hypertension: essential versus secondary hypertension, complications (e.g., cerebral vascular accidents, renal disease).
2. Common hematologic diseases (e.g., thrombocytopenia, clotting factor deficiencies, lymphoma, leukemia).
3. Valvular heart disease (e.g., mitral insufficiency, mitral regurgitation, aortic insufficiency, aortic regurgitation), including clinical presentation, associated murmurs, and cardiac catheterization results.
4. Thoracic and abdominal aortic aneurysms: similarities and differences.
5. Polycythemia: primary (polycythemia) and secondary (e.g., hypoxia) causes, clinical manifestations (e.g., pruritus, fatigue).

HIGH-YIELD FACTS

Pathology

General

1. Common clinical features of AIDS (e.g., CNS, pulmonary, GI, dermatologic manifestations).
2. Dermatologic manifestations of systemic disease (e.g., neoplasia, inflammatory bowel disease, meningococcemia, systemic lupus erythematosus).
3. Adult respiratory distress syndrome.
4. Geriatric pathology: diseases common in the elderly, normal physiologic changes with age.
5. Hypopituitarism: causes, manifestations.
6. Renal failure: acute versus chronic, features of uremia.
7. Acid–base disturbances, including renal tubular acidosis.
8. Wound repair.
9. Dehydration (e.g., hyponatremic vs. isotonic vs. hypernatremic), including appropriate treatment.

Pharmacology

Preparation for questions on pharmacology is straightforward. Memorizing all the key drugs and their characteristics (e.g., mechanisms, clinical use) is high yield. Focus on understanding the prototype drugs in each class. Avoid memorizing obscure derivatives. Learn the "classic" and distinguishing toxicities of the major drugs. Do not bother with drug dosages or trade names. There is a strong emphasis on autonomic nervous system, central nervous system, antimicrobial, and cardiovascular agents. Much of the material is clinically relevant.

Antimicrobial
CNS
Cardiovascular
Cancer Drugs
Toxicology
Miscellaneous
High-Yield Topics

Antimicrobial therapy

Mechanism of action	Drugs
Block cell wall synthesis by inhibition of peptidoglycan cross-linking	Penicillin, cephalosporins, imipenem, aztreonam
Block peptidoglycan synthesis	Bacitracin, vancomycin
Block protein synthesis at 50S ribosomal subunit	Chloramphenicol, erythromycin/macrolides, lincomycin, clindamycin
Block protein synthesis at 30S ribosomal subunit	Aminoglycosides, tetracyclines
Block nucleotide synthesis	Sulfonamides, trimethoprim
Block DNA topoisomerases	Quinilones
Block mRNA synthesis	Rifampin
Interrupt bacterial/fungal cell membranes	Polymyxins
Interrupt fungal cell membranes	Amphotericin B, nystatin, fluconazole/azoles
Unknown	Isoniazid, metronidazole, pentamidine

Penicillin

Penicillin G (IV form), penicillin V (oral):

Mechanism	1. Binds penicillin-binding proteins 2. Blocks transpeptidase cross-linking of cell wall 3. Activates autolytic enzymes
Clinical use	Bactericidal for gram-positive cocci, gram-positive rods, gram-negative cocci, and spirochetes. Not penicillinase resistant.
Toxicity	Hypersensitivity reactions.

Methicillin, nafcillin, dicloxacillin

Mechanism	Same as penicillin. Narrow spectrum, penicillinase resistant because of bulkier R group.
Clinical use	*Staphylococcus aureus.*
Toxicity	Hypersensitivity reactions; methicillin: interstitial nephritis.

Ampicillin, amoxicillin

Mechanism	Same as penicillin. Wider spectrum, penicillinase sensitive. Also, combine with clavulanic acid (penicillinase inhibitor) to enhance spectrum. Amoxicillin has greater oral bioavailability than ampicillin.
Clinical use	Extended-spectrum penicillin: certain gram-positive bacteria and gram-negative rods (*Haemophilus influenzae*, *Escherichia coli*, *Listeria monocytogenes*, *Proteus mirabilis*, *Salmonella*).
Toxicity	Hypersensitivity reactions; ampicillin: rash.

Coverage: ampicillin/amoxicillin "**HELPS**"

HIGH-YIELD FACTS

Pharmacology

Carbenicillin, ticarcillin

Mechanism	Same as penicillin. Extended spectrum.
Clinical use	*Pseudomonas* species and gram-negative rods.
Toxicity	Hypersensitivity reactions.

Cephalosporins

Mechanism	β-lactam drugs that inhibit cell wall synthesis but are less susceptible to penicillinases. Bactericidal.	
Clinical use	First generation: gram-positive cocci, *Proteus mirabilis,* *E coli,* *Klebsiella pneumoniae.*	1st generation: **PEcK**
	Second generation: gram-positive cocci, *Haemophilus influenzae,* *Enterobacter aerogenes,* *Neisseria* species, *Proteus mirabilis,* *E coli,* *K pneumoniae,* *Serratia marcescens.*	2nd generation: **HEN PEcKS**
	Third generation: serious gram-negative infections.	
	Cefot**ax**ime and ceftri**ax**one can penetrate the CNS (use for meningitis).	Think of an "**ax** to the head (CNS)."
Toxicity	Hypersensitivity reactions, increased nephrotoxicity of aminoglycosides, disulfiram-like reaction with ethanol (in cephalosporins with a methylthiotetrazole group, e.g., cefamandole).	

Aztreonam

Mechanism	A monobactam resistant to β-lactamases. Inhibits cell wall synthesis (binds to PBP3). Synergistic with aminoglycosides. No cross-allergenicity with penicillins.
Clinical use	Gram-negative rods: *Klebsiella* species, *Pseudomonas* species, *Serratia* species. No activity against gram-positives or anaerobes.
Toxicity	GI upset with possible superinfections, vertigo, headache.

Imipenem

Mechanism	A carbapenem. Wide spectrum. β-lactamase resistant. Always administered with cilastatin (inhibitor of renal dihydropeptidase I).
Clinical use	Gram-positive cocci, gram-negative rods, and anaerobes.
Toxicity	GI distress, skin rash, and CNS toxicity (at high plasma levels).

With imipenem, "the kill is **lastin** with cilastatin."

Vancomycin

Mechanism	Inhibits cell wall mucopeptide formation. Bactericidal.
Clinical use	Used for serious, gram-positive multidrug-resistant organisms, including *Staphylococcus aureus* and *Clostridium difficile* (pseudomembranous colitis).
Toxicity	**N**ephrotoxicity, **O**totoxicity, **T**hrombophlebitis, diffuse flushing—"red man syndrome" (can largely prevent by pretreatment with antihistamines and slow infusion rate). Well tolerated in general. Does **NOT** have many problems.

Protein synthesis inhibitors

30S inhibitors:

A = Aminoglycosides (streptomycin, gentamicin, tobramycin, amikacin) [bactericidal]

T = Tetracyclines [bacteriostatic]

50S inhibitors:

C = Chloramphenicol [bacteriostatic]

E = Erythromycin [bacteriostatic]

L = Lincomycin [bacteriostatic]

L = cLindamycin [bacteriostatic]

"Buy **AT 30, CELL** at 50"

Aminoglycosides

Gentamicin, streptomycin, tobramycin, amikacin

Mechanism	Bactericidal, inhibits formation of initiation complex and causes misreading of mRNA. Requires O_2 for uptake, therefore ineffective against anaerobes.
Clinical use	Severe gram-negative rod infections.
Toxicity	**N**ephrotoxicity (especially when used with cephalosporins), **O**totoxicity (especially when used with loop diuretics). Ami**NO**glycosides.

Tetracyclines

	Tetracycline, doxycycline, demeclocycline, minocycline
Mechanism	Bacteriostatic, binds to 30S and prevents attachment of aminoacyl-tRNA, limited CNS penetration. Doxycycline fecally eliminated and can be used in patients with renal failure. Must NOT take with milk or antacids because divalent cations inhibit its absorption in the gut.
Clinical use	*Borrelia burgdorferi* (Lyme disease), *Chlamydia, Ureaplasma, Mycoplasma pneumoniae, Rickettsiae*, **A**cne, **T**ularemia, **C**holera (*Vibrio cholerae*)
Toxicity	GI distress, discolors teeth in children, inhibits bone growth in children, Fanconi's syndrome, photosensitivity.

Coverage: **B CUM RATC:** "Become rats."

Erythromycin

Mechanism	Inhibits protein synthesis by blocking translocation, binds to the 23S rRNA of the 50S ribosomal subunit. Bacteriostatic.
Clinical use	Gram-positive cocci, *Mycoplasma, Legionella, Chlamydia, Neisseria*.
Toxicity	Acute cholestatic hepatitis, eosinophilia, skin rashes, GI discomfort.

Chloramphenicol

Mechanism	Inhibits 50S peptidyl transferase. Bacteriostatic.
Clinical use	Meningitis (*H influenzae, Neisseria meningitidis, Streptococcus pneumoniae*).
Toxicity	Anemia, aplastic anemia, gray baby syndrome (overdose in premature infants lacking liver UDP-glucuronyl transferase).

Sulfonamides

Sulfamethoxazole (SMZ), sulfisoxazole, triple sulfas

Mechanism	PABA antimetabolites inhibit dihydropteroate synthase. Bacteriostatic.
Clinical use	Gram-positive, gram-negative, *Nocardia, Chlamydia*. Triple sulfas or SMZ for simple UTI.
Toxicity	Hypersensitivity reactions, hemolysis if G6PD deficient, nephrotoxicity, kernicterus in infants, displace other drugs from albumin.

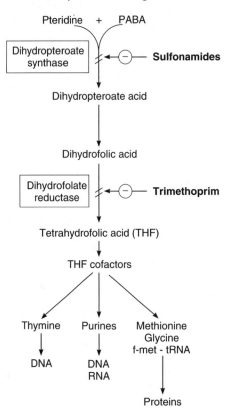

Trimethoprim

Mechanism	Inhibits dihydrofolate reductase. Bacteriostatic.	**T**rimethoprim = **TMP:**
Clinical use	Used in combination with sulfonamides (trimethoprim–sulfamethoxazole), causing sequential block of folate synthesis. Combination used for recurrent UTI, *Shigella, Salmonella, Pneumocystis carinii* pneumonia.	"**T**reats **M**arrow **P**oorly."
Toxicity	Megaloblastic anemia, leukopenia, granulocytopenia.	

Fluoroquinolones

Ciprofloxacin and norfloxacin (fluoroquinolones), nalidixic acid (a quinolone).

Mechanism	Inhibits DNA gyrase (topoisomerase II). Bactericidal.
Clinical use	Gram-negative rods (including *Pseudomonas*), *Neisseria,* some gram-positive organisms.
Toxicity	GI upset, superinfections, skin rashes, headache, dizziness. Contraindicated in pregnant women and in children because of animal studies showing damage to cartilage. Tendonitis and tendon rupture in adults.

Metronidazole

Mechanism	Forms toxic metabolites in the bacterial cell. Bactericidal.
Clinical use	Antiprotozoal, trichomoniasis, giardiasis, amebiasis, *Gardnerella vaginalis,* anaerobes (*Bacteroides, Clostridium*). Used with bismuth and amoxicillin or tetracycline for "triple therapy" against *H pylori.*
Toxicity	Disulfiram-like reaction with alcohol, vestibular dysfunction, headache.

"I took the **metro,** which made me dizzy (vestibular dysfunction) and made me vomit (disulfiram-like reaction with alcohol)."

Polymyxins

Polymyxin B, polymyxin E

Mechanism	Bind to cell membranes of bacteria and disrupt their osmotic properties. Polymyxins are cationic, basic proteins that act like detergents.
Clinical use	Resistant gram-negative cocci, gram-negative rods.
Toxicity	Neurotoxicity, acute renal tubular necrosis.

Isoniazid (INH)

Mechanism	Decreases synthesis of mycolic acids.
Clinical use	*Mycobacterium tuberculosis.* The only agent used as solo prophylaxis against TB.
Toxicity	Hemolysis if G6PD deficient, neurotoxicity, hepatotoxicity. Pyridoxine (vit. B_6) can prevent neurotoxicity.

INH:
Injures **N**eurons and **H**epatocytes.

Rifampin

Mechanism	Inhibits DNA-dependent RNA polymerase.
Clinical use	*M tuberculosis,* delays resistance to dapsone when used for leprosy. Always used in combination with other drugs except in the treatment of meningococcal carrier state, and chemoprophylaxis in contacts of children with *H influenzae* type B.
Toxicity	Increased elimination of HIV protease inhibitors, anticoagulants and methadone, hepatotoxicity, thrombocytopenia, skin rashes, flu response, decreased antibody responses.

Rifampin's **4 R's:**
RNA polymerase inhibitor
Revs up microsomal P450
Red/orange body fluids
Rapid resistance if used alone

TB drugs:
Rifampin (oral)
Ethambutol (oral)
Streptomycin (IM)
Pyrazinamide (oral)
Isoniazid (oral)
R
E

Amphotericin B

Mechanism	Binds ergosterol (unique to fungi), forms membrane pores that disrupt homeostasis.
Clinical use	*Cryptococcus, Blastomyces, Coccidioides, Histoplasma, Candida, Mucor* (systemic mycoses). Intrathecally for fungal meningitis; does not cross blood–brain barrier.
Toxicity	Fever, chills, hypotension, nephrotoxicity, arrhythmias ("amphoterrible").

Amphotericin "tears" holes in the fungal membrane by forming pores.

Fluconazole, ketoconazole, clotrimazole, miconazole

Mechanism	Inhibit fungal steroid synthesis.
Clinical use	Fluconazole for cryptococcus in AIDS patients and candidal infections of all types. Ketoconazole for *Blastomyces, Coccidioides, Histoplasma, C albicans.*
Toxicity	Hormone synthesis inhibition (gynecomastia), liver dysfunction (inhibits cyt. P450), fever, chills.

Griseofulvin

Mechanism	Interferes with microtubule function, disrupts mitosis. Deposits in keratin-containing tissues (e.g., nails).
Clinical use	Oral treatment of superficial infections, inhibits growth of dermatophytes (tinea, ringworm) and *C albicans.*
Toxicity	Teratogenic, carcinogenic, confusion, headaches, ↑ coumarin metabolism.

Antiviral chemotherapy

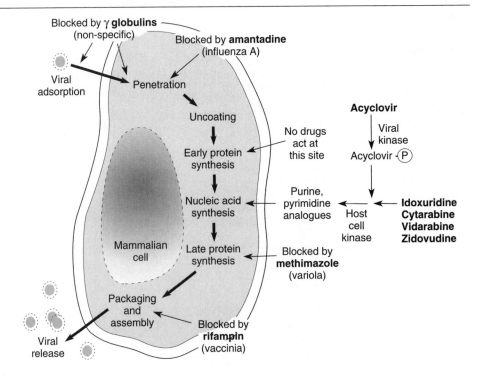

Amantadine

Mechanism	Blocks viral penetration/uncoating; may buffer pH of endosome. Also causes the release of dopamine from intact nerve terminals.
Clinical use	Prophylaxis for influenza A and rubella. Parkinson's disease.
Toxicity	Ataxia, dizziness, slurred speech.

Amantadine blocks influenza **A** and rubell**A** and causes problems with the cerebell**A**.

Acyclovir

Mechanism	Preferentially inhibits viral DNA polymerase when phosphorylated by viral thymidine kinase.
Clinical use	HSV, VZV, EBV. Mucocutaneous and genital herpes lesions. Prophylaxis in immunocompromised patients.
Toxicity	Delirium, tremor, renal crystals.

Ganciclovir

DHPG (dihydroxy-2-propoxymethyl guanine)

Mechanism	Phosphorylation by viral kinase preferentially inhibits CMV DNA polymerase.
Clinical use	CMV, especially in immunocompromised patients.
Toxicity	Leukopenia, thrombocytopenia, renal toxicity.

Foscarnet

Mechanism	Viral DNA polymerase inhibitor that binds to the pyrophosphate binding site of the enzyme. Does not require activation by viral kinase.
Clinical use	CMV retinitis in immunocompromised patients when ganciclovir fails.
Toxicity	Nephrotoxicity.

Zidovudine (AZT)

Mechanism	Preferentially inhibits reverse transcriptase of HIV.	**AZT: A**lways **Z**aps **T**hrombocytes.
Clinical use	HIV-infected patients.	
Toxicity	Thrombocytopenia, granulocytopenia, anemia.	

α **Blockers**	Application	Toxicity
Nonselective		
Phenoxybenzamine (irreversible)	Pheochromocytoma	Orthostatic hypotension, reflex tachycardia
Phentolamine (reversible)	Pheochromocytoma	Orthostatic hypotension, reflex tachycardia
α_1-selective		
Prazosin, terazosin, doxazosin	Hypertension, urinary retention in BPH	First-dose orthostatic hypotension, dizziness, headache
α_2-selective		
Yohimbine	Impotence (effectiveness is controversial)	

β **Blockers**	Propranolol, metoprolol, atenolol, nadolol, timolol, pindolol, esmolol, labetalol	
Application	**Effect**	
Hypertension	↓ cardiac output, ↓ renin secretion	
Angina pectoris	↓ heart rate and contractility, resulting in decreased oxygen consumption	
SVT (propranolol, esmolol)	↓ AV conduction velocity	
Glaucoma (timolol)	↓ secretion of aqueous humor	
Toxicity	Impotence, exacerbation of asthma, cardiovascular adverse effects (bradycardia, AV block, CHF), CNS adverse effects (sedation, sleep alterations)	
Selectivity	Nonselective ($\beta_1 = \beta_2$): propranolol, timolol, pindolol, nadolol, and labetalol (also blocks α_1 receptors)	
	β_1 selective ($\beta_1 > \beta_2$): metoprolol, atenolol, esmolol (short-acting)	

Barbiturates	Phenobarbital, pentobarbital, thiopental, secobarbital	BarbiDURATe (↑ DURATion). Contraindicated in porphyria.
Mechanism	Facilitate GABA action by ↑ **duration** of Cl⁻ channel opening.	
Clinical use	Anxiety, seizures, insomnia, induction of anesthesia (thiopental).	
Toxicity	Dependence, additive CNS depression effects with alcohol, respiratory or cardiovascular depression, drug interactions owing to induction of liver microsomal enzymes (cyt. P450).	

Benzodiazepines	Diazepam, lorazepam, triazolam, temazepam, chlordiazepoxide	FREnzodiazepines (↑ FREquency)
Mechanism	Facilitates GABA action by ↑ **frequency** of Cl⁻ channel opening. Most have long half-lives and active metabolites.	
Clinical use	Anxiety, spasticity, status epilepticus (diazepam), detoxification (especially alcohol).	
Toxicity	Dependence, additive CNS depression effects with alcohol. Treat overdose with flumazenil.	

Antipsychotics (neuroleptics)

Thioridazine, haloperidol, chlorpromazine.

Mechanism	Most antipsychotics block dopamine D_2 receptors (excess dopamine effects connected with schizophrenia).
Clinical use	Schizophrenia, psychosis.
Toxicity	Extrapyramidal system side effects, sedation, endocrine side effects, and side effects arising from blocking muscarinic, α, and histamine receptors. Retinal deposits from thioridazine. Neuroleptic malignant syndrome: rigidity, autonomic instability, hyperpyrexia (treat with dantrolene and dopamine agonists). Tardive dyskinesia: stereotypic oral–facial movements probably due to dopamine receptor sensitization; results of long-term antipsychotic use.

Evolution of EPS side effects:

4 h acute dystonia
4 d akinesia

4 wk akathisia
4 mo tardive dyskinesia (irreversible).

Clozapine

Mechanism	Atypical—blocks dopamine D_4 receptors.
Clinical use	2nd line drug for treatment of schizophrenia, psychosis.
Toxicity	Less sedation, anticholinergic, and extrapyramidal symptoms than typical antipsychotics. Causes agranulocytosis requiring weekly WBC monitoring.

Lithium

Mechanism	Not established; possibly related to inhibition of phosphoinositol cascade.
Clinical use	Mood stabilizer for bipolar affective disorder, blocks relapse and acute manic events.
Toxicity	Tremor, hypothyroidism, polyuria (ADH antagonist causing nephrogenic DI), teratogenesis. Narrow therapeutic window requiring close monitoring of serum levels.

Tricyclic antidepressants

Imipramine, amitriptyline, desipramine, nortriptyline, clomipramine, doxepin

Mechanism	Block reuptake of norepinephrine and serotonin.
Clinical use	Endogenous depression, bedwetting (imipramine), obsessive–compulsive disorder (clomipramine).
Side effects	Sedation, α-blocking effects, atropine-like (anticholinergic) side effects (tachycardia, urinary retention). Tertiary TCAs (amitriptyline) have more anticholinergic effects than secondary TCAs (nortriptyline). Desipramine is the least sedating.
Toxicity	Convulsions, coma, respiratory depression, hyperpyrexia, arrhythmias. Confusion and hallucinations in elderly.

SSRIs

Fluoxetine, sertraline, paroxetine

Mechanism	Serotonin-specific reuptake inhibitors.
Clinical use	Endogenous depression.
Toxicity	Anxiety, insomnia, tremor, anorexia, nausea, and vomiting.

It normally takes 2–3 wk for antidepressants to have an effect.

Anti-anginal therapy

Goal: Reduction of myocardial O_2 consumption (MVO_2) by decreasing one or more of the determinants of MVO_2: end diastolic volume, blood pressure, heart rate, contractility, ejection time.

Component	Nitrates	β Blockers	Nitrates + β blockers
End diastolic volume	↓	↑	No effect or ↓
Blood pressure	↓	↓	↓
Contractility	↑ (reflex response)	↓	Little/no effect
Heart rate	↑ (reflex response)	↓	↓
Ejection time	↓	↑	Little/no effect
MVO_2	↓	↓	↓↓

Calcium channel blockers
 —**N**ifedipine is similar to **n**itrates in effect
 —Verapamil is similar to β blockers in effect

Calcium channel blockers

Nifedipine, verapamil, diltiazem

Mechanism
Block voltage-dependent calcium channels of cardiac and smooth muscle and thereby reduce muscle contractility.
 Vascular smooth muscle: nifedipine > diltiazem > verapamil.
 Heart: verapamil > diltiazem > nifedipine.

Clinical use
Hypertension, angina, arrhythmias.

Toxicity
Cardiac depression, peripheral edema, flushing, dizziness, and constipation.

ACE inhibitors

Captopril, enalapril, lisinopril

Mechanism
Inhibit angiotensin-converting enzyme, reducing levels of angiotensin II and preventing inactivation of bradykinin, a potent vasodilator. Renin release is ↑d due to loss of feedback inhibition.

Clinical use
Hypertension, congestive heart failure, diabetic renal disease.

Toxicity
Cough, angioedema, proteinuria, taste changes, hypotension, fetal renal damage, rash.

Losartan is a new angiotensin II receptor antagonist. It is **not** an ACE inhibitor and does not cause cough.

Furosemide

Mechanism	Sulfonamide loop diuretic. Inhibits cotransport system $(Na^+, K^+, 2 Cl^-)$ of thick ascending limb of loop of Henle. Abolishes hypertonicity of medulla, preventing concentration of urine. Increases Ca^{2+} excretion.
Clinical use	Edematous states (CHF, cirrhosis, nephrotic syndrome, pulmonary edema), HTN, hypercalcemia.
Toxicity	**O**totoxicity, **H**ypokalemia, **D**ehydration, **A**llergy (sulfa), **N**ephritis (interstitial), **G**out.

Loops Lose calcium.

Toxicity: OH DANG!

Ethacrynic acid

Mechanism	Phenoxyacetic acid derivative (NOT a sulfonamide). Essentially same action as furosemide.
Clinical use	Diuresis in patients allergic to sulfa drugs.
Toxicity	Similar to furosemide except no hyperuricemia, no sulfa allergies.

Hydrochlorothiazide

Mechanism	Thiazide diuretic. Inhibits NaCl reabsorption in early distal tubule, reducing diluting capacity of the nephron. Decreases Ca^{2+} excretion.
Clinical use	Hypertension, congestive heart failure, calcium stone formation, nephrogenic diabetes insipidus.
Toxicity	Hypokalemic metabolic alkalosis, hyponatremia, hyper**G**lycemia, hyper**L**ipidemia, hyper**U**ricemia, and hyper**C**alcemia. "Hyper**GLUC**."

Acetazolamide

Mechanism	Carbonic anhydrase inhibitor. Causes self-limited $NaHCO_3$ diuresis and reduction in total-body HCO_3^- stores. Acts at the proximal convoluted tubule.
Clinical use	Glaucoma, urinary alkalinization, metabolic alkalosis.
Toxicity	Hyperchloremic metabolic acidosis, neuropathy, NH_3 toxicity.

K$^+$-sparing diuretics

	Spironolactone, **T**riamterene, **A**miloride
Mechanism	Spironolactone is a competitive aldosterone antagonist. Triamterene and amiloride act at same site by blocking Na^+ channels.
Clinical use	Hyperaldosteronism, K^+ depletion.
Toxicity	Hyperkalemia, endocrine effects (gynecomastia, anti-androgen effects).

The K$^+$ STAys.

Diuretics: electrolyte changes

Urine NaCl	$\uparrow$ (all diuretics: carbonic anhydrase inhibitors, loop diuretics, thiazides, K$^+$-sparing diuretics)
Urine K$^+$	$\uparrow$ (all except K$^+$-sparing diuretics)
Blood pH	$\downarrow$ (acidosis): carbonic anhydrase inhibitors, K$^+$-sparing diuretics $\uparrow$ (alkalosis): Loop diuretics, thiazides

Myocardial action potential

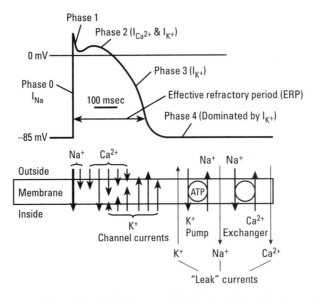

Occurs in atrial and ventricular myocytes and Purkinje fibers.

Phase 0 = Rapid upstroke—voltage-gated Na^+ channels open.

Phase 1 = Partial repolarization—inactivation of voltage-gated Na^+ channels. Voltage-gated K^+ channels begin to open.

Phase 2 = Plateau—Ca^{2+} influx from voltage-gated Ca^{2+} channels balances K^+ efflux. Ca^{2+} influx triggers myocyte contraction.

Phase 3 = Rapid repolarization—massive K^+ efflux due to opening of voltage-gated slow K^+ channels and closure of voltage-gated Ca^{2+} channels.

Phase 4 = Resting potential—high K^+ permeability through K1 channels.

Cardiac output

Fick principle:

Cardiac output = (stroke volume) (heart rate)

$$CO = \frac{\text{rate of } O_2 \text{ consumption}}{\text{arterial } O_2 \text{ content} - \text{venous } O_2 \text{ content}}$$

$$\frac{\text{Mean arterial}}{\text{pressure}} = \left(\frac{\text{cardiac}}{\text{output}}\right) \times \left(\frac{\text{total peripheral}}{\text{resistance}}\right)$$

During exercise, CO increases primarily as a result of increased HR. If HR is too high, CO drops (e.g., ventricular tachycardia).

Cardiac output variables	Stroke volume affected by **C**ontractility, **A**fterload, and **P**reload.	SV **CAP**
	Contractility (and SV) increased with:	Stroke volume increases in anxiety, exercise, and pregnancy.
	1. Catecholamines ($\uparrow$ activity of Ca^{2+} pump in sarcoplasmic reticulum).	
	2. $\uparrow$ extracellular calcium	Pulse pressure is proportional to stroke volume.
	3. $\downarrow$ extracellular sodium	
	4. Digitalis ($\uparrow$ intracellular Na^+)	
	Contractility (and SV) decreased with:	A failing heart has decreased stroke volume.
	1. β_1 blockade	Myocardial O_2 demand is $\uparrow$ by:
	2. Heart failure	$\uparrow$ afterload ($\propto$ diastolic BP)
	3. Acidosis	$\uparrow$ contractility
	4. Hypoxia/hypercapnea	$\uparrow$ heart rate
		$\uparrow$ heart size ($\uparrow$ wall tension)

Pacemaker action potential	Occurs in the SA and AV nodes. Key differences from the myocardial action potential include:
	Phase 0 = slow upstroke—opening of voltage-gated Ca^{2+} channels. These cells lack fast voltage-gated Na^+ channels. Results in a slow conduction velocity that is utilized by the AV node to prolong transmission from the atria to ventricles.
	Phase 4 = diastolic depolarization—membrane potential spontaneously depolarizes as K^+ conductance decreases and as Na^+ conductance increases. Accounts for automaticity of SA and AV nodes. Rate of diastolic depolarization in the SA node determines heart rate. Acetylcholine decreases and catecholamines increase the slope of this phase, thus decreasing or increasing heart rate, respectively.

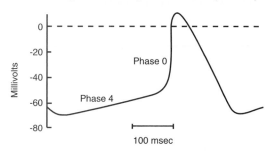

Preload and afterload	Preload = ventricular end-diastolic volume.	Preload increases with exercise (slightly), extra blood (overtransfusion), and excitement (sympathetics).
	Afterload = peripheral resistance.	
	Venous dilators (e.g., nitroglycerin) decrease preload.	
	Vasodilators (e.g., hydralazine) decrease afterload.	Preload pumps up the heart.
	$\uparrow$ SV when $\uparrow$ preload or $\downarrow$ afterload.	

Electrophysiologic differences between skeletal and cardiac muscle

In contrast to skeletal muscle:

1. Cardiac muscle action potential has a plateau, which is due to Ca^{2+} influx
2. Cardiac nodal cells spontaneously depolarize, resulting in automaticity
3. Cardiac myocytes are electrically coupled to each other by gap junctions
4. Cardiac muscle contraction is dependent on extracellular calcium, which stimulates calcium release from the cardiac muscle sarcoplasmic reticulum (calcium-induced calcium release)

Fetal circulation

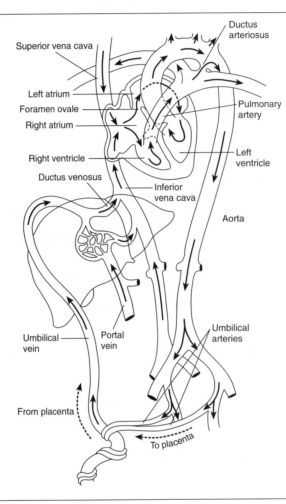

Blood in umbilical vein is ≈ 80% saturated with O_2.

Most oxygenated blood reaching the heart via IVC is diverted through the foramen ovale and pumped out the aorta to the head.

Deoxygenated blood from the SVC is expelled into the pulmonary artery and ductus arteriosus to the lower body of the fetus.

Control of mean arterial pressure

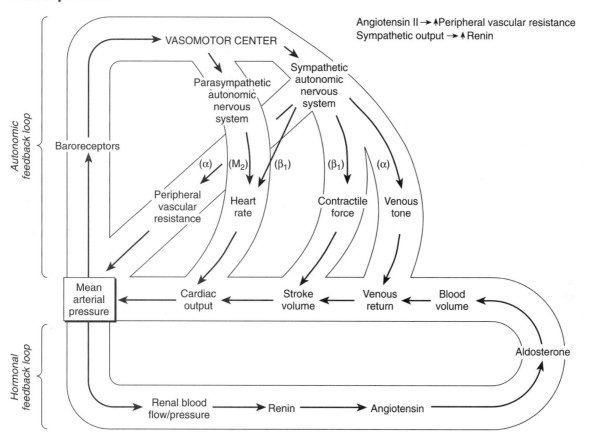

Angiotensin II → ↑Peripheral vascular resistance
Sympathetic output → ↑Renin

Circulation through organs	Liver: largest share of systemic cardiac output. Kidney: highest blood flow per gram of tissue. Heart: large arteriovenous O_2 difference. Increased O_2 demand is met by increased coronary blood flow, not by increased extraction of O_2.

Autoregulation	Sites: brain, kidney, heart Mechanism: in the brain and heart, blood flow is altered to meet demands of tissue via local metabolites (e.g., nitric oxide, adenosine). In the kidney, local metabolites maintain renal artery pressure constant.	The pulmonary vasculature is unique in that hypoxia causes vasoconstriction (in other organs hypoxia causes vasodilation).

PHYSIOLOGY—RESPIRATORY

Response to high altitude	1. Acute increase in ventilation by 65% 2. Chronic increase in ventilation 3. ↑ erythropoietin → ↑ hematocrit and hemoglobin (chronic hypoxia) 4. Increased 2,3-DPG (shifts curve to right so that Hb releases O_2 more readily) 5. Cellular changes (increased mitochondria) 6. Increased renal excretion of bicarbonate to compensate for the respiratory alkalosis

Important lung products	1. **S**urfactant: ↓ alveolar surface tension, ↑ compliance 2. **P**rostaglandins 3. **H**istamine 4. **A**ngiotensin converting enzyme (ACE): AI → AII; inactivates bradykinin (ACE inhibitors ↑ bradykinin and cause cough, angioedema) 5. **K**allikrein: activates bradykinin	Even the lungs get a big **SPHAK** attack! Surfactant: dipalmitoyl phosphatidylcholine (lecithin) deficient in neonatal RDS.
Particle size and lung entrapment	Diameter of: > 10 μm: Trapped by nostril hairs or settle on mucous membranes in nose and pharynx. 2–10 μm: Fall on bronchial walls → reflex bronchial constriction and coughing. Also removed by cilia. 0.5–2 μm: Reach alveoli → ingested by macrophages. < 0.5 μm: Remain suspended in air.	**Kartagener's syndrome** = immotile cilia due to a dynein arm defect. Bacteria and particles not pushed out (also sperm cilia inactive). Results in bronchiectasis, situs inversus, sterility, and recurrent sinusitis.

Physiology

Lung volumes

1. Residual volume (RV) = air in lung at maximal expiration
2. Expiratory reserve volume (ERV) = air that can still be breathed out after normal expiration
3. Tidal volume (TV) = air that moves into lung with each inspiration
4. Inspiratory reserve volume (IRV) = air in excess of tidal volume that moves into lung on maximum inspiration
5. Vital capacity (VC) = TV + IRV + ERV
6. Functional reserve capacity (FRC) = RV + ERV
7. Inspiratory capacity (IC) = IRV + TV
8. Total lung capacity = TLC

Vital capacity is everything but the residual volume.

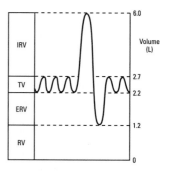

Pulmonary flow volume loops

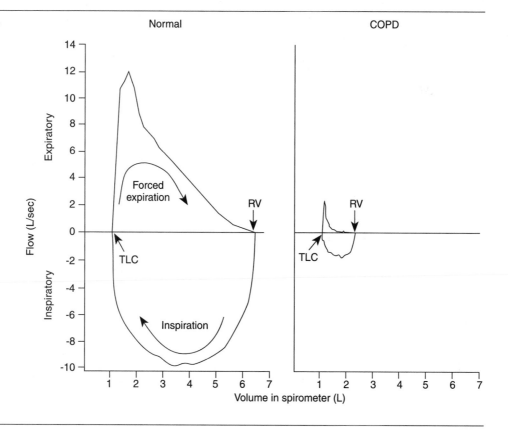

HIGH-YIELD FACTS

Physiology

Oxygen dissociation curve

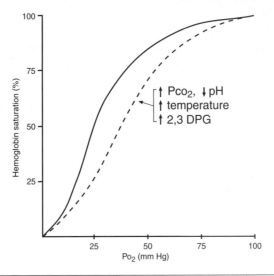

When curve shifts to the right, ↓ affinity of hemoglobin for O_2 (facilitates unloading of O_2 to tissue).

An ↑ in all factors (except pH) causes a shift of the curve to the right.

Acid-base physiology

	pH	Pco_2	$[HCO_3^-]$	Cause	Compensatory response
Metabolic acidosis	↓	↓	↓	Diabetic ketoacidosis; diarrhea	Hyperventilation
Respiratory acidosis	↓	↑	↑	COPD; airway obstruction	Renal $[HCO_3^-]$ reabsorption
Respiratory alkalosis	↑	↓	↓	High altitude	Renal $[HCO_3^-]$ secretion
Metabolic alkalosis	↑	↑	↑	Vomiting	Hypoventilation

Pulmonary circulation

Normally a low-resistance, high-compliance system keeps pulmonary blood pressure low. With increased Pco_2 (e.g., exercise), a low pulmonary blood pressure is maintained by vasodilating normally closed apical capillaries, thereby lowering pulmonary resistance.

A consequence of pulmonary hypertension is corpulmonale and subsequent right ventricular failure (jugular venous distension, edema, hepatomegaly).

V/Q mismatch

Ideally, ventilation is matched to perfusion (i.e., V/Q = 1) in order for adequate oxygenation to occur efficiently.

Lung zones:
Apex of the lung: V/Q = 3 (wasted ventilation)
Base of the lung: V/Q = 0.6 (wasted perfusion)
Both ventilation and perfusion are greater at the base of the lung than at the apex of the lung.

With exercise (increased cardiac output), there is vasodilation of apical capillaries, resulting in a V/Q ratio that approaches unity.

Certain organisms that thrive in high O_2 (e.g., TB) flourish in the apex.

V/Q → ∞ = dead space
V/Q → 0 = shunt

CO₂ transport	Carbon dioxide is transported from tissues to the lungs in 3 forms:

CO$_2$ transport   Carbon dioxide is transported from tissues to the lungs in 3 forms:

1. Bicarbonate (65%)

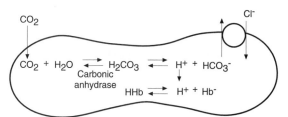

Deoxyhemoglobin binds H+ more actively than does oxyhemoglobin (Bohr effect).

2. Bound to hemoglobin as carbaminohemoglobin (25%)
3. Dissolved CO_2 (10%)

Obstructive lung disease   Obstruction of air flow, resulting in air trapping in the lungs. Pulmonary function tests: decreased FEV_1/FVC ratio (hallmark).

Types:

1. Chronic bronchitis ("blue bloater")—productive cough for greater than 3 consecutive months in two or more years. Reid index > 50% (hypertrophy of mucus-secreting glands in the bronchioles). Leading cause is smoking. Findings: wheezing, crackles, cyanosis.
2. Emphysema ("pink puffer")—enlargement of air spaces and decreased recoil resulting from destruction of alveolar walls. Caused by smoking (centroacinar emphysema) and α_1-antitrypsin deficiency (panacinar emphysema and liver cirrhosis) → ↑ elastase activity. Findings: dyspnea, ↓ breath sounds, tachycardia, ↓ I/E ratio.
3. Asthma—Bronchial hyperresponsiveness causes reversible bronchoconstriction. Can be triggered by viral URIs, allergens, and stress. Findings: cough, wheezing, dyspnea, tachypnea, hypoxemia, ↓ I/E ratio, pulsus paradoxus.
4. Bronchiectasis—chronic necrotizing infection of bronchi → dilated airways, purulent sputum, recurrent infections, hemoptysis. Associated with bronchial obstruction, cystic fibrosis, poor ciliary motility.

Restrictive lung disease   Decreased lung volumes (decreased VC and TLC).

Types:

1. Poor breathing mechanics (extrapulmonary):
   a. Poor muscular effort: polio, myasthenia gravis.
   b. Poor apparatus: scoliosis.
2. Poor lung expansion (pulmonary):
   a. Defective alveolar filling: pneumonia, ARDS, pulmonary edema.
   b. Interstitial fibrosis: causes increased recoil, thereby limiting alveolar expansion. PFTs reveal an FEV_1/FVC ratio > 90%. Complications include cor pulmonale. Can be seen in diffuse interstitial pulmonary fibrosis and bleomycin toxicity. Symptoms include gradual progressive dyspnea and cough.

Pancreatic exocrine secretion

Secretory acini synthesize and secrete zymogens, stimulated by acetylcholine and CCK. Pancreatic ducts secrete mucus and alkaline fluid when stimulated by secretin.

Pancreatic enzymes

Alpha-amylase: starch digestion, secreted in active form.

Lipase, phospholipase A, colipase: fat digestion.

Proteases (trypsin, chymotrypsin, elastase, carboxypeptidases): protein digestion, secreted as proenzymes.

Trypsinogen is converted to active enzyme trypsin by enteropeptidase, a duodenal brush-border enzyme. Trypsin then activates the other proenzymes and can also activate trypsinogen (positive-feedback loop).

Pancreatic insufficiency is seen in CF and other conditions. Patients present with malabsorption, steatorrhea (greasy, malodorous stool). Limit fat intake, monitor for signs of fat-soluble vitamin (A, D, G, K) deficiency.

Stimulation of pancreatic functions

Secretin	Stimulates flow of bicarbonate-containing fluid.
Cholecystokinin	Major stimulus for zymogen release, weak stimulus for alkaline fluid flow.
Acetylcholine	Major stimulus for zymogen release, poor stimulus for bicarbonate secretion.
Somatostatin	Inhibits the release of gastrin and secretin.

Physiology

Bilirubin   Product of heme metabolism, actively taken up by hepatocytes. Conjugated version is water soluble. Jaundice (yellow skin, scleral icterus) results from elevated bilirubin levels.

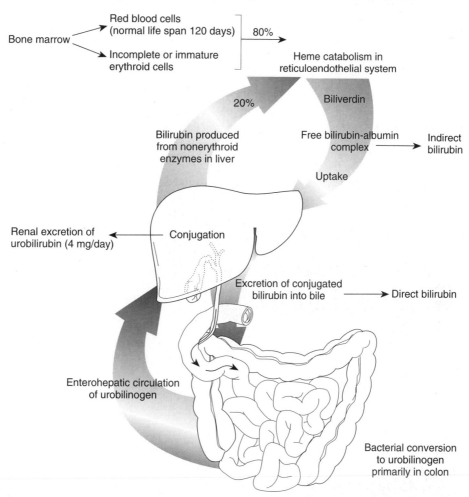

Bile   Secreted by hepatocytes. Composed of bile salts, phospholipids, cholesterol, bilirubin, water (97%). Bile salts are amphipathic (hydrophilic and hydrophobic domains) and solubilize lipids in micelles for absorption.

Carbohydrate digestion   Only monosaccharides are absorbed.

Salivary amylase   Starts digestion, hydrolyzes alpha-1,4 linkages to give maltose, maltotriose, and α-limit dextrins.

Pancreatic amylase   Highest concentration in duodenal lumen, hydrolyzes starch to oligosaccharides, maltose, and maltotriose.

Oligosaccharide hydrolases   At brush border of intestine, is the rate-limiting step in carbohydrate digestion, produces monosaccharides (glucose, galactose, fructose).

Salivary secretion

Source	Parotid, submandibular, and sublingual glands.
Function	1. Alpha-amylase (ptyalin) begins starch digestion
	2. Neutralizes oral bacterial acids, maintains dental health
	3. Mucins (glycoproteins) lubricate food

Salivary secretion is stimulated by both sympathetic and parasympathetic activity.

Glucose absorption

Occurs at duodenum and proximal jejunum.

Absorbed across cell membrane by sodium-glucose-coupled transporter.

Stomach secretions

	Purpose	Source
Mucus	Lubricant, protects surface from H^+	Mucous cell
Intrinsic factor	Vitamin B_{12} absorption (in small intestine)	Parietal cell
H^+	Kills bacteria, breaks down food, converts pepsinogen	Parietal cell
Pepsinogen	Broken down to pepsin (a protease)	Chief cell
Gastrin	Stimulates acid secretion	G cell

GI secretory products

	Source	Function	Regulation	Notes
Intrinsic factor	Parietal cells (stomach)	Vitamin B_{12} binding protein required for vitamin's uptake in terminal ileum		Autoimmune destruction of parietal cells → chronic gastritis → pernicious anemia
Gastric acid	Parietal cells	Lowers pH to optimal range for pepsin function. Sterilizes chyme	Stimulated by histamine, ACh, gastrin. Inhibited by prostaglandin	Not essential for digestion. Inadequate acid → ↑ risk of *Salmonella* infections
Pepsin	Chief cells (stomach)	Begins protein digestion; optimal function at pH 1.0–3.0	Stimulated by vagal input, local acid	Inactive pepsinogen converted to pepsin by H^+
Gastrin	G cells of antrum and duodenum	1. Stimulates secretion of HCl, IF and pepsinogen 2. Stimulates gastric motility	Stimulated by stomach distention, amino acids, peptides, vagus (via GRP); inhibited by secretin and stomach acid pH < 1.5	Hypersecreted in Zollinger–Ellison syndrome → peptic ulcers. Phenylalanine and tryptophan are potent stimulators.
Bicarbonate	Surface submucosal cells of stomach and duodenum	Neutralizes acid; forms an unstirred layer with mucus on luminal surface, preventing autodigestion	Stimulated by secretin (potentiated by vagal input, CCK)	
Cholecystokinin (CCK)	I cells of duodenum and jejunum	1. Stimulates gallbladder contraction 2. Stimulates pancreatic enzyme secretion 3. Inhibits gastric emptying	Stimulated by fatty acids, amino acids	In cholelithiasis, pain worsens after eating fatty foods due to CCK release
Secretin	S cells of duodenum	Nature's antacid: 1. Stimulates pancreatic HCO_3^- secretion 2. Inhibits gastric acid secretion	Stimulated by acid and fatty acids in lumen of duodenum	Alkaline pancreatic juice in duodenum neutralizes gastric acid, allowing pancreatic enzymes to function
Somatostatin	D cells in pancreatic islets, gastrointestinal mucosa	**Inhibits:** 1. Gastric acid and pepsinogen secretion 2. Pancreatic and small intestine fluid secretion 3. Gallbladder contraction 4. Release of both insulin and glucagon	Stimulated by acid; inhibited by vagus	Very inhibitory hormone; anti-growth hormone effects (↓ digestion and ↓ absorption of substances needed for growth)

Regulation of gastric acid secretion

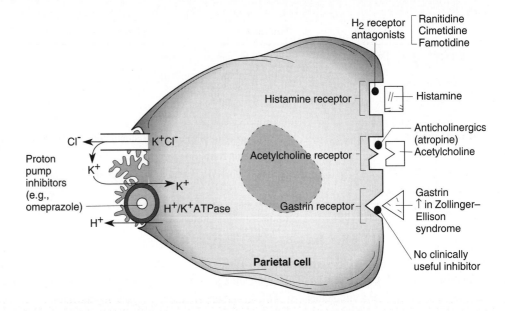

Filtration fraction

$FF = GFR/RPF$

$GFR = C_{inulin} \approx C_{creatinine}$

$RPF = C_{PAH}$

Renal clearance

$C_x = U \times V / P_x$ = volume of plasma from which the substance is cleared completely per unit time.

If $C_x <$ GFR, then there is net tubular reabsorption of X.

If $C_x >$ GFR, then there is net tubular secretion of X.

If $C_x =$ GFR, then there is no net secretion or reabsorption.

Glomerular filtration rate

$GFR = U_{Inulin} \times V / P_{Inulin} = C_{Inulin}$

$= K_f [(P_{GC} - P_{BS}) - (\pi_{GC} - \pi_{BS})]$

(GC = glomerular capillary; BS = Bowman's space)

Inulin is freely filtered and is neither reabsorbed nor secreted.

Effective renal plasma flow

$ERPF = U_{PAH} \times V / P_{PAH} = C_{PAH} = RBF (1 - Hct)$

PAH is filtered and secreted.

PAH

Secreted in proximal tubule.

Active transport process, requires ATP, inhibited by cyanide.

Mediated by a carrier system for organic acids, competitively inhibited by probenecid.

Glucose clearance

Glucose at normal level is completely reabsorbed (99% in proximal tubule, 1% in collecting ducts). Mechanism is saturable. Glucosuria is an important clinical clue to diabetes mellitus.

Renal threshold is 200 mg/dl of arterial plasma.

Amino acid clearance	Reabsorption by at least 3 distinct carrier systems, with competitive inhibition within each group. Active transport occurs in proximal tubule and is saturable.	

Electrolyte clearance

Sodium	>99% of filtered load is absorbed. Reabsorption is active throughout most of nephron.	
Chloride	Reabsorption is passive, driven by electrochemical gradients maintained by sodium reabsorption (except at thick ascending loop of Henle).	

Measuring fluid compartments

Compartment	**Direct measurement**
Total body water (TBW)	Antipyrine, tritium
Extracellular fluid (ECF) (⅓ TBW)	Inulin, mannitol
Plasma (¼ ECF, ½ TBW)	Evans blue, I^{131}-albumin
	Indirect measurement
Interstitial fluid (¾ ECF, ¼ TBW).	ECF − plasma
Intracellular fluid (⅔ TBW)	TBW − extracellular fluid

Kidney endocrine functions	Endocrine functions of the kidney: 1. Endothelial cells of peritubular capillaries secrete erythropoietin in response to hypoxia 2. Conversion of 25-OH vit. D to 1,25-(OH)$_2$ vit. D by 1α-hydroxylase, which is activated by PTH 3. JG cells secrete renin in response to ↓ renal arterial pressure and ↑ renal nerve discharge 4. Secretion of prostaglandins that vasodilate the afferent arterioles to increase GFR	NSAIDs can cause renal failure by inhibiting the renal production of prostaglandins, which normally keep the afferent arterioles vasodilated to maintain GFR.
Glomerular filtration barrier	Composed of: 1. Fenestrated capillary endothelium (size barrier) 2. Fused basement membrane with heparan sulfate (negative charge barrier) 3. Epithelial layer consisting of podocyte foot processes	The charge barrier is lost in nephrotic syndrome, resulting in albuminuria, hypoproteinemia, generalized edema, and hyperlipidemia.
Renal failure	Failure to make urine and excrete nitrogenous wastes. Consequences: 1. Anemia (failure of erythropoietin production) 2. Renal osteodystrophy (failure of active vit. D production) 3. Hyperkalemia, which can lead to cardiac arrhythmias 4. Metabolic acidosis due to ↓ acid excretion and ↓ generation of buffers 5. Uremia (increased BUN/creatinine) 6. Sodium and H$_2$O excess → CHF and pulmonary edema	Two forms of renal failure: acute renal failure (often due to hypoxia) and chronic renal failure.

HIGH-YIELD FACTS

Physiology

Hormones acting on kidney

	Stimulus for secretion	Action on kidneys
Vasopressin (ADH)	↑ plasma osmolarity ↓↓ blood volume	↑ H_2O permeability of principal cells in collecting ducts
Aldosterone	↓ blood volume (via AII) ↑ plasma [K^+]	↑ Na^+ reabsorption, ↑ K^+ secretion, ↑ H^+ secretion in distal tubule
Angiotensin II	↓ blood volume (via renin)	Contraction of mesangial cells → ↓ GFR ↑ Na^+ and HCO_3^- reabsorption in proximal tubule
Atrial natriuretic peptide (ANP)	↑ atrial pressure	↓ Na^+ reabsorption ↑ GFR
PTH	↓ plasma [Ca^{2+}]	↑ Ca^{2+} reabsorption, ↓ PO_4^{3-} reabsorption, ↑ $1,25 (OH)_2$ vitamin D production

Renin–angiotensin system

Mechanism
Renin is released by the kidneys upon sensing ↓ BP and serves to cleave angiotensinogen to angiotensin I (AI) (a decapeptide). AI is then cleaved by angiotensin-converting enzyme (ACE) in the lung capillaries to angiotensin II (AII, an octapeptide).

Actions
1. Potent vasoconstriction
2. Release of aldosterone from the adrenal cortex
3. Release of ADH from posterior pituitary
4. Stimulates hypothalamus → ↑ thirst

Overall, AII serves to ↑ intravascular volume and ↑ BP.

ANP may act as a "check" on the renin-angiotensin system (e.g., in heart failure).

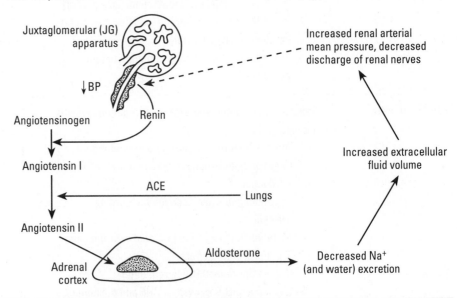

Hyperaldosteronism

Primary hyperaldosteronism (Conn's syndrome).
Caused by an aldosterone-secreting tumor, resulting in hypertension, hypokalemia, hypernatremia, metabolic alkalosis, and **low** plasma renin.

Secondary hyperaldosteronism.
Due to renal artery stenosis, chronic renal failure, CHF, cirrhosis, or nephrotic syndrome. Kidney misperception of low intravascular volume, resulting in an overactive renin-angiotensin system. Therefore, it is associated with **high** plasma renin.

Treatment includes spironolactone, a diuretic that works by acting as an aldosterone antagonist.

Nephron physiology

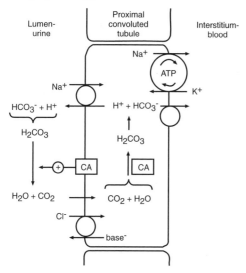

Proximal convoluted tubule—"workhorse of the nephron." Reabsorbs all of the glucose and amino acids and most of the bicarbonate, sodium, and water. Secretes ammonia, which acts as a buffer for secreted H^+.

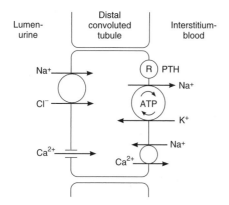

Distal convoluted tubule—actively reabsorbs Na^+, Cl^-. Reabsorption of Ca^{2+} is under the control of PTH.

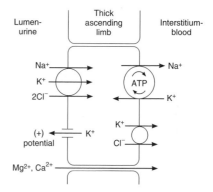

Thin descending loop of Henle—passively reabsorbs water via medullar hypertonicity (impermeable to sodium).

Thick ascending loop of Henle—actively reabsorbs Na^+, K^+, Cl^- and indirectly induces the reabsorption of Mg^{2+} and Ca^{2+}.

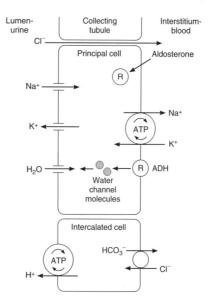

Collecting tubules—reabsorb Na^+ in exchange for secreting K^+ or H^+ (regulated by aldosterone). Reabsorption of water is regulated by ADH. Osmolarity of medulla can reach 1200–1400 mOsm.

HIGH-YIELD FACTS

Physiology

Steroid/thyroid hormone mechanism

The need for gene transcription and protein synthesis delays the onset of action of these hormones.

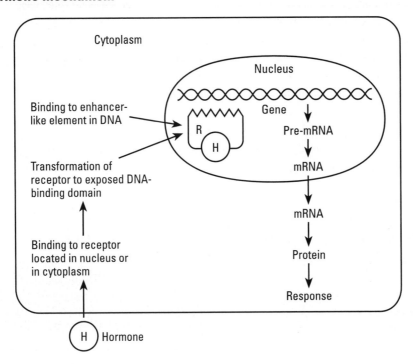

Cytoplasm

Nucleus

Binding to enhancer-like element in DNA

Gene

R

Pre-mRNA

H

Transformation of receptor to exposed DNA-binding domain

mRNA

mRNA

Binding to receptor located in nucleus or in cytoplasm

Protein

Response

H Hormone

Insulin-independent organs

Muscle and adipose tissue depend on insulin for glucose uptake. Brain and RBCs take up glucose independent of insulin levels.

Brain and RBCs depend on glucose for metabolism under normal circumstances. Brain uses ketone bodies in starvation.

Pituitary glycoprotein hormones

Anterior pituitary glycoprotein hormones are TSH, LH, FSH.

α subunit – common subunit to TSH, LH, FSH and hCG.

β subunit – determines hormone specificity.

T.S.H. and **TSH** = **T**he **S**ex **H**ormones and **TSH**

PTH

Source   Chief cells of parathyroid.

Function
1. Increase bone resorption of calcium
2. Increase kidney reabsorption of calcium
3. Decrease kidney reabsorption of phosphate
4. Increase 1,25 (OH)$_2$ vit. D production (cholecalciferol) by stimulating kidney 1α-hydroxylase

Regulation   Increases in serum Ca^{2+} decrease secretion.

PTH: increases serum Ca^{2+}, decreases serum PO$_4^{3-}$, increases urine PO$_4^{3-}$.

PTH stimulates both osteoclasts and osteoblasts.

Calcitonin

Source	Parafollicular cells (C cells) of thyroid.
Function	1. Decrease bone resorption of calcium 2. Increase urinary excretion of calcium
Regulation	Increases in serum Ca^{2+} increase secretion.

Calcitonin rhymes with **"bone in."**

Calcitonin opposes actions of PTH and acts faster than PTH. It is probably not important in normal calcium homeostasis.

Vitamin D

Source	Vitamin D_3 from sun exposure in skin. D_2 from plants. Both converted to 25-OH vit. D in liver and to 1,25-$(OH)_2$ vit. D (active form) in kidney.
Function	1. Increase absorption of dietary calcium 2. Increase absorption of dietary phosphate 3. Increase bone resorption of Ca^{2+} and PO_4^{3-}
Regulation	Increased PTH causes increased 1,25-(OH_2) vit. D conversion. Decreased phosphate causes increased 1,25-$(OH)_2$ vit. D conversion. 1,25-$(OH)_2$ vit. D feedback inhibits its own production.

If you do not get vit. D, you get rickets (kids) or osteomalacia (adults).

24,25-$(OH)_2$ vit. D is the inactive form of vit. D.

Estrogen

Source	Ovary (estradiol), placenta (estriol), blood (aromatization), testes.
Function	1. Growth of follicle 2. Endometrial proliferation, myometrial excitability 3. Genitalia development 4. Stromal development of breast 5. Fat deposition 6. Libido 7. Hepatic synthesis of transport proteins 8. Feedback inhibition of FSH 9. LH surge (estrogen feedback on LH secretion switches to positive from negative just before LH surge).

Potency: estradiol > estrone > estriol

Estrogen hormone replacement therapy after menopause: ↓ risk of heart disease, ↓ hot flashes, and ↓ postmenopausal bone loss.

Unopposed estrogen therapy: ↑ risk of endometrial cancer and possibly ↑ risk of breast cancer; use of estrogen/progesterone ↓ those risks.

Menstrual cycle

Follicular growth is fastest during second week of proliferative phase.

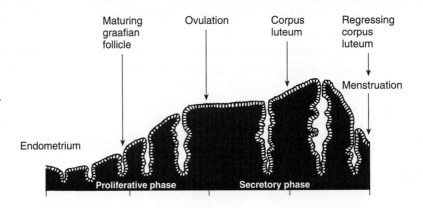

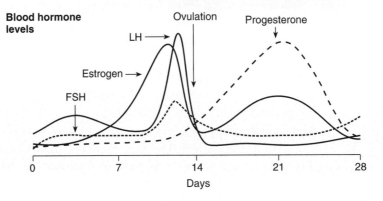

Menopause

Cessation of estrogen production with age-linked decline in number of ovarian follicles. Sx: vasomotor instability (hot flashes), vaginal atrophy (pain, infection), osteoporosis, ↑ CAD.

Average age of onset is 51 y (earlier in smokers). Hormonal changes: ↓ estrogen, ↑↑ FSH, ↑ LH (no surge).

Progesterone

Source — Corpus luteum, placenta, adrenal cortex, testes.

Function —
1. Stimulation of endometrial glandular secretions and spiral artery development
2. Maintenance of pregnancy
3. Decreased myometrial excitability
4. Production of thick cervical mucus, which inhibits sperm entry into the uterus
5. Increased temperature (0.5 degree)
6. Inhibition of gonadotropins (LH, FSH)
7. Uterine smooth muscle relaxation

hCG

Source	Trophoblast, placenta
Function	1. Maintains the corpus luteum for the 1st trimester because it acts like LH but is not susceptible to feedback regulation from estrogen and progesterone. In the 2nd and 3rd trimester, the placenta synthesizes its own estrogen and progesterone. As a result, the corpus luteum degenerates. 2. Used to detect pregnancy because it appears in the urine 8 days after successful fertilization (blood and urine tests available). 3. Elevated hCG in women with hydatidiform moles or choriocarcinoma.

Norepinephrine vs. epinephrine

	Epinephrine	Norepinephrine	
Predominant receptor effect	$\beta > \alpha$	$\alpha \gg \beta$	Adrenal medullary cells and some neurons contain the enzyme PNMT, which converts norepinephrine to epinephrine.
Total peripheral resistance	↓	↑	
Cardiac output	↑	↓	
Heart rate	↑	↓ (reflex)	
Blood pressure	↑ pulse pressure	↑	

Male spermatogenesis

Pituitary	Testes	Products	Functions of products

FSH → Sertoli cell → Androgen binding protein — Ensures that testosterone in seminiferous tubule is high

→ Inhibin — Inhibits FSH

LH → Leydig cell → Testosterone — Differentiates male genitalia, has anabolic effects on protein metabolism, maintains gametogenesis, maintains libido, inhibits LH, and fuses epiphyseal plates in bone

FSH → **S**ertoli cells → **S**perm production
LH → **L**eydig cells

Cardiovascular
1. Basic electrocardiographic changes (e.g., Q waves, ST segment elevation).
2. Effects of electrolyte abnormalities on the heart (e.g., potassium or calcium imbalances).
3. Physiologic effects of the Valsalva maneuver.
4. Cardiopulmonary changes with pregnancy.

Endocrine/Reproductive
1. Physiologic features of hypoparathyroidism, associated laboratory findings.
2. Clinical tests for endocrine abnormalities (e.g., dexamethasone suppression tests, glucose tolerance tests, TSH).
3. Diseases associated with endocrine abnormalities (e.g., Cushing's, Addison's, Conn's).
4. Sites of hormone production during pregnancy (e.g., corpus luteum, placenta).
5. Regulation of prolactin secretion.

Gastrointestinal
1. Sites of absorption of major nutrients (e.g., ileum: vit. B_{12}).
2. Bile production and enterohepatic circulation.
3. Glucose cotransport into cells of gut and peripheral tissues.

Pulmonary
1. Alveolar-arterial oxygen gradient and changes seen in lung disease.
2. Mechanical differences between inspiration and expiration.
3. Characteristic pulmonary function curves for common lung diseases (e.g., bronchitis, emphysema, asthma, interstitial lung disease).
4. Gas diffusion across alveolocapillary membrane.

Renal/Acid-Base
1. Differences among active transport, facilitated diffusion, and diffusion.
2. Differences between central and nephrogenic diabetes insipidus.

General
1. Role of calmodulin and troponin C, and tropomyosin in muscle contraction.
2. Role of ions (e.g., calcium, sodium, magnesium, potassium) in skeletal muscle, cardiac muscle, and nerve cells (e.g., muscle contraction, membrane and action potentials, neurotransmitter release).
3. The clotting cascade, including those factors which require vitamin K for synthesis (II, VII, IX, X).

Database of Basic Science Review Resources

Comprehensive
Anatomy
Behavioral Science
Biochemistry
Microbiology
Pathology
Pharmacology
Physiology

Commercial Review Courses
Publisher Contacts

This section is a database of current basic science review books, sample examination books, and commercial review courses marketed to medical students studying for the USMLE Step 1. At the end of this section is a list of publishers and independent bookstores with addresses and phone numbers. For each book, we list the **Title** of the book, the **First Author** (or editor), the **Series Name** (where applicable), the **Current Publisher,** the **Copyright Year,** the **Number of Pages,** the **ISBN Code,** the **Approximate List Price,** the **Format** of the book, and the **Number of Test Questions.** The entries for most books also include **Summary Comments** that describe their style and overall utility for studying. Finally, each book receives a **Rating.** The books are sorted into a comprehensive section as well as into sections corresponding to the seven traditional basic medical science disciplines (anatomy, behavioral science, biochemistry, microbiology, pathology, pharmacology, and physiology). Within each section books are arranged first by Rating, then by Title, and finally by Author.

For the 1997 edition of *First Aid for the USMLE Step 1,* the database of review books has been expanded and updated, with more than 30 new books and software and more in-depth summary comments. A letter rating scale with ten different grades reflects the detailed student evaluations. Each book receives a rating as follows:

A+	Excellent for boards review.
A A–	Very good for boards review; choose among the group.
B+ B B–	Good, but use only after exhausting better sources.
C+ C C–	Fair, but many better books in the discipline, or low-yield subject material.
D	Not appropriate.
N	Not rated.

The **Rating** is meant to reflect the overall usefulness of the book in preparing for the USMLE Step 1 examination. This is based on a number of factors, including:

- The cost of the book.
- The readability of the text.
- The appropriateness and accuracy of the book.
- The quality and number of sample questions.
- The quality of written answers to sample questions.
- The quality and appropriateness of the illustrations (e.g., graphs, diagrams, photographs).
- The length of the text (longer is not necessarily better).

- The quality and number of other books available in the same discipline.
- The importance of the discipline on the USMLE Step 1 examination.

Please note that the rating does **not** reflect the quality of the book for purposes other than reviewing for the USMLE Step 1 examination. Many books with low ratings are well written and informative but are not ideal for boards preparation. We have also avoided listing or commenting on the wide variety of general textbooks available in the basic sciences.

Evaluations are based on the cumulative results of formal and informal surveys of thousands of medical students at many medical schools across the country. The summary comments and overall ratings represent a consensus opinion, but there may have been a large range of opinion or limited student feedback on one particular book.

Please note that the data listed are subject to change in that:

- Publishers' prices change frequently.
- Individual bookstores often charge an additional markup.
- New editions come out frequently, and the quality of updating varies.
- The same book may be reissued through another publisher.

We actively encourage medical students and faculty to submit their opinions and ratings of these basic science review books so that we may update our database. (*See* How to Contribute, page xv.) In addition, we ask that publishers and authors submit review copies of basic science review books, including new editions and books not included in our database for evaluation. We also solicit reviews of new books or suggestions for alternate modes of study that may be useful in preparing for the examination, such as flashcards, computer-based tutorials, and commercial review courses.

Disclaimer/Conflict of Interest Statement

No material in this book, including the ratings, reflects the opinion or influence of the publisher. All errors and omissions will gladly be corrected if brought to the attention of the authors through the publisher. Please note that the book *Underground Step 1 Answers to the NBME Retired and Self-Test Questions* (p. 280) is an independent publication by the authors of this book; its rating is based solely on data from the student survey and feedback forms.

Retired NBME Basic Medical Sciences Test Items — Test/993 q

NBME

NBME, 1991, 136 pages, out of print

Contains "retired" questions in all seven areas of basic science. Excellent topics. Letter answers only with no explanations. Content still relevant, although format outdated (ignore the K-type question format). No clinical vignettes. High yield. Out of print. Try to find an old copy. Not available in bookstores. Explanatory study guide available as a separate publication (*Underground Step 1 Answers,* see later this section).

Review for USMLE Step 1 Examination $33.00 Test/1000+ q

NMS, Lazo

Williams & Wilkins, 1996, 348 pages, ISBN 068306276X

Very good source of practice questions and answers. Features updated clinical questions and vignettes. Some questions too picky or difficult. Occasional unnecessary detail. Good buy for the number of questions. Organized as four 200-question booklets; good for simulating the exam. Helpful color plates.

Appleton & Lange's Review for the USMLE Step I $34.95 Test/1200 q

Barton

Appleton & Lange, 1996, 331 pages, ISBN 0838502652

Good questions with very good answers. Many questions very picky. Seven subject-based tests and one 300+ question comprehensive exam. Good buy for the number of questions. Some clinical vignettes. A very good, straightforward, question-based review to assess your strengths and weaknesses. Revised anatomy section and some color plates. Compare closely with NMS/Lazo.

Self-Test in the Part I Basic Medical Sciences — Test/630 q

NBME

NBME, 1989, 91 pages, out of print

A very good source of questions, level of difficulty, and detail, although format very outdated. Ninety items per discipline. Letter answers with no explanations. No clinical vignettes. Out of print. Try to find an old copy. Not available in bookstores. Explanatory study guide available as a separate publication (*Underground Step 1 Answers,* see later this section).

Underground Step 1 Answers to the NBME Retired and Self-Test Questions

$22.95   Review/1600 a

Amin

S2S Medical, 1996, 387 pages, ISBN 1890061018

Concise explanatory study guide to 1600+ *NBME Retired* and *Self-Test* questions. Easy read. Useful with or without NBME questions (not included). Referenced to current textbooks. Second edition features expanded and updated explanations. Available in some bookstores or can be ordered at (800) 247-6553 or by fax at (419) 281-6883; fully refundable. Note that this book is by the authors of *First Aid for the USMLE Step 1.*

Medical Boards–Step 1 Made Ridiculously Simple

$21.95   Review

Carl

MedMaster, 1996, 260 pages, ISBN 0940780259

Quick reading. Table format is easy to learn and to memorize. Excellent pathology section. A good supplement to *First Aid.* High yield. Would rate an A– except 1st edition contained some errors, apparently corrected in a reprint. Limited student feedback.

MEPC USMLE Step 1 Review

$29.95   Test/1200 q

Fayemi

Appleton & Lange, 1996, 455 pages, ISBN 0838562698

New edition features questions with revised explanatory answers. Mixed-quality questions with some incomplete or inaccurate explanations. Includes new clinical vignettes.

Step 1 Success

$38.00   Test/720 q

Zaslau

FMSG, 1996, 240 pages, ISBN 1886468079

Full-length practice examination with four 180-question booklets with explanations (same as actual exam). Many clinically focused questions similar to USMLE format. Small number of black-and-white photographs of moderate quality but no color pictures. Some typographic and grammatical errors. Compare with Lazo (*Review for USMLE Step 1 Examination*) and Barton (*Appleton & Lange's Review for the USMLE Step 1*). Limited student feedback. Expensive for the number of questions.

B USMLE Success

$38.00   How-to/540 q

Zaslau

FMSG, 1995, 280 pages, ISBN 1886468095

Broad overview of preparation necessary for all three steps. Has a very useful "what to study" section with list of classic slides, x-rays, and gross specimens that have appeared on previous USMLE exams. Mnemonic section helpful. Includes 180-question mock Step 1 exam with explanations. This exam accurately represents format/clinical focus of USMLE exam but contains grammatical errors. Especially appropriate for the IMG student preparing for all three Step exams in a short time period. Expensive.

B⁻ Preparation for USMLE Step 1 Basic Medical Sciences, Volumes A, B, C

$14.00 ea   Test/315 q

Luder

Maval Medical Education, 1995, 70 pages, ISBN 1884083099 (Vol. A), 1884083102 (Vol. B), 1884083110 (Vol. C)

Well-written style questions with explanatory answers. Recently revised. Good color photographs. Poor editing. Some wrong answers in the key. Many typographic and grammatical errors and expensive for the number of questions.

B⁻ Preparation for the USMLE Step 1 Basic Medical Sciences, Volumes D, E

$14.00 ea   Test/210 q

Luder

Maval Medical Education, 1995, 54 pages, ISBN 1884083129

Same format and comments as for Volumes A, B, C, but even more expensive for the number of questions. Numerous errors. Poor editing.

B⁻ Rypin's Questions and Answers for Basic Science Review

$29.95   Test/1640 q

Frohlich

Lippincott, 1993, 211 pages, ISBN 0397512473

Questions with detailed answers to supplement *Rypin's Basic Sciences Review*. Decent overall question-based review of all subjects. Not referenced to a text. Requires time commitment. New edition expected December 1996.

C⁺ Basic Science Bank—"NBME"

$75.00   Test/3500 q

FMSG

FMSG, 1991, 301 pages

Advertised as questions "remembered" from past NBME exams. Variable-quality questions with letter answers only. Poor photo quality. Contains outdated K-type and C-type (A/B/both/neither) items. Not available in bookstores. Can be ordered at (800) 662-3244; nonrefundable.

Clinical Anatomy and Pathophysiology for the Health Professional

Stewart

MedMaster, 1994, 260 pages, ISBN 0940780062

Written for non-MD professionals. Not boards oriented. Simplistic, but may be a good place to start for some students. Good diagrams.

$17.95   Review only

 Future Test: USMLE Step 1

National Learning Corp.

Future Technologies, 1994, ISBN 0837394538

PC software features multiple ways to review and self-test from database of questions with explanations. Question styles not representative of current exam. Few clinical vignettes.

$49.95   Software

 Medical Student's Guide to Top Board Scores: USMLE Steps 1 and 2

Rogers

Little, Brown, 1995, 146 pages, ISBN 0316754366

Old edition, easy to read, but information is low yield and coverage of topics is spotty. Contains some good mnemonics in basic and clinical sciences, but not necessarily boards-relevant. Incomplete and very outdated list of recommended books for board review. **New edition not yet reviewed.**

$15.95   Review

 PASS USMLE Step 1: Practice by Assessing Study Skills

Schwenker

Little, Brown, 1995, 140 pages, ISBN 0316776009

Detailed review of study and testing strategies for standardized exams and medical school. Worth considering if you have study or testing difficulties. Includes diagnostic test.

$19.95   How-to/500 q

 Rypin's Basic Sciences Review, Vol. I

Frohlich

Lippincott, 1993, 856 pages, ISBN 0397512457

Multitopic textbook with very few figures and tables. A good general reference, but should be used with other subject-specific sources. Well priced for the number of pages and questions. Requires extensive time commitment.

$34.95   Review/1000+ q

Study Skills and Test-Taking Strategies for Medical Students

$17.95 How-to only

Oklahoma Notes, Shain

Springer-Verlag, 1995, 204 pages, ISBN 038794396X

Very detailed discussion of study skills for medical school. May be useful for some students seeking a structured approach, but probably not necessary for most medical students.

The Most Common Manual for Medical Students

$14.95 Review only

Grosso

Stephen Grosso, 1991, 487 pages, ISBN 0963335405

A compilation of more than 3500 "most common questions" of medicine. Well organized, compact. Useful for the wards, with some high-yield basic science material mixed in with the clinical material.

Year Book's Medical Licensure Review: Basic Sciences

$45.95 Review/250 q

Bollet

Mosby-Year Book, 1989, 510 pages, ISBN 0815110219

Detailed textbook approach to all subjects. Questions with letter answers only. Some good illustrations. Clinically correlated. Text needs updating. Worth considering, but requires time commitment.

How to Prepare for the USMLE Step 1

$15.95 How-to/575 q

Thornborough

McGraw-Hill, 1996, 261 pages, ISBN 0070645248

New edition not reviewed. A detailed but not very useful "how-to-prepare" book written for the new examination. Uses questions from other PreTest books. Sixteen 25-question practice tests divided by topic. Contains an alphabetic list of 2000 medical terms of dubious value.

New Rudman's Questions and Answers on the USMLE

$49.95 Test/280 q

Rudman

National Learning Corporation, 1991, 200 pages, ISBN 0837358043

Combines Step 1 and Step 2 questions but no explanations. Lacks clinical vignettes and references. Some errors. Very expensive. Limited review of anatomy and physiology at the end of the book.

C PreTest Step 1 Simulated Exam

$32.00 Test/420 q

Thornborough

McGraw-Hill, 1996, 178 pages, ISBN 0070520208

Typical PreTest questions, some repeated from PreTest book series. Letter answers only. Free computerized evaluation takes a long time to receive back from PreTest Center. Picky topics. Some poorly written questions. Also, beware of *Pretest "Customized Examinations"* offered at some individual medical schools. Students report similarly problematic questions.

C USMLE Step 1 Review: The Study Guide

$32.95 Review

Goldberg

Sage, 1996, 473 pages, ISBN 0803972849

A new comprehensive review that often reads like a textbook. Does not organize ideas in a way that is useful for review purposes. No mnemonics, no questions, very few diagrams or pictures. Requires a large commitment, but low yield.

NEW BOOKS—COMPREHENSIVE

N Ace Basic Sciences: USMLE Step 1

$29.95 Test/800 q

Ace, Mosby

Mosby-Yearbook, 1996, 206 pages, ISBN 081569043 (Windows),
   ISBN 081518669X (Mac)

Appropriate format questions; some clinically focused vignettes interspersed with basic science questions. Explanations to answers focus on why to choose correct answer, not on teaching main concept. Four comprehensive exams with 200 questions each. Money-back guarantee. Small type may be hard to read. Questions can be done in book or on diskette. Compare with Lazo (*Review for USMLE Step 1 Examination*) and Barton (*Appleton & Lange's Review for the USMLE Step 1*). Limited student feedback. Software not yet examined.

N Basic Science Bank—"USMLE"

$40.00 Test/1000 q

FMSG

FMSG, 1994, 176 pages

Combination of *Basic Science Update 1993* and *Basic Science Update 1994*. Mixed quality questions with letter answers only. Expensive. Includes extended matching questions.

Body Systems Reviews I, II, and III

$24.95 Test/650 q

Board Simulator Series, Gruber
Book I: Williams & Wilkins, 1996, 320 pages, ISBN 0683063294
Book II: Williams & Wilkins, 1996, 253 pages, ISBN 0683063324
Book III: Williams & Wilkins, 1996, 230 pages, ISBN 0683063286
Four exams with approximately 160 questions each. Follows new USMLE content outline (book I covers hematopoietic/lymphoreticular, respiratory and cardiovascular systems; book II tests GI, renal, reproductive, and endocrine systems; and book III tests nervous, skin/connective tissue, and musculoskeletal systems). Questions designed to reflect clinical slant of exam. Moderate number of black-and-white photographs that are integrated into questions in an appropriate manner. Explanations discuss important concepts. Limited student feedback.

Crashing the Boards: A Friendly Study Guide for the USMLE Step 1

$14.95 Review

Yeh

Lippincott, 1996, ISBN 0397584091
Expected October 1996.

General Principles in the Basic Sciences

$24.95 Test/650 q

Board Simulator Series, Gruber
Williams & Wilkins, 1996, 263 pages, ISBN 0683063308
Four exams with approximately 160 questions each. Follows USMLE content outline and tests basic science concepts with questions. Includes some clinical vignettes. Explanations highlight basic concept tested by each question. Motivated student willing to do the five books in this series may reap unique benefits. Some photographs (black and white). Limited student feedback.

Normal and Abnormal Processes in the Basic Sciences

$24.95 Test/650 q

Board Simulator Series, Gruber
Williams & Wilkins, 1996, 253 pages, ISBN 0683063316
Four exams with approximately 160 questions each. This is probably the one book in the series that students can do without using the other ones in the series. Questions cover all seven major subject areas. Many questions written as clinical vignettes. Limited student feedback.

Step 1 Update—Book A

$16.00 Test/180 q

Zaslau

FMSG, 1996, 66 pages, ISBN 1886468133
Questions and answers based on recent examinations. Not yet reviewed.

Anatomy: Review for New National Boards

$25.00 Test/506 q

Johnson

J & S, 1992, 217 pages, ISBN 0963287303

Easy reading. Questions with detailed explanations. Good, superficial overview of cell biology, histology, gross anatomy, embryology, and neuroanatomy. Discusses clnically relevant anatomic science with adequate explanations, illustrations, and pictures; also many clinically relevant genetic diseases. Several key topics not covered. Includes good photomicrographs and cross-sectional imaging-based questions.

High-Yield Neuroanatomy

$14.95 Review only

Fix

Williams & Wilkins, 1994, 111 pages, ISBN 0683032488

Clean outline format, easy to read. Straightforward text with excellent diagrams and illustrations. Just enough detail without anything extra. Some mislabeled diagrams. High-yield review. More comprehensive than *Clinical Neuroanatomy Made Ridiculously Simple.*

Clinical Anatomy Made Ridiculously Simple

$18.95 Review only

Goldberg

MedMaster, 1991, 187 pages, ISBN 094078002X

Easy reading, simple diagrams, lots of mnemonics, and "ridiculous" associations. Somewhat incomplete. This style does not appeal to all students, so browse before buying. Some students really love this book. Good review for the relatively low-yield subject of gross anatomy.

Clinical Neuroanatomy Made Ridiculously Simple

$12.95 Review/Few q

Goldberg

MedMaster, 1995, 89 pages, ISBN 0940780003

Easy to read, memorable, simplified, with clever hand-drawn diagrams. Very quick, high-yield review of clinical neuroanatomy. Good emphasis on clinically relevant pathways, cranial nerves, and neurologic diseases. Spotty coverage of some key boards topics. No USMLE-style questions.

MEPC Anatomy

$17.95 Test/700 q

Wilson

Appleton & Lange, 1995, 251 pages, ISBN 0838562183

Updated with many clinical vignettes followed by questions. Includes gross anatomy, neuroanatomy, cell biology, embryology. Worth considering as alternative to J&S *Anatomy.* Good value. Mixed-quality questions with concise answers.

REVIEW RESOURCES

Anatomy

B **Anatomy**

$17.95   Review/70 q

Oklahoma Notes, Papka

Springer-Verlag, 1995, 231 pages, ISBN 0387943951

Concise content review covers embryology, gross anatomy, neuroanatomy, and histology. Broad coverage, but format makes text somewhat difficult to read. Few illustrations and tables.

B **Cell Biology: Review for New National Boards**

$25.00   Review/524 q

Adelman

J&S, 1995, 203 pages, ISBN 0963287389

Question-based review format like other J&S books. Covers classic topics in cell biology. Contains some high quality micrographs. Recycles some questions and illustrations from J&S *Anatomy.*

B **Liebman's Neuroanatomy Made Easy & Understandable**

$30.00   Review/Few q

Gertz

Aspen, 1995, 176 pages, ISBN 0834207303

Old edition easy to read. Contains excellent diagrams. A fast, straightforward, high-yield review. Some humor and interesting facts to help remember pathways. Expensive. **New edition not yet reviewed.**

B⁻ **Clinical Anatomy: An Illustrated Review with Questions and Explanations**

$27.95   Review/500+ q

Snell

Little, Brown, 1996, 308 pages, ISBN 0316803073

Text is well organized. Great diagrams and tables. Questions incorporate radiographs, CT scans, and MRIs. Does not cover neuroanatomy or embryology. Neither text nor questions are as clinical as the title implies. Only some of the answers have explanations, most of which are too short.

B⁻ **Embryology**

$17.95   Review/500 q

BRS, Fix

Williams & Wilkins, 1995, 266 pages, ISBN 0683032437

Outline-based review of embryology that is typical for books in this series. Good review of important embryology, but too detailed. Good discussion of congenital malformations at end of each chapter. Comprehensive exam at the end of the book is the most high-yield part of book.

Essentials of Human Embryology $39.95   Review only
Moore
Mosby, 1988, 194 pages, ISBN 0941158977
Good illustrations, pretty fast reading. However, too expensive to justify for
boards alone, but useful for the course. Does not emphasize boards topics,
but students recommend looking up *First Aid* topics in this book. No prac-
tice questions. See also the companion book: Moore & Persaud, *Study
Guide and Review Manual of Human Embryology*.

 Neuroscience $17.95   Test/509 q
Pretest, Siegel
McGraw-Hill, 1996, 209 pages, ISBN 0070520828
Detailed questions and answers. Includes photographs of CT/MRIs and
drawings of brain sections. Useful after studying from other sources. For
the motivated student.

 Cell Biology & Histology $21.95   Review/500 q
BRS, Gartner
Williams & Wilkins, 1993, 377 pages, ISBN 068303426X
Nice format with good reproductions, but too detailed. Nineteen chapters
with detailed answers. For the motivated student.

 Histology QuizBank Vols. 1 & 2 $69.00   Software/800+ q
Downing
Keyboard Publishing, 1995, ISBN 1573493171 (Mac), ISBN 1573493198
(Windows)
Database of boards-style questions arranged by subject area. Explanations
on demand. Questions cross-referenced to Junqueira Text Stack (sold sep-
arately). Expensive for limited-yield topic.

 Molecular Biology QuizBank $59.00   Software/500+ q
Case Western Reserve
Keyboard Publishing, 1995, ISBN 1573493422 (Mac), ISBN 1573493430
(Windows)
Software database of board-style questions. Expensive for limited-yield
topic.

 Wheater's Functional Histology $54.95   Review only
Burkitt
Churchill-Livingstone, 1993, 407 pages, ISBN 0443046913
Color atlas with pictures of normal histology and accompanying text. Not
directed to boards-type review. May be more useful to skim through for
photomicrograph-based questions in the glossy booklets.

C Anatomy

$17.95 Test/500 q

PreTest, April
McGraw-Hill, 1996, 220 pages, ISBN 0070520909
Old edition has difficult questions with detailed answers. Some illustrations. Requires time commitment. **New edition not yet reviewed.**

C Basic Histology: Examination and Board Review

$29.95 Review/1000+ q

Paulsen
Appleton & Lange, 1996, 379 pages, ISBN 0838522823
Dense, thorough review, but low yield for boards. Good format with many questions. Designed to complement Junqueira's *Basic Histology* textbook. Requires time commitment.

C Blond's Anatomy

$17.99 Review only

Tesoriero
Sulzburger & Graham, 1994, 282 pages, ISBN 094581920X
Concise review of gross anatomy—a low-yield topic. Easy read. Good tables and illustrations. More appropriate for coursework than boards review.

C Gross Anatomy

$21.95 Review/500 q

BRS, Chung
Williams & Wilkins, 1995, 388 pages, ISBN 068301563X
Detailed, lengthy text in outline format with illustrations and tables. A good reference book, but should be used with other sources.

C Guide to Human Anatomy

$34.50 Review/350 q

Philo
Saunders, 1985, 335 pages, ISBN 0721612032
Contains excellent pictorial summaries of body regions, clinical comments, and a section of CTs of key body levels. Covers only gross anatomy. High volume, but low-yield topic. Very expensive. For the dedicated student.

C Histology & Cell Biology

$17.95 Test/500 q

PreTest, Klein
McGraw-Hill, 1995, 307 pages, ISBN 007052081X
Old edition similar to others in the PreTest series. A few good questions, but explanations often too detailed. Requires time commitment. **New edition not yet reviewed.**

C **Langman's Medical Embryology**
Sadler
Williams & Wilkins, 1995, 460 pages, ISBN 068307489X
Concise summary pages. Useful diagrams. **New edition not yet reviewed.**

$34.00   Review only

C **MedCharts: Anatomy**
Gest
ILOC, 1994, 309 pages, ISBN 1882531019
Tabular summaries of gross anatomy for course and board review. Chart overkill is low yield.

$17.95   Review only

C **Review of Gross Anatomy**
Pansky
McGraw-Hill, 1996, 688 pages, ISBN 0071054464
Outline format with pictures on opposite page. New color illustrations and imaging correlations. Very detailed review of only gross anatomy, so low overall yield. Contains good illustrations and a few tables. For the dedicated student.

$39.95   Review/500+ q

C **Review Questions: Gross Anatomy and Embryology**
Gest
Parthenon, 1993, 399 pages, ISBN 1850705038
Contains outdated K-type questions and has no matching questions or clinical vignettes. Huge collection of questions covers only gross anatomy and embryology.

$21.95   Test/2500+ q

C⁻ **Anatomy Study Guide**
Cobb
Lone Star, 1989, 131 pages, ISBN 0962667803
Typewritten, outline format with good summary pages at the end of each of its five sections. Low yield overall.

$14.95   Review/500+ q

C⁻ **Appleton & Lange's Review of Anatomy**
Montgomery
Appleton & Lange, 1995, 340 pages, ISBN 0838502466
Old edition has only gross anatomy, so low yield. High volume of questions with brief explanations, no text, and few diagrams. **1995 edition not yet reviewed.**

$29.95   Test/1000+ q

C⁻ **Cell Biology and Histology**
NMS, Johnson
Williams & Wilkins, 1991, 409 pages, ISBN 0683062107
Outline form. Questions with detailed answers.

$27.00   Review/500 q

Clinical Anatomy

$26.00   Review/500 q

NMS, April

Williams & Wilkins, 1996, 650 pages, ISBN 0683061992

Organized in outline form. Questions with detailed answers. Old edition was too in-depth and low yield. **New edition not yet reviewed.**

Essentials of Human Histology

$29.95   Review/100 q

Krause

Little, Brown, 1996, 452 pages, ISBN 0316503363

Review text with some boards-style questions and letter answers. May be more appropriate as a course text than as a review book. **New edition not yet reviewed.**

Gross Anatomy: A Review with Questions and Explanations

$28.95   Review/430+ q

Snell

Little, Brown, 1990, 345 pages, ISBN 0316801976

A preeminent author. Dense, thorough, and requires time commitment. Good diagrams. Some questions outdated. Very little clinical correlation. Still low yield.

Human Developmental Anatomy

$27.00   Review/450 q

NMS, Johnson

Williams & Wilkins, 1989, 447 pages, ISBN 0683062263

Outline form. Low yield.

Keyboard Histology Series Personal Edition

$149.00   Software/800+ q

Keyboard Publishing, 1995, ISBN 1573492973 (Mac), ISBN 1573492981 (Windows)

Includes Histology Quizbanks Vols. 1 & 2 (reviewed previously) and Junqueira Histology Text Stack. Quizbank questions linked to passages in Text Stack. Text can be exported to word processor. Very expensive for a limited-yield subject. Better if purchased by the library. Text Stack more appropriate for reference than for review.

MEPC Histology

$40.00   Review/300 q

Amenta

Appleton & Lange, 1995, 94 pages, ISBN 1572350695

Old edition very detailed for low-yield topic. Very expensive.

Neuroanatomy $26.00 Review/300 q
NMS, DeMyer
Williams & Wilkins, 1997, 380 pages, ISBN 068330075X
Outline form. Old edition was too detailed. Nice diagrams, but low yield.
New edition not yet reviewed.

Neuroanatomy $21.95 Review/500 q
BRS, Fix
Williams & Wilkins, 1995, 416 pages, ISBN 0683032496
Updated text. Covers anatomy and embryology of the nervous system. Still
low yield.

Neuroanatomy: A Review with Questions $29.95 Review/400+ q
and Explanations
Snell
Little, Brown, 1992, 298 pages, ISBN 0316802468
Reasonably easy to read, contains some clinical correlations. Length of the
book too long relative to the small portion of the exam related to neuroanatomy. New edition titled *Clinical Neuroanatomy: An Illustrated Review
with Questions and Explanations* expected in December 1997.

Student Aid to Gross Anatomy $19.50 Review only
Snell
Appleton & Lange, 1986, 514 pages, ISBN 0838586872
A pocket-sized handbook for quick reference. Written as an abstract of the
larger textbook, which covers gross anatomy by system. Good organization
but too detailed for the boards.

NEW BOOKS—ANATOMY

Ace Anatomy $29.95 Review/300+ q
Ace, Moore
Mosby-Year Book, 1996, 400 pages, ISBN 0815169051 (Windows), ISBN
0815186711 (Mac)
Expected in December 1996. Concise content review with boards-style
questions. Test software included with text. Money-back guarantee.

REVIEW RESOURCES

Anatomy

Ace Histology and Cell Biology

$26.95   Review/286 q

Ace, Burns

Mosby-Year Book, 1996, 250 pages, ISBN 0815113382 (Windows), ISBN 0815113358 (Mac)

Good diagrams of tissues, but no actual photomicrographs. Outline format and boldfaced key words facilitate quick review. Icons are more distracting than helpful. Review questions at the end of each chapter are not representative of USMLE examination format. Too much detail in some areas. Limited feedback on software.

Ace Neuroscience

$28.95   Review/235 q

Ace, Castro

Mosby-Year Book, 1996, 464 pages, ISBN 0815114796 (Windows), ISBN 081511480X (Mac)

Expected in late 1996. Concise content review with boards-style questions. Test software included with text. Money-back guarantee.

High-Yield Gross Anatomy

$14.95   Review only

Dudek

Williams & Wilkins, 1997, 170 pages, ISBN 0683182153

Expected in 1997.

High-Yield Histology

$14.95   Review only

Dudek

Williams & Wilkins, 1997, 95 pages, ISBN 0683027204

Expected in December 1996.

Histology

$26.00   Review/q

NMS, Henrickson

Williams & Wilkins, 1997, 350 pages, ISBN 0683062255

Expected in March 1997.

PreTest Anatomy Study Disk

$28.00   Software/500 q

April

McGraw-Hill, 1995, ISBN 0078641632 (Mac), ISBN 0078641624 (Windows)

Software test review based on *PreTest Anatomy* text. Includes questions with detailed answers and some illustrations. Program can custom-generate tests. Copy protection mechanism is inconvenient.

Behavioral Science Review

$21.95   Review/500 q

BRS, Fadem

Williams & Wilkins, 1994, 237 pages, ISBN 0683029533

Easy reading, outline format, boldfacing of key terms. Appropriate length and good, detailed coverage of high-yield topics. Great tables and charts. Short but complete statistics chapter. Good value.

High Yield Behavioral Science

$14.95   Review only

High Yield, Fadem

Williams & Wilkins, 1997, ISBN 0683029401

Clear, concise, very quick review of behavioral science. Logical presentation with charts, graphs, and tables. Limited student feedback. Compare to Fadem's other review text (*Behavioral Science Review*).

Behavioral Sciences in Psychiatry

$27.00   Review/300 q

NMS, Wiener

Williams & Wilkins, 1995, 375 pages, ISBN 0683062034

New edition retains detailed multidisciplinary outline, but with improved formatting. Neatly organized. Incorporates DSM-IV. Probably more detailed than necessary. For the motivated student starting early or to be used as a reference. New biostatistics chapter is inadequate.

Behavioral Sciences for the Boreds

$14.95   Review only

Sierles

MedMaster, 1993, 146 pages, ISBN 0940780194

Short, easy reading, reasonable yield, but can get lost in narrative format. Includes biostatistics, medical sociology, psychopathology. Not enough to achieve a high score. Must supplement with another text. Casual style does not appeal to all students. Appropriate if you have very limited time. New edition expected mid-1997.

High-Yield Biostatistics

$15.00   Review only

Glaser

Williams & Wilkins, 1995, 83 pages, ISBN 0683035665

Complete, well-written, illustrated book covering the biostatistics likely to be on the USMLE Step 1. Good review exercises. Still, limited-yield topic. For the motivated student, not for last-minute cramming.

REVIEW RESOURCES

Behavioral Science

B **Review of Epidemiology and Biostatistics** $21.95 Review
Hanrahan
Appleton & Lange, 1994, 109 pages, ISBN 083850244X
Excellent, concise overview of epidemiology with complete explanations
and diagrams. Does not include other behavioral science subtopics. Expen-
sive and limited yield. Good for the motivated student.

B⁻ **Behavioral Sciences** $17.95 Review/169 q
Oklahoma Notes, Krug
Springer-Verlag, 1995, 311 pages, ISBN 0387943935
Typewritten, easy reading. Outline format. Questions of mixed quality. Good
tables. For the motivated student.

B⁻ **Digging Up the Bones: Behavioral Sciences** $16.00 Review only
Linardakis
Michaelis Medical, 1995, 85 pages, ISBN 1884084117
Concise narrative review of behavioral sciences; disorganized format covers some high-yield topics. Probably too concise. Nevertheless, this book
may assist the student who needs a "last minute" review. Limited student
feedback.

C⁺ **Behavioral Sciences** $17.95 Test/500 q
PreTest, Pattishall
McGraw-Hill, 1996, 275 pages, ISBN 0070520844
Easy reading. Questions with detailed answers. Requires some time invest-
ment. **New edition not yet reviewed.**

C⁺ **Medical Biostatistics and Epidemiology: Examination** $29.95 Review
and Board Review
Essex-Sorlie
Appleton & Lange, 1995, 359 pages, ISBN 0838562191
Too in-depth for biostatistics. Requires time commitment. Sample questions
may not be representative of the USMLE Step 1.

C **Clinical Epidemiology and Biostatistics** $27.00 Review/300 q
NMS, Knapp
Williams & Wilkins, 1992, 435 pages, ISBN 0683062069
Overkill for a limited-yield topic.

Behavioral Science

A Review of Biostatistics

$22.95   Review only

Leaverton

Little, Brown, 1995, 117 pages, ISBN 0316518832

Review of biostatistics that does not focus on high-yield topics for the USMLE. Last two chapters cover material relevant to USMLE review. More appropriate for coursework than for USMLE review.

Psychiatry Made Ridiculously Simple

$12.95   Review only

Good

MedMaster, 1995, 90 pages, ISBN 0940780224

Easy reading. Includes epidemiology. Low basic science yield, but very good clinical material.

NEW BOOKS—BEHAVIORAL SCIENCE

Ace Behavioral Science

$27.95   Review/217+ q

Ace, Cody

Mosby-Year Book, 1996, 200 pages, ISBN 0815118449 (Windows), ISBN 0815114877 (Mac)

Concise content review with boards-style questions. Test software included with text. Money-back guarantee. Expected late 1996.

REVIEW RESOURCES

Behavioral Science

Lippincott's Illustrated Reviews: Biochemistry

$29.95   Review/250+ q

Champe

Lippincott, 1994, 443 pages, ISBN 0397510918

Excellent book, but requires time commitment, so must start early. Best used while taking the course. Excellent diagrams. Emphasizes concepts. Good clinical correlations. Comprehensive review of biochemistry, including low-yield topics. Not for cramming unless you skim many parts.

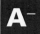

Biochemistry

$21.95   Review/500 q

BRS, Marks

Williams & Wilkins, 1994, 337 pages, ISBN 0683055976

Easy-to-read outline with very good boldfaced chapter summaries. More concise alternative to Lippincott. Outline format not ideal for some sections. Mixed-quality diagrams. High-yield clinical correlations at end of each chapter. Questions with short answers. Some questions too picky.

Biochemistry Review

$19.95   Review/600 q

Star, Roskoski

Saunders, 1996, 242 pages, ISBN 0721651755

Content review in outline format. First six chapters of book focus on basic concepts, while the rest of the book reviews metabolic pathways and molecular/cell biology. Chapters are short and include only relevant pathways. Excellent book for students who prefer outline-based review. Parallels a core text by the same authors. Comprehensive exam at the end of the book has some clinically focused questions. Compare to Champe (*Lippincott's Illustrated Reviews: Biochemistry*) and Marks (*Biochemistry*). Limited student feedback.

Biochemistry: Review for New National Boards

$25.00   Test/505 q

Kumar

J & S, 1993, 211 pages, ISBN 0963287311

Quick review of biochemistry consisting primarily of questions with detailed answers. Includes clinical vignettes and extended matching questions; few diagrams. Use in conjunction with other resources.

Digging Up the Bones: Biochemistry

$16.00   Review only

Wilson

Michaelis Medical, 1994, 124 pages, ISBN 1884084044

Collection of high-yield biochemistry facts. Use for last-minute review or in conjunction with another review book. Some lists are helpful. Choppy style.

REVIEW RESOURCES

Biochemistry

B Biochemistry

$17.95   Review/549+ q

Oklahoma Notes, Briggs

Springer-Verlag, 1995, 287 pages, ISBN 0387943986

Dense text retains many hand-drawn diagrams. Good chapter on medical genetics. Non-clinically oriented questions with brief explanations in the margin. Multiple authors, inconsistent style. Limited student feedback.

B Biochemistry

$17.95   Test/500 q

PreTest, Chlapowski

McGraw-Hill, 1996, 231 pages, ISBN 0070520895

Difficult questions with detailed, referenced explanations. Better than average for this series; best for the motivated student who uses this and a review book. New edition has some questions on biochemical diseases but no clinical vignettes.

B Biochemistry: An Illustrated Review with Questions and Explanations

$29.95   Review/220+ q

Friedman

Little, Brown, 1995, 220 pages, ISBN 0316294284

Good quality, concise text review. Metabolism section is well illustrated. Molecular biochemistry section fails to emphasize important concepts and has few illustrations. Too few pathways; too many structures. Boards-style questions favor basic biochemistry over clinical correlation. Letter answers with occasional short explanations.

B Biochemistry: Examination and Board Review

$31.95   Review/500+ q

Balcavage

Appleton & Lange, 1995, 433 pages, ISBN 0838506615

Comprehensive review of biochemistry. Requires time commitment. Appropriate as a course text. Has some clinical correlations.

B Biochemistry Illustrated

$34.95   Review only

Campbell

Churchill-Livingstone, 1994, 304 pages, ISBN 0443045739

Excellent diagrams with explanations but no questions. Good for students who prefer learning by diagrams. Readable. Very expensive. Requires time commitment.

B Blond's Biochemistry

$17.99   Review only

Guttenplan

Sulzburger & Graham, 1994, 269 pages, ISBN 0945819498

Easy reading. Moderate time commitment. Some topics covered only superficially. Not boards oriented; may be more appropriate with coursework.

B   Clinical Biochemistry Made Ridiculously Simple $22.95   Review only

Goldberg

MedMaster, 1993, 93 pages, ISBN 0940780100

Conceptual approach to clinical biochemistry, with humor. The casual style does not appeal to all students. A good overview and integration for all metabolic pathways. Includes a 23-page clinical review that is very high-yield and crammable. Contains a unique foldout "road map" of metabolism. Not adequate as sole study source. For students with firm biochemistry background. New edition expected March 1997 (ISBN 0940780305).

B   Metabolism at a Glance $24.95   Review only

Salway

Blackwell Science, 1994, 95 pages, ISBN 0632032588

Highly visual. Features diagrams with associated text. Illustrations pretty but complicated. Use as a supplement to traditional review books. Large-page format.

B⁻   Biochemistry $27.00   Review/500 q

NMS, Davidson

Williams & Wilkins, 1994, 584 pages, ISBN 0683062050

Very long, detailed outline. Questions with detailed answers. Good pathway illustrations but too much chemical structure detail. Concise review of genetics. Overall, too detailed to use as review text unless previously used during coursework. For the motivated student.

B⁻   Essentials of Biochemistry $32.95   Review/100 q

EBS, Schumm

Little, Brown, 1995, 382 pages, ISBN 0316775312

Review text with some boards-style questions and letter answers. May be more appropriate as a course text than review book.

B⁻   MEPC Biochemistry $17.95   Test/700 q

Glick

Appleton & Lange, 1995, 228 pages ISBN 0838557791

Picky questions with brief explanations. Revised edition has few clinical vignettes.

C⁺   Genetics $27.00   Review/300 q

NMS, Friedman

Williams & Wilkins, 1995, ISBN 0683062174

Old edition has detailed outline format supplemented by numerous charts and diagrams. Low yield. Some chapters not relevant for board review. For the very motivated student. **New edition not yet reviewed.**

C **Basic Concepts in Biochemistry:**
A Student's Survival Guide $25.95   Review only

Gilbert

McGraw-Hill, 1992, 298 pages, ISBN 0070234493

Presents concise summaries of difficult biochemical concepts and principles. Because it ignores much of the high-yield material, it is not very useful for boards review. Oriented toward undergraduate courses.

C **Genetics** $17.95   Test/500 q

PreTest, Finkelstein

McGraw-Hill, 1996, 206 pages, ISBN 0070520836

Old edition has detailed questions and answers. Questions of mixed quality.
Limited student feedback. **New edition not yet reviewed.**

NEW BOOKS—BIOCHEMISTRY

N **Ace Biochemistry** $29.95   Review/400+ q

Ace, Pelley

Mosby-Year Book, 1996, 400 pages, ISBN 0815186525 (Windows),
    ISBN 0815186681 (Mac)

Expected in December 1996. Concise content review with boards-style
questions. Test software included with text. Money-back guarantee.

N **Molecular Biology QuizBank Personal Edition** $59.00   Software

Keyboard Publishing, 1995, ISBN 1573493422 (Mac), ISBN 1573493430 (Windows)

Not yet reviewed.

N **PreTest Biochemistry Study Disk** $28.00   Software/500 q

Chlapowski

McGraw-Hill, 1995, ISBN 0078641659 (Mac), ISBN 0078641640 (Windows)

Software test review based on *PreTest Biochemistry*. Includes questions
with detailed answers and some illustrations. Program can custom-
generate tests. Copy protection mechanism is inconvenient.

Medical Microbiology & Immunology: Examination and Board Review   **$29.95**   Review/692 q

Levinson

Appleton & Lange, 1996, 523 pages, ISBN 0838562256

Clear, concise writing, with excellent diagrams and tables. Excellent readability for both text and questions. Forty-two page "Summary of Medically Important Organisms" very crammable. Requires time commitment. Sometimes too detailed. Best if started early with the course. Covers all topics, including low-yield ones. Good practice questions, but with letter answers only a disadvantage.

 Clinical Microbiology Made Ridiculously Simple   **$22.95**   Review

Gladwin

MedMaster, 1995, 268 pages, ISBN 0940780208

Very good chart-based review of microbiology. Clever and humorous mnemonics. Text easy to read. Excellent antibiotic review helps for pharmacology as well. "Ridiculous" style does not appeal to everyone. Does not cover immunology. Excellent if you have very limited time.

 Microbiology & Immunology   **$21.95**   Review/500 q

BRS, Johnson

Williams & Wilkins, 1996, 297 pages, ISBN 0683180053

Outline format, well organized. Good questions at the ends of chapters. Too few diagrams. Chapters on bacterial genetics and laboratory methods. Immunology section concise. Compare with Levinson *(Medical Microbiology & Immunology: Examination and Board Review)*.

 Microbiology: Review for New National Boards   **$25.00**   Test/507 q

Stokes

J & S, 1993, 194 pages, ISBN 096328732X

Easy reading. Covers many high-yield topics and includes case-based questions and extended matching questions. Very good question-and-answer–based review of clinically relevant microbiology and immunology, but lacking somewhat in detailed information. Excellent supplement to a review book.

 Ace Microbiology & Immunology   **$28.95**   Review/282+ q

Ace, Rosenthal

Mosby-Year Book, 1996, 320 pages, ISBN 0815173490 (Windows),
    ISBN 0815186703 (Mac)

Concise but comprehensive review of microbiology and immunology in outline format. Good diagrams and tables. Icons designed to help classify information, but overabundance may confuse some students. Boards-style questions at the end of each chapter. Test software included with text. Money-back guarantee. Limited student feedback.

REVIEW RESOURCES

Microbiology

Appleton & Lange's Review of Microbiology and Immunology for USMLE Step 1

$29.95   Test/995 q

Yotis

Appleton & Lange, 1997, 288 pages, ISBN 0838502733

Large number of questions with detailed answers. Updated for the USMLE. Well referenced. Inadequate as a primary source, but a very good supplement. For the motivated student. Limited feedback on new edition.

Microbiology

$27.95   Review only

Tof

Alert and Oriented, 1994, 243 pages, ISBN 0964012413

Chart format is well organized and easy to read and carry. Most relevant to microbiology topics. High-yield flash cards are a plus. Has a short immunology review.

B — Buzzwords in Microbiology

$19.95   Review only

Hurst

Bryan Edwards, 1994, 155 pages, ISBN 1878576089

Spiral-bound flash cards contain important facts about the most medically relevant bacteria and fungi. Directed to boards review. Bullet presentation of information affords easy and quick review. Excellent pictures and buzzwords. Useful as a speedy pocket-sized review after studying from a more complete text. Does not cover virology, parasitology, or immunology.

B — Essentials of Pathophysiology

$39.95   Review/69 q

EBS, Kaufman

Little, Brown, 1996, 650 pages, ISBN 0316484059

Review book with few questions. Features clinical descriptions of important diseases, but too detailed for high-yield review. Good diagrams, tables, and black-and-white photographs. More appropriate as a course text and reference. For the very motivated student. Limited student feedback.

B — Microbiology and Immunology

$17.95   Review/312+ q

Oklahoma Notes, Hyde

Springer-Verlag, 1995, 229 pages, ISBN 0387943927

Old edition easy to read, but not adequate as sole study source. Good summary statements at end of each chapter. Extended matching questions. Poor typeface and diagrams. Unequal coverage. **New edition not yet reviewed.**

B

Microbiology & Immunology: An Illustrated Review with Questions and Explanations

$29.95   Review/450+ q

Hentges

Little, Brown, 1995, 304 pages, ISBN 0316357847

Comprehensive review takes time commitment. Revised edition has updated tables and charts. Improved format and organization. Summation chapter at end of book is of limited value. Limited student feedback.

B⁻

Blond's Microbiology

$15.99   Review only

Alcamo

Sulzberger & Graham, 1994, 181 pages, ISBN 0945819412

Text review. Spotty coverage of some key topics. Below average for this series.

B⁻

Digging Up the Bones: Microbiology

$17.95   Review/Cards

Linardakis

Michaelis Medical, 1996, 99 pages and flash cards, ISBN 1884084192

Old edition easy to read. Brief collection of phrases and associations based on answers to assorted multiple-choice questions. A few tables and simple diagrams. Very expensive for the amount of material. New edition (October 1996) will feature improved organization and new flash cards.

B⁻

Essential Immunology Review

$19.95   Test/422 q

Roitt

Blackwell Scientific, 1995, 319 pages, ISBN 0865424586

Boards-style questions with explanations that also discuss the incorrect answers.

B⁻

Immunology at a Glance

$19.95   Review only

Playfair

Blackwell Scientific, 1992, 43 pages, ISBN 0632033150

Diagram-based synopsis of immunology. Text and figures on the left, with legends on the right. Expensive for length of book. New edition released in 1996 (ISBN 0865426775).

B⁻

MEPC Microbiology

$17.95   Test/700 q

Kim

Appleton & Lange, 1995, 257 pages, ISBN 0838563082

Updated with clinical vignettes. Good infectious disease questions. Variable quality questions. Easy read. Explanations are brief and direct.

REVIEW RESOURCES

Microbiology

Microbiology

$17.95   Test/500 q

PreTest, Tilton

McGraw-Hill, 1996, 191 pages, ISBN 0070520887

Mixed-quality questions with detailed explanations. Questions often too difficult and answers verbose. Bacteriology section better than immunology. Useful for additional question-based review in bacteriology and virology, but not high yield.

Microbiology and Infectious Disease

$26.00   Review/500 q

NMS, Virella

Williams & Wilkins, 1996, 575 pages, ISBN 0683062352

Outline form. Old edition was too detailed in some areas. Insufficient immunology; NMS has a separate immunology book. Lacks good explanation of bacterial genetics. Updated material on AIDS. Useful only if previously used as a textbook. **New edition not yet reviewed.**

Microbiology QuizBanks Vols. 2 & 3

$69.00   Software/800+ q

Gotts

Keyboard Publishing, 1995, ISBN 1573493252 (Mac), 1573493279 (Windows)

Computer-based questions with explanations. Questions electronically referenced to Sherris Microbiology Text Stack (sold separately). Expensive.

Immunology

$27.00   Review/300 q

NMS, Hyde

Williams & Wilkins, 1995, 316 pages, ISBN 068306231X

Outline form. Very detailed. Good figures and explanations of laboratory methods. Updated information on immune response, but lengthy for immunology alone. Requires time commitment.

Immunology QuizBank Vol. 1

$69.00   Software/400+ q

Roitt

Keyboard Publishing, 1995, ISBN 157349321X (Mac), 1573493236 (Windows)

Software database of boards-style questions with explanations. Questions electronically referenced to Roitt Immunology Text Stack (sold separately). Packaged with bonus case collection. Very expensive for number of questions.

The Keyboard Immunology Series Personal Edition
Roitt

$149.00   Software/400 q

Keyboard Publishing, 1995, ISBN 1573492035 (Mac), ISBN 1573492043 (Windows).

More appropriate for use with course work. Includes Histology QuizBank and *Essential Immunology* Text Stack by Roitt. Questions cross-linked to Text Stack. Text can be exported to a word processor. Available for PC and Macintosh. Limited student feedback. Good learning tool, but beyond the student budget. More appropriate as a library purchase.

The Keyboard Microbiology Series Personal Edition
Ryan

$149.00   Software/800 q

Keyboard Publishing, 1995, ISBN 1573492701 (Mac), ISBN 157349271X (Windows)

Includes two Microbiology QuizBanks and the electronic edition of *Sherris Medical Microbiology*. Questions cross-linked to Text Stack. Text can be exported to a word processor. More appropriate for use with course work and as a reference. Good learning tool but beyond the student budget. More appropriate as a library purchase.

Microbiology & Immunology Casebook
Barrett

$17.95   Review/185 q

Little, Brown, 1995, 262 pages, ISBN 0316081329

Uses case examples to cover major concepts. Cases do not resemble typical boards vignettes. Useful only as a supplement to a review book.

Immunology Illustrated Outline
Male

$19.95   Review only

Raven Press, 1991, ISBN 0397448252

Pocket-sized booklet, well organized, concise. Quick to read and review. Not targeted for boards review.

NEW BOOKS—MICROBIOLOGY

Lippincott's Illustrated Reviews: Microbiology
Strohl

—   Review

Lippincott, 1997

Expected in June 1997. Features a comprehensive, highly illustrated review of microbiology similar in style to Champe's *Lippincott's Illustrated Reviews: Biochemistry*.

Medical MicroCards $14.95 Review

Orlando

Medfiles, 1996, 150 pages, ISBN 0965537307

Not yet reviewed. High yield flash cards cover bacteriology, virology, mycology, and parasitology. Designed for fast review. Can be ordered at
(908) 286-1300.

 Microbiology Review $19.95 Review/600 q

STAR, Walker

Saunders, 1997, ISBN 0721646425

Will parallel core text by the same authors. Expected in late 1997.

 MicroCharts $24.95 Review only

Weiner

MRO MicroCharts, 1993, 116 pages

Not reviewed. Quick review of microbiology in tabular form.

PreTest Microbiology Study Disk $28.00 Software/500 q

Tilton

McGraw-Hill, 1995, ISBN 0078641551 (Mac), ISBN 0078641543 (Windows)

Software test review based on *PreTest Microbiology* text. Includes questions with detailed answers and some illustrations. Program can custom-
generate tests. Copy protection mechanism is inconvenient.

Pathology

$21.95   Review/500 q

BRS, Schneider

Williams & Wilkins, 1993, 412 pages, ISBN 0683076086

Excellent, concise review with appropriate emphasis. Outline-format chapters with boldfacing of key facts. Excellent questions with explanations at the end of each chapter and at the end of the book. Well-organized tables and diagrams. Good black-and-white photographs representative of classic pathology. Short on clinical details for vignette questions. Consistently high student recommendations. Must start early, but very worthwhile to master this book. Correlate with color photographs from an atlas.

Pathology: Review for New National Boards

$25.00   Test/509 q

Miller

J & S, 1993, 222 pages, ISBN 0963287338

Question-and-answer–based review of pathology. Includes many case-based questions. Focuses on high-yield topics. Good black-and-white photographs. Inadequate as sole source of review. Expensive for number of questions.

Pathophysiology of Disease: An Introduction to Clinical Medicine

$32.95   Review/Few q.

McPhee

Appleton & Lange, 1995, 521 pages, ISBN 0838578152

Interdisciplinary course text that students report is useful in dealing with the growing clinical slant of the boards. Excellent integration of basic sciences with mechanisms of disease. Great graphs, diagrams, and tables. Does not discuss pharmacotherapy. Few non–boards-style questions. Clinical emphasis nicely complements *BRS Pathology.*

Appleton & Lange's Review of General Pathology

$29.95   Test/896 q

Lewis

Appleton & Lange, 1993, 197 pages, ISBN 0838501613

Short text sections followed by lots of questions with answers. Some very useful high-yield tables at the beginning of each section. Good illustrations and photographs. Covers only general pathology (i.e., no organ-based pathology). Can be used as a supplement to more detailed texts. Reviewable in a short period.

Medical Exam Review: Pathology

$17.95   Test/600 q

A&L/MEPC, Fayemi

Appleton & Lange, 1994, 317 pages, ISBN 0838584411

Good-quality questions with explanations. Good case-study chapter. Use as a supplement to other review books.

Pathology: Examination and Board Review

$29.95   Review

Newland

Appleton & Lange, 1995, 314 pages, ISBN 0838577199

Short, to-the-point text review with many high-quality illustrations. Has some good charts and illustrations. Some overlap with microbiology. Limited student feedback.

Pathology Notes

$26.95   Review only

Chandrasoma

Appleton & Lange, 1992, 788 pages, ISBN 0838551645

Lengthy but well organized and easy to read. Requires considerable time commitment. Good tables. No photographs. Good line drawings. Compare the format with *Pocket Companion to Robbins'* as to which best suits your style. Companion to *Concise Pathology* by same authors.

Pocket Companion to Robbins' Pathologic Basis of Diseases

$25.00   Review only

Robbins

Saunders, 1995, 620 pages, ISBN 0721657427

Old edition was good for reviewing associations between keywords and specific diseases. Very condensed, easy to understand. Explains most important diseases and pathologic processes. No photographs or illustrations. Useful as a quick reference. **New edition not yet reviewed.**

Digging Up the Bones: Pathology

$17.95   Review only

Linardakis

Michaelis Medical, 1996, 130 pages, ISBN 1884084206

Old edition was easy reading. Brief collection of phrases and associations often based on answers to assorted multiple-choice questions. Very expensive for the amount of material. New edition expected in December 1996 will feature new photomicrographs (gross and microscopic).

Pathology

$17.95   Review/140 q

Oklahoma Notes, Holliman

Springer-Verlag, 1995, 279 pages, ISBN 0387943900

Dense text. Few diagrams and tables. No illustrations. Questions with letter answers only. Good when you have no time for comprehensive review books. **New edition not yet reviewed.**

B Pathology Illustrated

$54.95 Review only

Govan

Churchill-Livingstone, 1995, 843 pages, ISBN 0443050686

Lengthy, but fast reading. Well illustrated with many line drawings. User-friendly format. Worth considering despite price. **New edition not reviewed.**

B⁻ Neurology and Clinical Neuroscience

$17.95 Review/101 q

Oklahoma Notes, Brumback

Springer-Verlag, 1996, 186 pages, ISBN 0387946357

Utilizes organ system approach by integrating CNS anatomy, pathology, physiology, and some pharmacology. Easy to read. Good-quality line drawings. Use either with organ system review or as a supplement to a subject review. Limited student feedback.

B⁻ Pathologic Basis of Disease Self-Assessment and Review

$21.75 Test/1600+ q

Compton

Saunders, 1995, 239 pages, ISBN 0721640419

Old edition features huge number of good practice questions, some very difficult and detailed. A good buy for the number of questions. Includes outdated K-type question format. Very good for the dedicated student. **New edition not yet reviewed.**

B⁻ Pathology

$27.00 Review/500 q

NMS, LiVolsi

Williams & Wilkins, 1994, 508 pages, ISBN 0683062433

Outline form. Comprehensive review of large amount of material. Sometimes too detailed. Slow reading.

B⁻ Pathology Facts

$19.95 Review only

Harruff

Lippincott, 1994, 424 pages, ISBN 0397512589

A handbook-sized text database, organized by disease. Limited topic coverage. Worth considering.

B⁻ **Pathology QuizBank, Vol. 2** **$99.00** Software/1000+ q

Faculty UC Davis

Keyboard Publishing, 1995, ISBN 1573493295 (Mac), ISBN 1573493317 (Windows)

Expensive software database of board-style questions with explanations. Good, detailed explanations. Some repetitive questions. Requires time commitment. Electronically referenced to Robbins' *Pathology TextStack*. Quizzer has no timer or ability to custom-generate tests. Good for library acquisition.

B⁻ **Pathology** **$17.95** Test/500 q

PreTest, Brown

McGraw-Hill, 1996, 299 pages, ISBN 0070520860

Picky, difficult questions with detailed, complete answers. Often obscure or esoteric questions. Good-quality black-and-white photographs; no color photographs. Can be used as a supplement to other review books. For the motivated student who desires challenging exposure to lots of photographs.

C⁺ **The Keyboard Pathology Series Personal Edition** **$199.00** Software/1000+ q

Cotran

Keyboard Publishing, 1995, ISBN 1573492116 (Mac), ISBN 1573492124 (Windows)

Includes electronic edition of the 5th edition of Robbins' *Pathologic Basis of Disease* on CD-ROM and *Pathology QuizBank*. Very good if used as reference or with course. Beyond the student budget. More appropriate as a library purchase.

C **Basic Histopathology** **$54.95** Review only

Wheater

Churchill-Livingstone, 1991, 252 pages, ISBN 0443042373

Color atlas with text. Contains pictures of pathologic histology. Not directed to boards-type review. May be more useful for photomicrograph-based questions.

NEW BOOKS—PATHOLOGY

N **Ace Pathology** **$29.95** Text/600+ q

Ace, Wurzel

Mosby-Year Book, 1996, 400 pages, ISBN 0815192762 (Windows), ISBN 0815194285 (Mac)

Expected December 1996. Features a concise content review with boards-style questions. Test software included with text. Money-back guarantee.

PreTest Pathology Study Disk

$28.00   Software/500 q

Brown

McGraw-Hill, 1995, ISBN 0078641594 (Mac); ISBN 0078641586 (Windows)

Software test review based on *PreTest Pathology*. Includes questions with detailed answers and some illustrations. Program can custom-generate tests.

Lippincott's Illustrated Reviews: Pharmacology

$29.95 Review/230+ q

Harvey

Lippincott, 1997, 475 pages, ISBN 0397515677

Outline format with practice questions and many excellent illustrations and tables. Cross-referenced to Lippincott's *Biochemistry*. Good for the big picture. Good pathophysiologic approach. Detailed, so must start early. For the motivated student. New edition released November 1996 adds ten illustrated case studies with questions and answers in the appendix.

Pharmacology: Examination and Board Review

$28.95 Review/650+ q

Katzung

Appleton & Lange, 1995, 509 pages, ISBN 083858067X

Text is well organized and readable. Good charts and tables. Relevant and challenging questions with concise explanations. Good for drug interactions and toxicities. Text is quite detailed and requires large time commitment. Compare with new *Lippincott's Illustrated Reviews: Pharmacology.* Includes some low-yield/obscure drugs. Good diagrams. The 40-page (417–457) crammable list of "top boards drugs" is especially high yield.

Pharm Cards: A Review for Medical Students

$25.95 Review only

Johannsen

Little, Brown, 1995, 195 cards, ISBN 0316465496

Review in index-card format; very popular with students. Highlights important features of major drugs/drug classes. Perfect for class review; also offers a quick, focused review of pharmacology for the USMLE. Good charts and diagrams. Particularly useful for students who enjoy flash-card based review. Follow instructions on "sample pharmcard" regarding use of the cards for USMLE review.

Clinical Pharmacology Made Ridiculously Simple

$18.95 Review only

Olson

MedMaster, 1994, 162 pages, ISBN 0940780178

Includes general principles and many drug summary charts. Particularly strong in cardiovascular drugs and antimicrobials, incomplete in other areas. The casual style does not work for some students. Well organized, but occasionally too detailed. Effective as a chart-based review book but not as a sole study source. Must supplement with a more detailed text.

B+ Pharmacology: An Illustrated Review with Questions and Explanations

$29.95   Review/400+ q

Ebadi

Little, Brown, 1996, 336 pages, ISBN 0316199575

New edition with many more illustrations and tables. Comprehensive review of pharmacology, but the content and emphasis do not always reflect high-yield topics. Some emphasis on neuropharmacology. Good for the student who likes comprehensive chart/illustration–based review. Requires time commitment. Includes clinical case-based questions.

B+ Pharmacology: Review for New National Boards

$25.00   Test/539 q

Billingsley

J & S, 1995, 186 pages, ISBN 0963287370

Question-and-answer book, typical for this series. Good explanations cover many high-yield pharmacology topics. Easy, fast reading. Questions about drug structures probably low yield. Useful adjunct to a review book. Limited student feedback.

B Blond's Pharmacology

$19.99   Review only

Kostrzewa

Sulzburger & Graham, 1995, 398 pages, ISBN 094581948X

Concise review of pharmacology. Many good diagrams. Some key topics inadequately covered.

B Digging Up the Bones: Pharmacology

$17.95   Review/Cards

Linardakis

Michaelis Medical, 1996, 99 pages and 100+ flash cards, ISBN 1884084230

Old edition was easy reading. Brief collection of phrases and associations based on answers to assorted multiple-choice questions. Expensive for the amount of material. **New edition not yet reviewed.** Contains 100+ flash cards of top drugs.

B Essentials of Pharmacology

$29.95   Review/250+ q

EBS, Theoharides

Little, Brown, 1996, 444 pages, ISBN 0316839361

Review text with some boards-style questions and letter answers. May be more appropriate as a course text than as a review book. New edition has many good tables that summarize important drug mechanisms and toxicities. Too much boldface is distracting. Limited student feedback.

B | MEPC Pharmacology

$17.95 Test/700 q

Krzanowski

Appleton & Lange, 1995, 267 pages, ISBN 0838562272

Questions with brief, direct explanations. Well referenced. Answers recently updated.

B | Medical Pharmacology at a Glance

$24.95 Review only

Neal

Blackwell Science, 1992, 92 pages, ISBN 0632033738

Contains excellent figures followed by explanations. Visual synthesis of sites and mechanisms of drug actions. Occasionally, British terminology may be confusing. High yield for those with limited study time. Useful only as a supplement to a review text. May be hard to find.

B | Pharmacology

$17.95 Test/500 q

PreTest, DiPalma

McGraw-Hill, 1996, 253 pages, ISBN 0070520879

Typical for this series. Questions are picky and challenging with detailed answers. For the motivated student. New edition does reflect question types on USMLE Step 1.

B | Pharmacology

$27.00 Review/450+ q

NMS, Jacob

Williams & Wilkins, 1996, 373 pages, ISBN 0683062514

Outline format. More tables and diagrams in new edition. Often too detailed. Lacks emphasis on high-yield material. Has a lengthy USMLE-type exam. Requires time commitment. Typical for this series.

B | Pharmacology

$17.95 Review/560+ q

Oklahoma Notes, Moore

Springer-Verlag, 1995, 235 pages, ISBN 0387943943

Conceptual approach. Features USMLE-type questions with brief explanations. A concise and readable review book.

B⁻ | Med Charts, Pharmacology

$14.95 Review only

Rosenbach

ILOC, 1993, 171 pages, ISBN 1882531000

Contains tables and summaries. Good for quick review, but requires previous reading from other sources. May be helpful for students who prefer studying charts.

Pharmacology   **$21.00**   Review/450 q

BRS, Rosenfeld

Williams & Wilkins, 1993, 357 pages, ISBN 0683073613

Outline format. Good use of boldface, although few tables. Questions are of moderate difficulty with short answers. Worse than average for this series. New edition expected in June 1997 (ISBN 0683180509).

The Pharmacology Text Stack Personal Edition   **$135.00**   Software/200+ q

Theoharides

Keyboard Publishing, 1993, ISBN 1573492132 (Mac),
    ISBN 1573492140 (Windows)

Includes text of electronic pharmacology textbook by Theoharides. Questions linked to text. Good as reference or with course. Too expensive for students. More appropriate as a library purchase.

NEW BOOKS—PHARMACOLOGY

N

Basic Concepts in Pharmacology   **$24.95**   Review only

Stringer

McGraw-Hill, 1996, 288 pages, ISBN 0070631654

Presents summaries of "elusive" concepts in pharmacology, from simple to complex.

N

Mosby Ace Pharmacology   **$28.95**   Review/462 q

Ace, Enna

Mosby-Year Book, 1996, 394 pages, ISBN 0815131127 (Windows), ISBN 0815131526 (Mac)

Concise content review with boards-style questions. Test software included with text. Money-back guarantee. Not yet reviewed.

N

PreTest Pharmacology Study Disk   **$28.00**   Software/500 q

DiPalma

McGraw-Hill, 1995, ISBN 0078641616 (Mac), ISBN 0078641608 (Windows)

Software test review based on *PreTest Pharmacology*. Includes questions with detailed answers and some illustrations. Program can custom-generate tests. Copy protection mechanism is inconvenient.

Physiology

$21.95   Review/400 q

BRS, Costanzo

Williams & Wilkins, 1995, 288 pages, ISBN 0683021346

Clear, concise review of physiology. Fast, easy reading. Great charts and tables. Good practice questions with explanations with a clinically oriented final exam. Excellent review book, but may not be enough for in-depth coursework. Comparatively weak respiratory and acid–base sections.

B+

Clinical Physiology Made Ridiculously Simple

$18.95   Review only

Goldberg

MedMaster, 1995, 152 pages, ISBN 0940780216

Easy reading with many "ridiculous" associations. Style does not work for everyone. Not as well illustrated as the rest of series. Short length allows for quick review.

B+

Physiology: An Illustrated Review with Questions & Explanations

$29.95   Review/320 q

Tadlock

Little, Brown, 1995, 333 pages, ISBN 0316827649

New edition features updated text with superb illustrations and tables. Format and organization improved. Quite detailed. Best used with the course. Some questions include complex calculations not typical for the board. Requires time commitment.

B

Blond's Physiology

$20.00   Review only

Grossman

Sulzburger & Graham, 1995, 439 pages, ISBN 0945819420

Comprehensive but easy-to-read review text of physiology. Clear and simple classic diagrams and charts. Better than average for this series. Strong endocrine chapter. Good hormone list.

B

Color Atlas of Physiology

$29.00   Review only

Despopoulos

Georg Thieme Verlag, 1991, 369 pages, ISBN 0865773823

Compact, with more than 156 colorful but complicated diagrams on the right and dense explanatory text on the left. Some translation problems. A unique, highly visual approach worthy of consideration. Useful as an adjunct to other review books.

REVIEW RESOURCES

Physiology

B | Physiology $27.00   Review/300 q

NMS, Bullock

Williams & Wilkins, 1995, 641 pages, ISBN 068306259X

Very complete text in outline form. Often too detailed, but some good diagrams. Moderately difficult questions with detailed answers. Provides some pathophysiology. More useful if used as a course text and reference; too long as a review text. Inexpensive for the amount of material. For the motivated student.

B | Physiology $17.95   Test/500 q

PreTest, Ryan

McGraw-Hill, 1996, 228 pages, ISBN 0070520852

Questions with detailed, well-written explanations. Some questions too difficult or picky. May be useful for the motivated student following extensive review from other sources.

B | Physiology: A Review for the New National Boards $25.00   Test/506 q

Jakoi

J & S, 1994, 214 pages, ISBN 0963287346

Good review book, but inadequate as sole source of review. Quick reading. Below-average question quality for this series. Answer discussions cover many important topics.

B | MEPC Physiology $17.95   Test/700 q

Penney

Appleton & Lange, 1995, 257 pages, ISBN 0838562221

Questions with brief, direct answers. Recently revised. Reflects USMLE Step 1 format. Compare with *PreTest Physiology*. Good as an adjunct to other review texts. Limited student feedback.

B⁻ | Essentials of Physiology $35.95   Review/100 q

EBS, Sperelakis

Little, Brown, 1996, 680 pages, ISBN 0316806285

Dense review text with some boards-style questions and letter answers. Numerous diagrams, including some that are not particularly helpful. May be more appropriate as a course text than as a review book. Significant time commitment.

B⁻ | Physiology $17.95   Review/345 q

Oklahoma Notes, Thies

Springer-Verlag, 1995, 280 pages, ISBN 0387943978

Dense text. Inconsistent quality of sections. Emphasizes general concepts. Boards-type questions with short answers. Some errors.

N | **Ace Physiology** | **$28.95** | Review/250 q

Ace, Ackermann

Mosby-Year Book, 1996, 285 pages, ISBN 081510054X (Windows), ISBN 0815109334 (Mac)

Not yet reviewed. Concise content review with boards-style questions. Test software included with text. Money-back guarantee.

N | **Appleton & Lange's Review of Physiology** | **$24.95** | Test/1000 q

Penney

Appleton & Lange, 1997, ISBN 0838502741

Boards-style questions with letter answers and explanations. Expected May 1997.

N | **Linardakis' Illustrated Review of Physiology** | **$37.95** | Review/200+ q

Linardakis

Michaelis Medical, 1997, 340 pages, ISBN 1884084176

Expected in December 1996. Comprehensive, illustration-based review of medical physiology. Integrated text and color illustrations.

N | **PreTest Physiology Study Disk** | **$28.00** | Software/500 q

Ryan

McGraw-Hill, 1995, ISBN 0078641578 (Mac), ISBN 007864156X (Windows)

Software test review based on *PreTest Physiology*. Includes questions with detailed answers and some illustrations. Program can custom-generate tests. Copy protection mechanism is inconvenient.

Commercial Review Courses

Compass Medical Education
  Network
Kaplan Educational Center
National Medical School Review
NMS Prep
Northwestern Learning Center
Postgraduate Medical Review
  Education
The Princeton Review
Youel's Prep, Inc.
Zaslau/FMSG Live-Lecture
  Course

Commercial preparation courses can be helpful for some students, but these courses are expensive and require significant time commitment. They are usually effective in organizing study material for students who feel overwhelmed by the volume of material. Note that the multiweek courses may be quite intense and thus leave limited time for independent study. Note that some commercial courses are designed for first-time test takers while other courses focus on students who are repeating the examination. Some courses focus on foreign medical graduates who want to take all three Steps in a limited amount of time. Student experience and satisfaction with review courses are highly variable. We suggest that you discuss options with recent graduates of review courses you are considering. Course content and structure can evolve rapidly. Some student opinions can be found in discussion groups on the World Wide Web.

Compass Medical Education Network

Compass Medical Education Network, formerly known as ArcVentures Medical Education Services, offers a series of live-lecture preparation courses for all three Steps of the USMLE. Compass is an ArcVentures company, an affiliate of Rush–Presbyterian–St. Luke's Medical Center in Chicago, Illinois.

Compass' 1997 Step live-lecture schedule includes the IntensePrep, 7-week, and 15-week courses. Courses are offered in all Compass locations—Chicago; Detroit; Houston; Los Angeles; Miami; Clifton, New Jersey; New York City; and Washington, DC—as well as in San Juan, Puerto Rico; Guadalajara, Mexico; and London, England. In addition, IntensePrep Step 1 courses will be offered at 25 US medical school locations in 1997.

The IntensePrep Step 1 course is designed exclusively for second-year medical students who are first-time takers of the exam. The structured USMLE Step 1 courses review the seven basic sciences, with emphasis on material most likely to be found on the exam. The course provides a concise review of the material most likely to appear on the USMLE Step 1. Through live lectures, course notes, and hundreds of practice questions (including a computer-scored diagnostic exam), students receive a structured review of the basic sciences. Compass recruits US medical school faculty, including authors of basic science and medical board review books, to teach its programs.

Students enrolled in the 7- and 15-week Step 1 courses undergo an extensive review of the basic sciences and participate in small group sessions designed to supplement the lectures and help students retain more information through discussion of USMLE-type practice questions. With the help of the Compass' diagnostic exam, students identify areas for improvement and sharpen their test-taking skills.

Costs range from $900 for the IntensePrep course to $5500 for the 15-week course. To receive an application and more information on tuition and course locations, call 1-800-818-9128 or write to:

Compass Medical Education Network
820 W. Jackson Blvd., Suite 750
Chicago, IL 60607

Kaplan Educational Center

Kaplan's comprehensive USMLE Step 1 course is a multi-modal program with live and video lecture review. With the help of diagnostic exams and computerized feedback, students are guided through the course materials and can study at their own pace. Some students enroll in their first year of medical school so that they can use the program to supplement their regular course work.

For 1997, Kaplan is introducing new organ-system review books that contain the basic science material organized around the USMLE Step 1 content outline. Also included in the course are thousands of USMLE-style review questions grouped by subject area and organ system, subject-area final exams, and 3-hour simulated exams with computerized feedback. A complete set of video lectures taught by US medical school faculty is available in all Kaplan Medical centers. Live-lecture series are available in select locations throughout the United States. A full course syllabus integrates all of the materials and provides study suggestions and test-taking strategies.

There are more than 100 Kaplan Medical centers nationwide and around the world. The price of the course varies with length of study. For more information, call 1-800-KAP-TEST or write to:

Kaplan Medical
810 Seventh Avenue, 22nd Floor
New York, NY 10019

Kaplan Educational Center can also be found online: http://www.kaplan.com/usmle

National Medical School Review

National Medical School Review (NMSR) offers comprehensive, 100% live-lecture review programs for the USMLE Steps 1, 2, 3, and SPEX. NMSR faculty are experts on USMLE material and are chosen from U.S. medical school faculty. Many are authors of USMLE review books. Each program is designed to emphasize the current high-yield information tested on the USMLE. Besides subject lectures, the programs offer diagnostic testing, test-taking skills and stress-reduction workshops, faculty-reviewed subject tests, and extensive up-to-date written notes and published review books.

To better meet an individual student's need, NMSR offers three Step 1 review programs. The 3-Week Program is primarily designed for U.S. medical students taking Step 1 for the first time. The 7-Week Program covers material in greater depth for students who need more time for review or who have had an initial failure. The 13-Week Program is designed for students who have been away from the content for an extended period of time, who have scored less than 156 on a previous examination, or who have had multiple failures.

In addition to review programs, NMSR offers *"Startup Study Kits"* which are sent to all students before programs begin. Except for the 3-Week Programs, each Step 1 program's *Startup Study Kit* includes the 5-volume *Board Simulator Series* and instructions on how the books can be utilized as a preview.

Fees for the Step 1 programs are: 3 Week, $1,000; 7 Week, $2,700; 13 Week, $5,000. Substantial discounts are available for enrollment in multiple programs, and NMSR's *Quality+Plus Guarantee* allows a student to repeat a program at a significantly reduced rate. The programs are available at several sites in the United States. To receive an application and/or more information, call 1-800-533-8850 or 1-714-476-6282, Fax 1-714-476-6286, or write:

National Medical School Review
4500 Campus Drive, Suite 201
Newport Beach, CA 92660

E-mail should be sent to: nmsr@nmsr.com
The NMSR can also be found online: http://www.nmsr.com

NMS Prep

NMS Prep specializes in helping examinees prepare for the USMLE Step I exam. NMS Prep is a joint program of Williams & Wilkins (NMS), a publisher in USMLE Review, and Columbia Review, a test preparation company. NMS Prep programs offer intensive and complete preparation courses for the USMLE, utilizing USMLE study materials from Williams & Wilkins and the NMS preparation library. NMS Prep programs are taught by USMLE experts, medical school faculty, and book authors.

NMS Prep offers an intensive live-lecture program and intensive home study programs. The live course emphasizes strategies, content review, and in-class analysis of USMLE-style questions. The live program lasts 10 weeks, and includes lectures, discussions, and USMLE practice testing. Live lectures emphasize clinical correlations, organ system interrelationships, and the basic science content most likely to be found on the actual exam. The live course includes USMLE review books and up to 100 topical USMLE practice tests. Home study courses offer students USMLE review books, a study planner, study strategies, up to 75 topical USMLE practice tests, and optional USMLE software. All courses provide students practice tests from the extensive NMS question bank of thousands of practice USMLE-style questions. Course fees range from $395 for the home-study course to $1950 for the live course. Travel discounts and partial scholarships are available. Live-course enrollment is limited.

For course information, call 1-800-NMS-7123 or 1-415-337-1955, Fax 1-415-337-1781, or write to:

NMS Prep
Main Office
220 Madison Avenue
San Francisco, CA 94134

E-mail should be sent to: nmsprep@aol.com
NMS Prep can also be found online: http://www.wwilkins.com/sor/NMS_Prep.html

Northwestern Learning Center

Northwestern Learning Center offers live-lecture review camps in preparation for both the USMLE Step 1 and the NBOME Part 1 examinations. Two programs are available: NBI 300 (*Intensive Care for the Boards*) and NBI 100 (*Primary Care for the Boards*). NBI 300 is offered in 9-, 14-, and 21-day review camp formats immediately prior to each scheduled National Board Examination. NBI 300 courses include live lectures taught by faculty from various universities and/or authors of review board texts. It also includes extensive printed lecture notes, Multimedia TALLP[97], simulated exams, and organized group activities. Review camps are held at resorts, convention centers, and universities throughout the country. Costs for the programs range from $780 to $1300. NBI 100 is an on-site, 2-day workshop that uses TALLP[97] techniques in conjunction with the review of high-yield boards-related facts and concepts. NBI 100 is available only to groups of students or sponsoring medical schools. The cost ranges from $80 to $120 per student. TALLP[97] is a multimedia presentation that is offered as an integral part of the Center's courses. It incorporates medical test-taking techniques and provides a system of choosing answers based on their logical structures and holistic patterns. For more information, call 1-800-837-7737 or 1-517-332-0777, or write to:

Northwestern Learning Center
4700 S. Hagadorn
East Lansing, MI 48823

E-mail should be sent to: testbuster@aol.com or northwestern@voyager.net.

The Northwestern Learning Center may also be found online:
http://www.northwesternlearning.com/nw

Postgraduate Medical Review Education (PMRE)

Postgraduate Medical Review Education (PMRE) offers live and videotaped classes for the USMLE Steps 1, 2, 3, and SPEX on a monthly basis in Miami Beach, Florida. Once a year, classes are also offered in Los Angeles, New York City, and New Jersey. Tuition ranges from $1000 for the "crash" course to $3500 for the full course. Complete home-study courses in the form of books and audiotapes are available for all three USMLE exams as well as the SPEX. For more information, call 1-800-433-3539 or write to:

PMRE
407 Lincoln Road, Suite 12E
Miami Beach, FL 33139

The Princeton Review

All USMLE Step 1 review courses offered by The Princeton Review are live and taught by instructors who have scored above the 80th percentile on Step 1. Courses of varying lengths and prices are available in more than 35 cities in the United States. Many courses are held directly on medical school campuses to prepare second-year students for the June Step 1 exam. Schedules are customized to meet the needs of individual schools. Scoring software analyzes both individual and collective performance on all exams taken in the program and produces a Diagnostic Score Report (DSR) for each student.

Students first take a placement exam that simulates one 3-hour Step 1 booklet. Each student is placed in a small class with students closely matching his or her profile. During workshops, trained instructors review the most important principles and topics for Step 1 through a combination of lectures, discussions, and homework review. After completing instruction, students take a subject assessment exam and receive a DSR. Instructors then go over the entire test. Additional 3-hour integrated exams are given during each course.

All course materials are prepared jointly by medical school faculty and Princeton Review instructors. A Step 1 review manual deals with difficult basic sciences concepts as well as the clinical context now prevalent throughout the Step 1 exam. The review manual is accompanied by gross, microscopic, and radiographic image appendices, a Step 1 workbook with practice items and more clinical cases, a booklet of test-taking tips, multiple mock boards booklets and subject assessment exams, and wrap-up materials to use in the final week before the exam. Course tuition ranges from $345 to $2600. Tuition varies by location and course option. To find the Princeton Review location nearest you, call 1-800-USMLE84 or write to:

The Princeton Review
2315 Broadway, Third Floor
New York, NY 10024

E-mail should be sent to: info.tpr@review.com.

The Princeton Review may also be found online:
   World Wide Web: http://www.review.com
   America Online: keyword "princeton"
   Microsoft Network: go to "Princeton Review"

Youel's Prep, Inc.

Youel's Prep offers a live-lecture and discussion test preparation program for the USMLE Steps 1, 2, and 3 and for NBOMLE COMLEX 1, 2, and 3. The lectures are given by Dr. Youel at various sites and dates throughout the United States. The Step 1 course format is a 1-week, 8-hour-per-day program. Tuition is $375 and is discounted to $175 for those purchasing the $600, 3000-page, 8-book Home Study Program. Tuition is further discounted to $75 for medical students of host medical schools. There is no charge for repeating the same-level examination as many times as desired.

The programs emphasize highlights from the Home Study Program books and practice examinations. The focus is what to study, how to remember it, and how to use high-yield facts at test time.

The Home Study Program is formatted and written to engage active learning. Facts are clustered in question-relevant boxes: grouping together facts with language links, mnemonic links, and logic links. Fact clusters relevant to only one examination are labeled by the relevant number. The program is designed to focus and improve preparation for regular medical school examinations. The program is also for any student or physician who has failed the boards or has done poorly on medical school examinations.

Shorter versions are available for the individual examinations: PREP NOTES, the FUNdaMENTALS (for Step 1), and PREP NOTES, the Clinical Books (for Steps 2 and 3). Each is a two-book set, and each set sells for $400. The Step 1 set is 1325 pages and the Step 2–3 set is 1200 pages. All of the information in both PREP NOTES sets is included in the Home Study Program.

Appearing in fall 1996 are the shorter versions: QUICK FIX #1 for Step 1/Part I and QUICK FIX #2 for Step 2/Level 2. Each will be approximately 700 pages and will sell for $275. These books are designed for students who are reasonably well prepared and who are preparing for only a single examination. For more information and materials, call 1-800-645-3985, fax 1-561-795-0169, or write to:

Youel's Prep, Inc.
P.O. Box 273685
Boca Raton, FL 33427

Zaslau/FMSG Live-Lecture Course

Dr. Zaslau is introducing a 2-day live-lecture course featuring 12 hours of review of "high-yield" concepts in all subjects. Courses will be available for Step 1 and Step 2/3 combined. The cost is $395, which includes lecture materials and several of Dr. Zaslau's books. For more information, call 1-800-662-3244 or write to:

FMSG
P.O. Box 3454
Apopka, FL 32703

Publisher Contacts

If you do not have convenient access to a medical bookstore, consider ordering directly from the publisher.

Appleton & Lange
P.O. Box 120041
Stamford, CT 06912
(800) 423-1359
Fax: (203) 406-4602

Blackwell Science
238 Main Street
Cambridge, MA 02142
(800) 759-6102
Fax: (617) 876-7022

Churchill Livingstone
300 Lighting Way
Secaucus, NJ 07094
(800) 553-5426
Fax: (201) 319-9659

FMSG Inc.
P.O. Box 3454
Apopka, FL 32703
(800) 662-3244
(407) 869-7330
Fax: (407) 869-7844

ILOC Inc.
P.O. Box 232
Granville, OH 43023
(800) 495-4562
(614) 587-2658
Fax: (614) 587-2679

J&S Publishing
1300 Bishop Lane
Alexandria, VA 22302
(703) 823-9833
Fax: (703) 823-9834
Jandspub@ix.netcom.com
www.jandspub.com

Lippincott-Raven Publishers
P.O. Box 1580
Hagerstown, MD 21741
(800) 777-2295
Fax: (301) 824-7390

Little, Brown and Company
P.O. Box 1580
Hagerstown, MD 21741
(800) 777-2295
Fax: (301) 824-7390

McGraw-Hill Customer Service
P.O. Box 545
Blacklick, OH 43004
(800) 262-4729
Fax: (614) 755-5645
www.mghmedical.com

MedMaster, Inc.
P.O. Box 640028
Miami, FL 33164
(800) 335-3480
(305) 653-3480
Fax: (305) 653-9678
stgoldberg@aol.com

Michaelis Medical Publishing
2274 South 1300 East
Suite G8-288
Salt Lake City, UT 84106
(800) 557-6672 (Tel/Fax)

Mosby-Year Book
11830 Westline Industrial Drive
St. Louis, MO 63146
(800) 325-4177 ext. 5017
Fax: (800) 535-9935
www.mosby.com

National Learning Corporation
212 Michael Drive
Syosset, NY 11791
(800) 645-6337
Fax: (516) 921-8743

Springer-Verlag, NY Inc.
Attention: Service Center
333 Meadowlands Parkway
Secaucus, NJ 07094
(800) 777-4643
Fax: (201) 348-5405
www.Springer-NY.com
orders@Springer-NY.com

W.B. Saunders
6277 Sea Harbor Drive
Orlando, FL 32887
(800) 545-2522
Fax: (800) 874-6418

Williams & Wilkins
P.O. Box 1496
Baltimore, MD 21298-9724
(800) 638-0672
Fax: (800) 477-8438
www.wwilkins.com

Data in Section III were verified by Discount Medical Books & Supplies and Reiter's Professional Books—independent bookstores that are able to ship books from multiple publishers at list price both domestically and internationally.

Discount Medical Books & Supplies
345 Judah Street
San Francisco, CA 94122
(415) 664-5555
Fax: (415) 664-7810
medical@discmedbooks.com

Reiter's Scientific & Professional Books
2021 K Street, N.W.
Washington, DC 20006-1003
(800) 537-4314
(202) 223-3327
Fax: (202) 296-9103
books@reiters.com

Abbreviations and Symbols

Abbreviation	Meaning
Ab	antibody
ACE	angiotensin-converting enzyme
ACh	acetylcholine
ACTH	adrenocorticotropic hormone
AD	autosomal dominant
ADA	adenosine deaminase
ADH	antidiuretic hormone
Ag	antigen
AIDS	acquired immunodeficiency syndrome
ALA	aminolevulinate synthase
ALL	acute lymphocytic leukemia
ALS	amyotrophic lateral sclerosis
ALT	alanine transaminase
AML	acute myelogenous leukemia
ANA	antinuclear antibody
ANOVA	analysis of variance
ANP	atrial natriuretic peptide
ANS	autonomic nervous system
AP	arterial pressure
ARDS	acute respiratory distress syndrome
ASD	atrial septal defect
ASO	antistreptolysin O
AST	aspartate transaminase
ATP	adenosine triphosphate
ATPase	adenosine triphosphatase
AV	atrioventricular
AVM	arteriovenous malformation
AZT	azidothymidine
BAL	British anti-Lewisite (dimercaprol)
BP	blood pressure
BPG	bis phosphoglycerate
BPH	benign prostatic hyperplasia
CAD	coronary artery disease
cAMP	cyclic adenosine monophosphate
CCK	cholecystokinin
CD	cluster of differentiation
CDC	Centers for Disease Control
CDP	cytidine diphosphate
cGMP	cyclic guanosine monophosphate
ChAT	choline acetyltransferase
CHF	congestive heart failure
CJD	Creutzfeldt–Jakob disease
CL	clearance
CML	chronic myelogenous leukemia
CMV	cytomegalovirus
CN	cranial nerve
CNS	central nervous system
CO	cardiac output
CoA	coenzyme A
COMT	catechol-O-methyltransferase
COPD	chronic obstructive pulmonary disease
C_p	concentration in plasma
CPK-MB	creatine phosphokinase, MB fraction
CSF	cerebrospinal fluid

Abbreviation	Meaning
CT	computed tomography
DAG	diacylglycerol
DEA	Drug Enforcement Agency
DES	diethylstilbestrol
DIC	disseminated intravascular coagulation
DIMS	disorder in initiating and maintaining sleep
DMD	Duchenne muscular dystrophy
DMN	dorsal motor nucleus
2,4-DNP	2,4-dinitrophenol
DOES	disorder of excessive somnolence
DPG	diffuse proliferative glomerulonephritis; diphosphoglycerate
DPPC	dipalmitoyl phosphatidylcholine
ds	double stranded
dTMP	deoxythymidine monophosphate
DTR	deep tendon reflex
DTs	delirium tremens
EBV	Epstein–Barr virus
ECF	extracellular fluid
ECT	electroconvulsive therapy
EDRF	endothelium-derived relaxing factor
EDTA	ethylenediamine tetraacetic acid
EDV	end-diastolic volume
EEG	electroencephalogram
EF-2	elongation factor 2
EGF	epidermal growth factor
EM	electron microscopy
EMB	eosin–methylene blue
EPS	extrapyramidal symptoms
ER	endoplasmic reticulum; emergency room
ERP	effective refractory period
ERV	expiratory reserve volume
ESR	erythrocyte sedimentation rate
ESV	end-systolic volume
EtOH	ethyl alcohol
FAD	oxidized flavin adenine dinucleotide
$FADH_2$	reduced flavin adenine dinucleotide
FDA	Food and Drug Administration
FEV	forced expiratory volume
FF	filtration fraction
FFP	fresh frozen plasma
FH_x	family history
FMN	flavin mononucleotide
FSH	follicle-stimulating hormone
FTA-ABS	fluorescent treponemal antibody—absorbed
FVC	forced vital capacity
G3P	glucose-3-phosphate
G6PD	glucose-6-phosphate dehydrogenase
GABA	γ-aminobutyric acid
GFAP	glial fibrillary acidic protein
GFR	glomerular filtration rate
GI	gastrointestinal
G_i	G protein, inhibitory

Abbreviation	Meaning	Abbreviation	Meaning
GM-CSF	granulocyte-macrophage colony-stimulating factor	MMR	measles, mumps, rubella
		MPTP	1-methyl-4-phenyl-1, 2, 3, 6-tetrahydro-pyridine
GMP	guanosine monophosphate		
GN	glomerulonephritis	MRI	magnetic resonance imaging
GnRH	gonadotropin-releasing hormone	MTP	metatarsal–phalangeal
GRP	gastrin-releasing peptide	NAD	oxidized nicotinamide adenine dinucleotide
G_s	G protein, stimulatory	NADH	reduced nicotinamide adenine dinucleotide
GTP	guanosine triphosphate	NADP	oxidized nicotinamide adenine dinucleotide phosphate
HAV	hepatitis A virus		
Hb	hemoglobin	NADPH	reduced nicotinamide adenine dinucleotide phosphate
HBV	hepatitis B virus		
hCG	human chorionic gonadotropin	NE	norepinephrine
HCV	hepatitis C virus	NIDA	National Institute on Drug Abuse
HDL	high-density lipoprotein	NREM	non–rapid eye movement
HDV	hepatitis D virus	NSAID	nonsteroidal anti-inflammatory drug
HEV	hepatitis E virus	OAA	oxaloacetic acid
HGPRT	hypoxanthine-guanine phosphoribosyltransferase	OBS	organic brain syndrome
		PABA	para-aminobenzoic acid
HIV	human immunodeficiency virus	PAH	para-aminohippuric acid
HLA	human leukocyte antigen	PALS	periarterial lymphoid sheath
HMG	human menopausal gonadotropin	PAN	polyarteritis nodosa
HMG-CoA	hydroxymethylglutaryl-CoA	PAS	periodic acid–Schiff (stain)
HMP	hexose monophosphate	PCl_2	prostacyclin I_2
HPV	human papillomavirus	PCAT	phosphatidylcholine-cholesterol acyltransferase
HSV	herpes simplex virus		
HTLV	human T-cell lymphotropic virus	PCP	*Pneumocystis carinii* pneumonia; phencyclidine hydrochloride
HTN	hypertension		
ICF	intracellular fluid	PCR	polymerase chain reaction
ICU	intensive care unit	PDA	patent ductus arteriosus
IDL	intermediate-density lipoprotein	PDE	phosphodiesterase
IF	intrinsic factor	PDGF	platelet-derived growth factor
IFN	interferon	PEP	phosphoenolpyruvate
Ig	immunoglobulin	PFK	phosphofructokinase
IHSS	idiopathic hypertrophic subaortic stenosis	PFT	pulmonary function tests
IL-1	interleukin-1	PGE	prostaglandin E
IM	intramuscular	PID	pelvic inflammatory disease
IMP	inosine monophosphate	PIP_2	phosphatidylinositol 4,5-bisphosphate
IND	investigational new drug	PK	pyruvate kinase
INH	isonicotine hydrazine (isoniazid)	PKU	phenylketonuria
IP_3	inositol triphosphate	PML	progressive multifocal leukoencephalopathy
IRV	inspiratory reserve volume		
IVC	inferior vena cava	PMN	polymorphonuclear
JCV	JC virus	PNH	paroxysmal nocturnal hemoglobinuria
JGA	juxtaglomerular apparatus	PNS	peripheral nervous system
KSHV	Kaposi's sarcoma–associated herpesvirus	POMC	pro-opiomelanocortin
		PP	pyrophosphate
LA	left atrium	PPRF	parapontine reticular formation
LAD	left anterior descending; left atrial defect	PR	pulmonic regurgitation
		PRPP	phosphoribosylpyrophosphate
LCAT	lecithin-cholesterol acyltransferase	PSA	prostate-specific antigen
LDH	lactate dehydrogenase	PSS	progressive systemic sclerosis
LDL	low-density lipoprotein	PT	prothrombin time
LFT	liver function test	PTH	parathyroid hormone
LH	luteinizing hormone	PTT	partial thromboplastin time
LMN	lower motor neuron (signs)	RA	right atrium
LPS	lipopolysaccharide	RBC	red blood cell
LT	leukotriene; long thoracic	RCA	right coronary artery
MC	musculocutaneous	REM	rapid eye movement
MAC	*Mycobacterium avium–intracellulare* complex; membrane attack complex	RER	rough endoplasmic reticulum
		RES	reticuloendothelial system
M-CSF	macrophage colony-stimulating factor	RPF	renal plasma flow
		RSV	respiratory syncytial virus
MAO	monoamine oxidase	RV	residual volume
MEN	multiple endocrine neoplasia	RVH	right ventricular hypertrophy
MHC	major histocompatibility complex		
MI	myocardial infarction		

Abbreviation	Meaning
SA	sino-atrial
SAM	*S*-adenosylmethionine
SC	sickle cell, subcutaneous
SCID	severe combined immunodeficiency disease
SEM	standard error of the mean
SER	smooth endoplasmic reticulum
SES	socioeconomic status
SGOT	serum glutamic oxaloacetic transaminase
SGPT	serum glutamic pyruvate transaminase
SLE	systemic lupus erythematosus
SRS-A	slow-reacting substance of anaphylaxis
ss	single stranded
SSPE	subacute sclerosing panencephalitis
STD	sexually transmitted disease
SV	stroke volume
SVT	supraventricular tachycardia
$t_{1/2}$	half-life
TAT	thematic apperception test
TB	tuberculosis
TBW	total body water
TCA	tricarboxylic acid
TGF	transforming growth factor
TGV	transposition of great vessels
TLC	total lung capacity
TMP-SMX	trimethoprim-sulfamethoxazole
TNF	tissue necrosis factor
ToRCH	toxoplasmosis, rubella, CMV, herpes
tPA	tissue plasminogen factor
TPP	thiamine pyrophosphate

Abbreviation	Meaning
TSH	thyroid-stimulating hormone
TSST	toxic shock syndrome
TV	tidal volume
TxA_2	thromboxane A_2
UDP	uridine diphosphate
UMN	upper motor neuron (signs)
URI	upper respiratory infection
UTI	urinary tract infection
VC	vital capacity
V_d	volume of distribution
VDRL	Venereal Disease Research Laboratory
VF	ventricular fibrillation
VLDL	very low-density lipoprotein
VMA	vanillylmandelic acid
V/Q	ratio of ventilation to perfusion
VSD	ventricular septal defect
VZV	varicella-zoster virus
WBC	white blood cell

Symbol	Meaning
↑	increase(s)
↓	decrease(s)
→	leads to
1°	primary
2°	secondary
3°	tertiary
≈	approximately; homologous
≡	defined as
⊖	negative effect
⊕	positive effect

Index

Anesthetics
    inhaled, 225
    intravenous, 225
    local, 226
Aneurysms
    aortic, 207
    berry, 189
Angelman's syndrome, 109
Angina, 190
Angina pectoris, 228
Angiosarcoma, 176
Angiotensin converting enzyme, 258
Angiotensin converting enzyme inhibitors, 227–228
Angiotensin II, 54, 113, 245, 268
Angular stomatitis, 126
Anion gap, 239
Anisocytosis, 52
Anisoylated plasminogen-streptokinase-activator complex, 240
Anistreplase, 240
Ankylosing spondylitis, 174
Annular pancreas, 59
Anopsia, 75
Anosognosia, 92
ANOVA. See Analysis of variance
ANP. See Atrial natriuretic peptide
Anterograde amnesia, 73, 93
Anti-anginal therapy, 228
Antiarrhythmics, 232–234
Antibody structure, 160
Anticholinergic agents, 237
Anticholinesterases, 220, 237
Anticipation, 109
Antidiuretic hormone, 113
Antidiuretic hormone antagonists, 230
Antidotes, 237
Antigenic variation, 134
Antigen-presenting cell(s) (APC), 53
Antihypertensive drugs, 227
Antimicrobial pharmacology, high-yield facts, 210–218
Antimicrobial prophylaxis, nonsurgical, 245
Antimicrobial therapy, 210
Antimuscarinic(s), 220, 236, 245
Antiparasitic(s), 218
Antipsychotic(s), 223
Antischkow's cells, 200
Antisocial personality disorder, 96
Antithrombin III, 239–240
α_1-Antitrypsin, 177
Aorta, 63
    ascending, 58
    coarctation of, 170
Aortic aneurysm, 207
Aortic arch, 56
Aortic arch derivatives, 56
Aortic bodies, 255
Aortic insufficiency, 199
Aortic outflow tract, 58
Aortic regurgitation, 254
Aortic stenosis, 254
APC. See Antigen-presenting cell(s)
APC gene, 177
APGAR (mnemonic), 85
Apgar score, 85
Apocrine secretion, 69
Apolipoproteins, 120
Appendix, 65

Arachidonate, 123
Arachidonic acid products, 122, 243
Arboviruses, 157
Arcuate artery, 65
Arcuate vein, 65
ArcVentures Medical Education Services. See Compass Medical Education Network
ARDS. See Adult respiratory distress syndrome
Arenaviruses, 155
Argyll-Robertson pupil, 199
Arnold-Chiari malformation, 186
ARP (mnemonic), 199
Arsenic, 237
Arterial baroreceptors, 255
Arteriole(s)
    afferent, 65
    efferent, 65
Arteritis
    Takayasu's, 195
    temporal, 195
Arthritis, rheumatoid, 174, 187
Arthus reaction hypersensitivity, 165
Arylcyclohexylamines, 225
Arytenoids cartilage, 57
3 As (mnemonic), 145
4 As (mnemonic), 97
Asbestosis, 197
Aschoff body, 194, 200
Ascorbic acid. See Vitamin C
Aspartate aminotransferase, 191, 203
Aspergillus fumigatus, 146
Aspirin, 237, 243
Association areas, 72
Associative auditory cortex, 72
Asteroid bodies, 188
Asthma, 261
    drugs for, 242
Astrocytes, 71
Astrocytoma, 176–177
Ataxia-telangiectasia, 166
Atenolol, 222
Atheromata, 200
Atherosclerosis, 190, 206
Athetosis, 72
Atonic seizures, 186
Atopic hypersensitivity, 165
ATP. See Adenosine triphosphate
Atracurium, 241
Atresia, 58
Atria, primitive, 58
Atrial natriuretic peptide (ANP), 113, 245, 268
Atrial septal defect, 170
Atrioventricular block, 255
Atrium, right, 58
Atrophic glossitis, 176
Atropine, 220
Attorney, durable power of, 88
Auditory cortex, 72
    associative, 72
    primary, 72
Auditory hallucinations, 97

Auditory meatus
    external, 57
    internal, 74
Auerbach's plexus. See Myenteric plexus
Auer bodies (rods), 200
AUG codon, 104
Auricular appendages, 58

Autism, 97
Autoimmune pathology, high-yield facts, 187–189, 207
Autonomic drugs, 219
Autonomic innervation, of male sexual response, 65
Autonomic nervous system, 55
Autonomic second messengers, 219
Autonomy, 87
Autopagnosia, 92
Autoregulation, 257
Autosomal dominant diseases, 173
Autosomal dominant inheritance, 108
Autosomal recessive inheritance, 108
Autosomal trisomies, 171
Autotroph, 132
Auxotroph, 132
Avoidant personality disorder, 96
Axillary nerves, injuries to, 60
Axoles, 210
AZT. See Zidovudine
AZT (mnemonic), 217
Aztreonam, 210–211
Azygous vein, 63

B
Babinski reflex, 78
Bacillus anthracis, 135
Bacillus cereus, 141
Bacitracin, 210
Bacteria. See also Bugs
    encapsulated, 147
    α-hemolytic, 138
    β-hemolytic, 138
    lactose-fermenting enteric, 142
    pigment-producing, 136
    zoonotic, 142
Bacterial endocarditis, 193
Bacterial genetic transfer, 134
Bacterial growth curve, 132
Bacterial structures, 133
Bacteroides, 132
BAGS (mnemonic), 69
Barbiturates, 222, 225, 237
Barrett's esophagus, 176, 179
Basal cell carcinoma, 176, 178
Basal ganglia
    degenerative diseases of, 185
    lesions of, 72
Basal ganglion tremor, 72
Basement membrane, 65
Basophils, 52
B-cell deficiency, 166
B-cell lymphomas, 176
bcl-2 (oncogene), 177
Becker's muscular dystrophy, 172
Bedwetting, 91
Behavioral science
    high-yield facts, 81–101
    high-yield topics, 101
    review resources, 295–297
Bell's palsy, 78, 188
Bell's phenomenon, 78
Beneficence, 88
Benzathine, 245
Benzodiazepines, 91, 222, 225, 237
Benztropine, 220, 245
Bepridil, 233
Ber1Ber1 (mnemonic), 126
Berger's disease, 196
Beriberi, 126
Berry aneurysms, 189
BEST (mnemonic), 77

Hemorrhoids, 63
  external, 64
  internal, 64
HEN PEcKS (mnemonic), 211
Hepadnavirus, 154
Heparan sulfate, 67
Heparin, 52, 237, 240
Hepatitis
  alcoholic, 183
  serologic markers, 153
  transmission, 152
Hepatitis A virus, 151–152, 155
Hepatitis B virus, 151–152, 178
Hepatitis C virus, 152
Hepatitis D virus, 152
Hepatitis E virus, 152, 155
Hepatocellular carcinoma, 176, 181
Hepatocytes, 68
Hepatoma. See Hepatocellular carcinoma
Hepatomegaly, 193
Hereditary spherocytosis, 194
Hernias
  direct, 62
  indirect, 62
  inguinal, 62
Heroin, 224
Heroin addiction, 85
Herpes simplex virus
  type 1, 151, 154, 157
  type 2, 151, 154, 157
Herpesvirus(es), 151, 154, 157
Heterochromatin, 104
Heterotroph, 132
Heterozygosity, loss of, 109
Hexamethonium, 220
Hexokinase, 113
Hexokinase deficiency, 110
High altitude, respiratory response to, 257
High-density lipoprotein(s), functions of, 120
Hirschsprung's disease, 182
Histamine, 52, 258
Histamine H$_2$-receptor blockers, 239
Histology
  high-yield facts, 66–70
  high-yield topics, 79–80
Histoplasmosis, 146
Histrionic personality disorder, 96
Hodgkin's disease, 201
Hollingshead determinants of socioeconomic status, 85
Holocrine secretion, 69
Homatropine, 220
Homicidal patient, 88
Homocystinuria, 110
Homonymous hemianopsia, 75
Hopelessness, factors in, 99
Hormones, acting on kidney, 268
Horner's syndrome, 180, 186
Hot T bone stEAk (mnemonic), 163
Hull hypothesis, 84
Human chorionic gonadotropin, 270, 273
  β-subunit (β-hCG), 177
Human immunodeficiency virus infection, 151, 155. See also Acquired immunodeficiency syndrome
  diagnosis, 157

in microglia, 54
  time course, 158
Human leukocyte antigen(s), 174
  HLA-A3, 174
  HLA-B27, 174
  HLA-DR2, 174
  HLA-DR3, 174
  HLA-DR4, 174
  HLA-DRY, 174
Human papillomavirus, 178
Human T cell leukemia virus, 151
Human T-lymphotropic virus-1, 178
Huntington's disease, 72, 173, 185
  neurotransmitter changes with, 90
Hyaline casts, 200
Hyalinosis, 196
Hydatidiform mole, 197
Hydralazine, 227, 237
Hydrocephalus, 207
Hydrochlorothiazide, 227, 229
Hydrocortisone, 243
Hydrogen ions, 264
Hyoid
  greater horn of, 56
  lesser horn of, 56
Hyoid artery, 56
Hyperbilirubinemia, 121, 184
  hereditary, 184
Hypercalcemia, 181
Hypercholesterolemia, familial, 173
Hyperlipidemia signs, 200
Hyperorality, 73
Hyperplasia, 175
Hypersensitivity, 165
  type I, 165
  type II, 165
  type III, 165
  type IV, 165
Hypersexuality, 73
Hypertension, 69, 207
Hyperthyroidism, 199, 244
Hypertrophic cardiomyopathy, 192
Hyperuricemia, 187
Hypnagogic hallucinations, 92, 97
Hypnopompic hallucinations, 92, 97
Hypoaldosteronism, 269
  primary, 269
  secondary, 269
Hypocalcemia, 184
Hypocalcemic tetany, 128
Hypochondriasis, 95
Hypochromic anemia, 202
Hypoglossal canal, 74
Hypoglossal nerve, 62, 74
Hypomanic episode, 94
Hypopituitarism, 208
Hypospadias, 59, 170
Hypothalamic nuclei, 91
Hypothalamus, 74
  functions of, 71
Hypothesis
  alternative, 84
  hull, 84
Hypothyroidism, 199

I

Ibuprofen, 237, 242
IC. See Inspiratory capacity
Id, 98
Identification, as ego defense, 98
Idiotype, 161
Ig. See Immunoglobulin
IGAD! (mnemonic), 99

IgA nephropathy, 196
Illusion, 96
I loVe Lucy (mnemonic), 110
Imipenem, 210, 212
Imipramine, 91, 223
Immune complex hypersensitivity, 165
Immune deficiencies, 166
Immunity
  active, 165
  passive, 165
Immunizations, 86
Immunodeficiency states, 176
Immunoglobulin(s), 160
  epitopes, 161
  IgA, 160
    nephropathy, 196
    production, 70
    proteases, 137
  IgD, 160
  IgE, 160
  IgG, 160
  IgM, 160
Immunology, high-yield topics, 167
Impetigo, 139
Implied consent, 87
Imprinting, 109
Incidence, 82
Incomplete penetrance, 109
Incus, 56–57
India ink stain, 66
Indomethacin, 242
Infant(s)
  deprivation effects, 89
  developmental milestones, 90
Infarcts
  pale, 189
  red, 189
Inferior vena cava, 63
Infertility, 244
Inflammatory bowel disease, 174
Influenza immunizations, 86
Influenza virus, 151, 155–156
Informed consent, 87
  exceptions to, 87
Infraspinatus muscles, 62
Inguinal hernias, 62
INH. See Isoniazid
INH (mnemonic), 215
Inhaled anesthetics, 225
Inheritance, modes of, 108
Inhibitors
  competitive, 123
  noncompetitive, 123
Inner ear, 67
Inspiratory capacity, 259
Inspiratory reserve volume, 259
Insulin, 69, 113, 122
Insulin-dependent (type I) diabetes mellitus (IDDM), 174, 198
Insulin-independent organs, 270
Intelligence testing, 100
Interferons
  γ-INF, 53, 163
  mechanism of, 164
Interleukins. See also Cytokines
  IL-1, 163
  IL-2, 163
  IL-3, 163
  IL-4, 163
  IL-5, 163
Interlobular artery, 65
Interlobular vein, 65
Intermediate filament, 68

New from the authors of *First Aid for the USMLE Step 1*

First Aid for the Wards

Le, Bhushan, & Amin

This high-yield student-to-student guide is designed to help students make the transition from the basic sciences to the hospital wards and succeed on their clinical rotations. The book features an orientation to the hospital environment, tips on being an effective and efficient junior medical student, student-proven advice tailored to each rotation, a database of high-yield clinical facts, and recommendations for clinical pocket books, texts, and references. Expected in early 1997. ISBN 0-8385-2595-4, A2595-5.

First Aid for the Match

Le, Bhushan, & Amin

The student-to-student guide helps medical students effectively and efficiently navigate the residency application process. Students make the most of their limited time, money, and energy. The book draws on the advice and experiences of successful student applicants as well as residency directors. Features application and interview tips tailored to each specialty, successful personal statements and CVs with analyses, current trends, and common interview questions with suggested strategies for responding. Available in bookstores. ISBN 0-8385-2596-2, A2596-3.

About the Authors

Vikas Bhushan, MD, completed residency training in diagnostic radiology at the University of California at Los Angeles. He is currently working part-time *locum tenens* in radiology while taking time off to travel and write. His interest in medical education led to the development and publication of the original *First Aid for the USMLE Step 1* in 1992. He is active in medical informatics and digital radiology. Vikas earned his MD with Thesis from the University of California at San Francisco. Vikas is single and resides in the Beverly Glen area of Los Angeles. He can be reached at vbhushan@aol.com

Tao Le, MD, recently earned his medical degree from the University of California at San Francisco. He has been involved in major writing and editing projects over the past five years. As a medical student he was editor-in-chief of *Synapse,* a campus-wide student-run newspaper with a weekly circulation of 5000. He recently entered residency training in internal medicine at Yale–New Haven Hospital. He is recently married and lives in New Haven with his wife, Thao, a resident in pediatrics. Tao can be reached at taotle@aol.com

Chirag Amin, MD, recently graduated from medical school at the University of Miami and has begun residency training in orthopedic surgery at Orlando Regional Medical Center. Chirag has been involved extensively in teaching and in writing books. He recently led the completion of *Jump Start MCAT: A High-Yield Student-to-Student Guide* (Williams & Wilkins). Chirag is single and lives in Orlando, Florida. He can be reached at chiragamin@aol.com

Ross Levine is a third-year medical student at the Johns Hopkins University School of Medicine. He helped coordinate the 1997 revision of *First Aid for the USMLE Step 1* and was a contributor to *Jump Start MCAT: A High Yield Student-to-Student Guide*. He has been involved in medical research, including clinical research and molecular biology, and hopes to pursue a career in academic medicine. Ross is single and lives in the Fells Point area of Baltimore. He can be reached at rlevine@welchlink.welch.jhu.edu

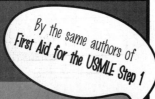
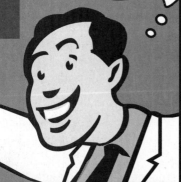
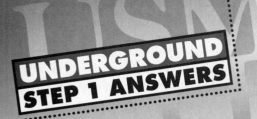
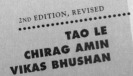
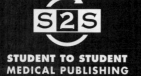